STRENGTH
AND
CONDITIONING
FOR
FEMALE ATHLETES

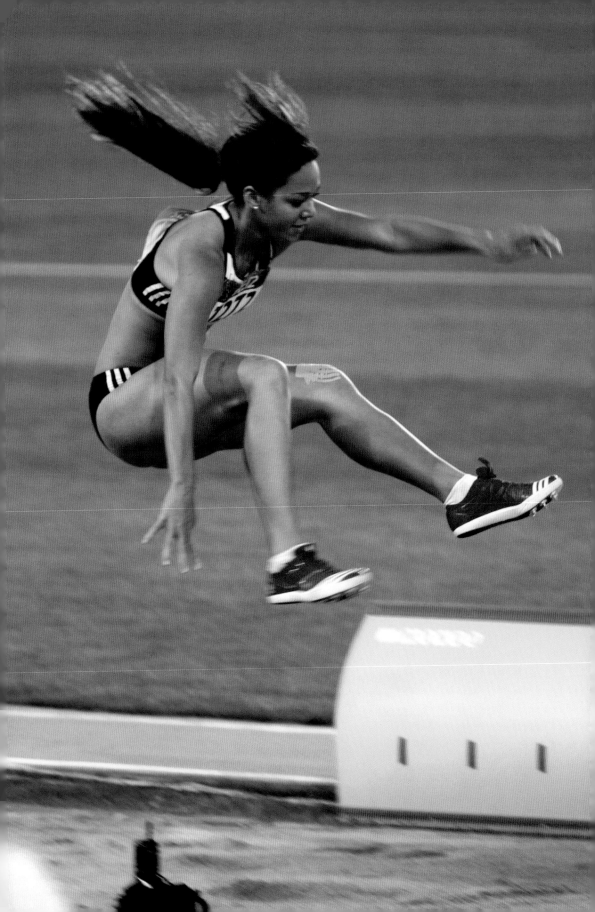

STRENGTH
AND
CONDITIONING
FOR
FEMALE ATHLETES

KEITH BARKER AND
DEBBY SARGENT

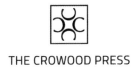

THE CROWOOD PRESS

First published in 2018 by
The Crowood Press Ltd
Ramsbury, Marlborough
Wiltshire SN8 2HR

www.crowood.com

© Keith Barker and Debby Sargent 2018

British Library Cataloguing-in-Publication Data
A catalogue record for this book is available from the British Library.

ISBN 978 1 78500 409 4

Frontispiece: Shutterstock

Typeset by Sharon Dainton Design
Printed and bound in India by Replika Press Pvt Ltd

Contents

CHAPTER 1
CONSIDERATIONS FOR PROGRAMME DESIGN: NEEDS ANALYSIS

Rodrigo Aspe MSc, ASCC

PART ONE – INTRODUCTION

Successful sports performance is a combination of skill and athleticism; athletes need to demonstrate technical and tactical mastery with the optimal application of force during performance. As performance is multifactorial, elite athletes are often resourced with extensive technical staff to develop each quality. These may include a technical coach, physiologist, nutritionist, sport psychologist and strength and conditioning coach. Although each staff member has their own performance metrics within their specific area of expertise, they have a unified goal to enhance performance. Therefore it is important that the coaching staff work together and appreciate the input of others and how this may impact their own work. For example during periods of extensive training led by the technical coach, the strength and conditioning coach should alter their training and the nutritionist should modify calorie intake to fulfil the demand of the total training load. These alterations from each coach provide the athlete with the best platform to achieve the unified goal. The strength and conditioning coach is primarily tasked with enhancing athletic qualities that are key determinants to sporting success. A secondary goal is to create a robust athlete who is able to continually train and be available for competition. Creating a strength and conditioning programme that enhances specific physical qualities is a complex process

that must consider the physiological adaptation process and thus address the basic training principles: overload, specificity and variation (Stone *et al.*, 2000; Kraemer *et al.*, 2002; ACSM 2009). This is achieved by systematic manipulation of the acute programme variables: muscle action, loading and volume, exercise selection and order, rest periods, repetition velocity and frequency (Bird *et al.*, 2005).

Principles Of Training – Overload

The principle of overload refers to providing an appropriate stimulus for eliciting a desired physiological adaptation and athletic outcome. To promote physiological adaptations the training intensity imposed on an athlete must be greater than what they are accustomed to in normal training. Thus applying overload in a training programme is completed by systematically increasing the training stimulus imposed on the athlete. The most common method of applying an overload stimulus is by manipulation of the training intensity. Within a resistance training environment, intensity refers to the amount of weight employed within an exercise and is typically expressed as repetition maximum (RM), the greatest amount of weight that can be lifted with proper form for a desired number of repetitions, or as a percentage of one repetition maximum (1-RM). As the RM method does not require establishing a 1-RM it is often the preferred load prescription method in practice. Depending on the goal of training (power, strength, hypertrophy or muscular endurance) the repetition maximum continuum identifies the RM range. Relatively heavy loads should be used for power (1–3RM) and strength (3–8RM), moderate loads for hypertrophy (8–15RM), and light loads for muscular endurance (20>RM) (Bird et al., 2005). Although the repetition maximum continuum suggests specific adaptations from each RM, the training benefits are blended, as moderate loads will also incur strength adaptations (Sheppard and Triplett, 2016). For example, at the beginning of a training programme the stimulus for a back squat 5RM might be 100kg, an appropriate repetition range to elicit and increase in strength. During the initial stages of the programme this training stimulus will cause acute fatigue and a temporary reduction in performance due to the muscle damage caused by the overload (Chiu and Barnes, 2003). However, as the programme progresses, continual exposure to the stimulus of 5RM with 100kg elicits physiological adaptations and the athlete becomes accustomed to the training load and may be able to squat this load for a higher amount of repetitions. At this point the training stimulus becomes insufficient and a greater load is required for 5RM to promote further adaptations and an increase in strength. If the training stimulus is not increased, no further positive adaptations in muscle strength will occur. Whatever the focus of training, applying overload is necessary to promote physiological adaptations. If the goal is to increase aerobic capacity, intensity can be prescribed as a percentage of the lowest running velocity (velocity at VO_2max) that elicits maximal oxygen uptake during a volume of oxygen maximum (VO_2max) test or average running speed from a 5-minute time trial (Clarke et al., 2016). For example, overload would be applied using an interval session with a training intensity prescribed as a percentage of the average velocity in metres per second ($m\cdot s^{-1}$) obtained from a 5-minute time trial.

The adaptive response of the human body is integral in the application of overload. The adaptive response of the human body in regards to training enables adaptation provided there is sufficient time to recover. General adaptation syndrome (GAS) has been adapted to describe the body's response to training stimuli or stress (Buckner et al., 2017; Seyle, 1950). Training stress provokes an alarm response in the body, which has an acute detrimental effect on muscle function post-training (Fig. 1.1). Mechanistically the acute decline in muscle function is caused by depletion of energy sources and alterations in intra- and extra-cellular metabolite concentrations that are caused by the mechanical tension and metabolic stress (Schoenfeld, 2010). This can be substantially reduced with rest and appropriate nutrition within a few hours (Schoenfeld, 2010). Muscle damage can have a longer lasting effect on muscle function as this promotes an inflammatory response from the muscle, a phenomenon known as delayed onset muscle soreness (DOMS) which can last up to several days (Howatson and Van Someren, 2008). The culmination of these physiological responses takes time to dissipate as the body undergoes a resistive response and adapts to the training stress. The final stage of the resistive response is supercompensation where the training adaptation surpasses the pre-training level. Understanding of the recovery and adaptation process is essential when creating a strength and conditioning programme; frequent training sessions with insufficient recovery will not enable supercompensation. In fact, a chronic exhaustive state may manifest and could result in injury, illness or overtraining (Carfagno and Hendrix, 2014). Conversely, infrequent training sessions will not provide the athlete with frequent exposure to overload and the

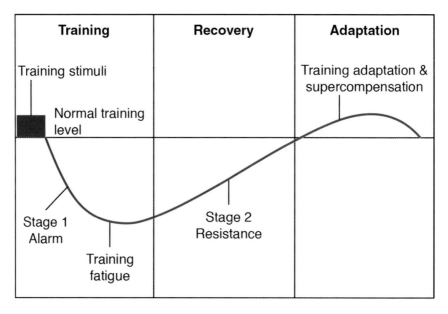

Fig. 1.1 An illustration of general adaptation-syndrome theory explaining response to training. Adapted from Seyle, H., 1956, The Stress of Life (London: Longmans Green).

supercompensation adaptation from the initial training stimuli will return to that of the habitual pre-training level. It should be noted that the level of fatigue experienced and subsequent recovery required after a training session is highly dependent on the level of stress created within training. For example, the after-effects of an interval session utilizing shuttle runs with frequent accelerations, change of direction and decelerations is markedly different from a training session that includes a continuous linear run at 70 per cent maximum heart rate (MHR). Finally, the summation of several training sessions may exacerbate training fatigue and increase the time required to reach supercompensation. Therefore, to optimize the recovery and adaptation process it is important to plan appropriately within programme design

micro and mesocycles. This further highlights the importance of communication and training integration between staff; to promote positive physiological adaptation each member of support staff has to consider the unifed goal of the training block and the amount of total training volume the athlete is experiencing.

Principles Of Training – Specificity

To successfully transfer training into performance it is important that the principle of specificity is realized. The principle of specificity alludes that the physiological adaptions from training are specific to the selected programme variables. These include the muscle actions involved (Roig et al., 2009), velocity of movement (Cormie *et al.*, 2007), muscles recruited and direction of force application (Loturco *et al.*, 2015). The most effective strength and conditioning programmes carefully consider acute training variables to produce specific physiological adaptations. For example, accelerative sprinting necessitates force production via triple extension of the lower limbs with a key emphasis on horizontal force production (Morin *et al.*, 2011). In this instance, the inclusion of horizontal jump squats compared to the barbell back squat or vertical jump squat may be more prudent as this closer matches the contraction velocity, direction of force application and muscle recruitment patterns of performance should the key goal be transfer of training (Loturco *et al.*, 2015). However, this does not mean that the back squat and vertical jump should be permanently excluded from training as these exercises could be employed to provide alternate training stimulus and desired physiological adaptations within other phases of training. For example the back squat may be utilized during a phase where the goal is to enhance lower-body strength and a stimulus of >80 per cent 1-RM is required to stimulate the appropriate neuromuscular mechanism (Shepard and Triplett, 2016). In this scenario both the vertical and horizontal jump squats would be inefficient exercise choices.

Athletes are permanently completing highly specific training by playing and training for their sport. While technical and tactical training is completed with the goal of improving skill, the intensity and volume of the session may cause a physiological training stimulus. Therefore, it is important that the technical and strength and conditioning coaches work collectively and do not attempt to promote diverse physiological adaptation or repeat training stimuli. Reilly and White (2005) demonstrated that twice-weekly small-sided

games for six weeks produced similar improvements in both the 6 × 30 second anaerobic shuttle test and multistage fitness test compared with matched interval training in youth premiership football club players. Therefore small side games may be used to simultaneously develop technical skill or tactical plays and aerobic capacity, provided certain parameters such as pitch size, number of players, game duration and work:rest ratios are met (Hill-Haas, *et al.*, 2011). In addition it is important that the strength and conditioning coach understands and appreciates the technical and tactical movements but ultimately carefully considers programme design and exercise selection to apply overload and develop athletic qualities. While the notion of specificity is fundamental to transfer of training it is important that exercise specificity is progressive throughout a training programme; during preseason athletes may train non-specific movements that promote muscle and tissue adaptation whilst improving general athleticism. This general training will serve the athlete well, creating a solid foundation whilst providing appropriate physiological adaptations to facilitate the increased training intensity as the season approaches. Creating a strength and conditioning programme that only meets the training principle of specificity will provide limited opportunities to apply overload and variation, and thus a sufficient training stimulus to enhance physical qualities such as maximal strength.

Principles Of Training – Variation

The principle of variation is the deliberate alteration of the strength and conditioning programme over time; this ensures the training stimulus remains optimal throughout a season. Basic periodization separates the seasonal plan into three main subdivisions: 1) preparatory, 2) competitive and 3) transitional, which facilitates systematic variation of the acute training variables within seasonal planning (Haff and Haff, 2012). Typically strength and conditioning sessions progress from moderate-intensity high-volume training within the preparatory phase, which is achievable due to the absence of competition and reduced technical and tactical sessions, to high-intensity moderate-volume in the competitive phase due to the additional demands of competition and technical and tactical training sessions. As well as manipulation of volume and intensity, periodization enables variation of exercise selection. Within the preparatory phase the primary focus is on muscle recruitment and action. However, as the competitive phase approaches consideration must also be given to velocity of movement and direction of force application, thus progressing from general to more specific exercises.

The amount of variation required is partly dictated by the training experience of the athlete. The law of diminishing returns suggests the magnitude of physiological adaptation is related to the initial starting point, with greater developments in relatively novice athletes due to the large potential for adaptation (Appleby et al., 2012). Therefore basic overload coupled with concurrent technical and tactical training may provide enough stimuli and transfer of training to enhance performance in novice athletes. However, when it comes to advanced athletes, creating a programme requires more astute manipulation of overload, specificity and variation as their window for adaptation is small and requires more attention to detail with regards to transfer of training.

PART TWO – INTRODUCTION

Along with knowledge of the basic training principles, it is important to complete a needs analysis prior to programme design. To enhance performance, the strength and conditioning coach must delineate specific physical qualities that are key determinants to performance and determine the strengths and weaknesses of the athlete (Read et al., 2016). Therefore, before designing a strength and conditioning programme it is paramount that the strength and conditioning coach has coherent knowledge of both the sport and the athlete in question. The process of a needs analysis provides the strength and conditioning coach with a method that enables exercise prescription based on informed choices of the acute programme variables achieved by means of essential knowledge of the sport and athlete in question. The process of a needs analysis has four central components:

- Determination of the physiological demands
- The biomechanical characteristics of the movements involved
- Injury epidemiology of the sport
- Evaluation of the athlete.

Finally, completion of a needs analysis is essential to create a test battery that is relevant to the sport and identifies athlete strength and weakness that may need to be addressed within training. The process of a needs analysis and results from a testing battery provide the strength and conditioning coach with the important information required to create an evidence-based programme to achieve predetermined goals.

Needs Analysis – Physiological Demands

Understanding the physiological demands of the sport considers several aspects of performance. Firstly it is important to determine the predominant metabolic pathway. When a muscle or group of muscles are recruited to produce force, the magnitude and duration of force determines the energy system (Herda and Cramer, 2016). For example, netball has a total duration of sixty minutes and elite runners will regularly complete the half marathon distance in less than sixty-five minutes. However, both sports have distinctly different energy demands; the half marathon is a continuous linear race and elite athletes will work at 75–85 per cent Vo2max, a pace that does not evoke Vo2max (Joyner and Coyle, 2008). Therefore it is no surprise that female champion endurance athletes display extremely high Vo2max values between 63–76.5 ml^{-1} min-1 (Joyner and Coyle, 2008). Conversely netball is intermittent and players will transition between walking, jogging, shuffling, running, sprinting and jumping (Fox et al., 2013). The actions can be separated into maximal intensity explosive actions such as multidirectional accelerations, declarations and jumps that require high amounts of concentric and eccentric force production; and submaximal intensity actions of walking, jogging and shuffling which provide opportunity for aerobic recovery (Thomas et al., 2016). Additionally, within netball players have multiple opportunities for recovery whether it is during in-game rest periods as play moves from one area of the court to another or via the 3 minutes afforded to breaks between quarters. These brief recovery periods enable repeated maximal intensity explosive actions that are commonly seen within intermittent sports, such as tennis, football, field hockey and rugby. Moreover the work-to-rest periods are specific to each sport and the metabolic pathway contribution differs consequently. A strength and conditioning programme must address the specific energy system demands and force production profiles for each sport.

It is also important to determine the key physical fitness qualities that are associated with the sport; these could include aerobic capacity, anaerobic capacity, strength, power, max velocity, acceleration, deceleration and/or change of direction. If the sport in question has several fitness qualities then they should be ranked in order of importance and coupled with athlete testing results to systematically determine goals of training that are most likely to have a positive effect on performance. For example within netball, centres have been reported to perform an average of 57.7±10 sprints, 90±11.1 runs, 53.7±6.7 jumps and 134.7±16.8 passes with the average duration of a high intensity lasting 1 to 3 seconds (Fox et al., 2013). While this data suggests anaerobic capacity is an important fitness quality to consistently perform throughout a game, it is equally important that players have sufficient aerobic capacity to efficiently recover during submaximal activities and breaks in play. This is further highlighted by the 75–85 per cent maximum heart rate reported during match play, as the game progresses greater demand will be placed on the aerobic energy system (Thomas et al., 2017b). Therefore it is important to determine the fitness qualities that are determinants of performance and then identify if this is a strength or weakness for the athlete. For example a netball player with a high anaerobic capacity but low aerobic capacity may be able to perform frequent repeated high-intensity activities during the first and second quarters. However, as the duration of the game increases and greater contribution is placed on their aerobic capacity, their ability to frequently perform repeated high-intensity actions will gradually decline. This example highlights the importance of being able to determine the physical requirements of the sport and identifiy the strength and weakness of the athlete; as developing the aerobic capacity of this athlete will be more beneficial compared to developing their anaerobic capacity to improve performance. Finally, it should be noted that the physical qualities required within a sport may be different, depending on playing position. Time-motion analysis data from Fox *et al.* (2013) identifies that defensive, mid-court and attacking positions all display different game statistics with regards to time spent walking, jogging, shuffling, running, sprinting and jumping.

Slightly more complex analysis necessitates knowledge, and understanding of the physiological undergoing of each fitness quality. For example, physiological mechanisms that contribute toward acceleration are leg extension strength, trunk stability, leg stiffness, stretch-shortening cycle capabilities and rate of force development (RFD) (Morin *et al.*, 2011: Read *et al.*, 2016). Therefore if acceleration is a target fitness quality it is important to determine which mechanism is limiting performance. Thomas *et al.* (2016) established that stronger netball players, determined by isometric mid-thigh pull, performed more favourably in 5- and 10-metre sprints than their weaker academy counterparts. Furthermore the stronger athletes also demonstrated better scores in change of direction (COD) assessment and measures of lower-body leg power. This demonstrates the importance of strength within performance of explosive movements that involve concentric and eccentric muscle actions. It is likely that netball players routinely perform jumping, acceleration, deceleration and change of direction patterns whilst training for their sport. Therefore a strength and conditioning coach should evaluate technical training and establish which physical qualities are routinely trained, as strength training coupled with netball training may provide greater improvement to speed and COD performance. Moreover it is important to include a variety of assessments within a testing battery to evaluate which physical qualities and underpinning mechanism the strength and conditioning programme should target.

Needs Analysis – Biomechanical Demands

The biomechanical analysis of the sport can be split into two sections, kinematics and kinetics. Kinematics refers to the characteristic of motion from a spatial and temporal perspective without reference to the forces causing the movements (Hamill *et al.*, 2015). Angular kinematics is of particular interest when designing a strength and conditioning programme, as this is an observation of joint movement sequences or segmental velocities within a specific movement pattern. Additionally the planes of motion (sagittal, frontal and transverse) should be considered together with muscle recruitment and coordination. During performance of a netball shoulder pass, the arm movement is initiated with shoulder flexion culminating with elbow extension, wrist flexion and rotation of the torso (Hetherington *et al.*, 2009). Therefore to enhance this movement, exercise selection should consider the key kinematic factors such as muscle recruitment, joint movement sequences and planes of motion. Programming a unilateral dumbbell bench press compared to a barbell bench press may better satisfy the kinematic requirements of the sporting moment whilst targeting strength development. However when targeting RFD, a standing one-arm medicine ball throw will closer match muscle contraction velocity whilst providing movement on the transverse plane with torso rotations that are evident during performance of the netball shoulder pass.

Kinetic movement analysis examines the forces causing movement or maintaining static body positions that have no movement (Hamill *et al.*, 2015). Kinetic analysis is more difficult to

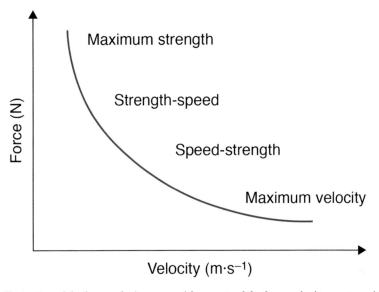

Fig. 1.2 An illustration of the force-velocity curve with aspects of the force-velocity spectrum identified.

perform, as forces cannot be accurately evaluated without specialist equipment (Kraemer *et al.*, 2012). Acceleration of the body or limb will generally be accomplished by a concentric muscle action and deceleration will be achieved by an eccentric action (Hamill *et al.*, 2015). This is important to consider as the forces experienced during jump landing can be in excess of four times body weight and muscles should be conditioned to tolerate these forces to prevent injury (Thomas *et al.*, 2017b). For the strength and conditioning coach, kinetic analysis should be considered as maximizing force production within the body. However it is important that maximal force is developed within the spectrum of high and low contraction velocities (Fig. 1.2). Moreover, the rate at which force can be developed is of greater interest than the amount of force that can be achieved due to the limited time to apply force in a sporting context. McBride *et al.* (1999) demonstrated strength adaptations are specific to training history and contraction velocity, as Olympic weightlifters outperformed sprinters and powerlifters in a range of assessments across the force–velocity curve.

Needs Analysis – Injury Epidemiology

Within sport, athletic injury can be classified as contact injuries or non-contact injuries, the difference being the mechanism as to how the injury occurred. A contact injury comes from the body being exposed to an external force or excessive load. Within field hockey, a contact injury may come from being struck with the ball and in rugby during contact within a tackle. Non-contact injuries generally occur during accelerative or decelerative movement patterns, and it is likely that there are a variety of predisposing factors such as insufficient range of motion about a joint, muscle weakness, previous injury, strength imbalance between agonist and antagonist muscles and fatigue (Small *et al.*, 2010). For example sprinting is the primary mechanism for a hamstring strain within soccer due to the hamstring being a biarticular muscle (crosses two joints) and thus working simultaneously during the late stage swing phase to eccentrically decelerate the limb whilst controlling knee extension (Small *et al.*, 2009). Couple this with fatigue, muscle imbalance or previous injury and the likelihood of injury is high. Moreover, within a sporting context sprinting is usually performed in a series of movements that contain a subsequent action such as a deceleration, change of direction or jump, which places considerable demand on the muscles, ligaments and tendons to produce and tolerate force. It is at this point that tissue around the limb or joint fails to meet the demand imposed and becomes injured by way of muscle or ligament damage.

Playing and training for particular sports may increase the probability of injury due to overuse. Overuse injuries are specific to youth athletes and occur due to repetitive submaximal musculoskeletal actions with insufficient time for recovery and adaptation between training sessions (DiFiori et al., 2014). Again there are multiple factors that can contribute to overuse injuries such as growth spurts, high training volumes, previously injury and amenorrhea. Therefore special consideration should particularly be given to youth female athletes (DiFiori et al., 2014). An example of overuse injury may be the repetitive bowling action in cricket or freestyle swimming where a high volume of shoulder circumduction is performed within sport-specific training. Consequently in sports where overuse injuries are a potential risk, such as bowling and freestyle, the strength and conditioning coach should consider strengthening the shoulder stabilizers and antagonist muscle groups, whilst all the coaching staff work together to manage total training volume.

Information from the biomechanical analysis should be utilized within the injury analysis to help establish mechanisms for injury. When this is complete, exercise and training intensity can be considered in a strength and conditioning programme to match the demands of performance and injuries inherent to the sport or movement patterns within this sport. This information should be communicated to other technical staff, such as the physiotherapist and technical coach, so that they are aware of the potential injury risk and plan accordingly within their own work, or integrated with the work of other technical staff. Regardless of the sport there are often multiple related factors that eventually lead to injury; fatigue impairs kinematics, which causes improper loading or uncontrollable movement that increases the probability of injury (Kraemer et al., 2012; Small et al., 2010). It is the role of the strength and conditioning coach to determine how the athlete may encounter injury during performance, and subsequently target the underlying mechanisms within the strength and conditioning programme.

Needs Analysis – Evaluation Of The Athlete

The final part of the needs analysis is evaluation of the athlete; this should include the athlete's needs and goals. Firstly it is important to establish training status as this may impact the basic training principles and influence exercise selection during programme design. This includes the training age and history of the athlete; this will determine the volume, intensity and frequency of training. Novice athletes respond favourably to basic training principles whereas well-trained athletes require a much larger training stimulus and astute consideration to specificity, variation and the acute programme variables (Appleby et al., 2012). Likewise training history will normally indicate the modes of exercises the athlete has encountered and level of competence. Dysfunctional movement patterns should not be loaded regardless of the experience of the athlete and technical competence should be assured in all exercises that are selected within the strength and conditioning programme (Lloyd and Oliver, 2012). For example the level of skill and coordination required to complete a weighted vest countermovement jump and hang power clean are distinctly different, despite eliciting similar training adaptations with regards to RFD. Programming a hang power clean for a novice athlete over a weighted vest countermovement jump has questionable training efficacy. In addition to training age and history, information regarding illness and injury history should also be obtained as this is a key factor in injury reoccurrence (Small *et al.*, 2010). Finally details regarding the athlete's personal life should be collected, these include stress level, sleep patterns and quality of sleep, nutritional information and employment details. Discovering irregularities in any of these topics may impact the recovery adaptation process and the desired physiological outcomes of the strength and conditioning programme.

Needs Analysis – Gender Specificity

There are some specific considerations when creating a strength and conditioning programme for females in comparison with males:

- Physiological differences such as menstruation and hormonal profile between males and females, specifically the production of testosterone (Vingren *et al.*, 2010)
- Anthropometrical differences; there are obvious differences between males and females with regards to body fat percentage, muscle mass and hip width in relation to the waist and shoulders (Lloyd and Faigenbaum, 2016)
- Joint laxity is more apparent in females compared to males and this seems to be exacerbated after puberty (Myer *et al.*, 2008)
- Level and intensity of competition and training history relating to the slower development and professionalism of female sport compared to male sport

(Zatsiorsky and Kraemer, 2006)
- Coach/athlete relationship and environment may need to be considered with female athletes as there seems to be different perceptions on nutritional intake, body mass and body shape required to succeed in sport between males and females (Adams *et al.*, 2016; McMahon and Barker-Ruchti, 2017).

For example, females who participate in sports such as soccer, netball and basketball suffer anterior cruciate ligament (ACL) injury at a four- to six-fold greater rate than men (Myer *et al.*, 2008). The mechanisms that may contribute to this are multifactorial and may include physiological differences, anthropometrical differences, joint laxity and total training volume (Lloyd and Faigenbaum, 2016; Myer *et al.*, 2008; Zatsiorsky and Kraemer, 2006). This not only highlights the specific considerations required within a strength and conditioning programme for females but also the importance of athlete adherence to minimize the potential for injury with appropriate conditioning. Moreover promoting a positive training environment for female athletes may necessitate a different coaching style compared to males (Adams *et al.*, 2016; McMahon and Barker-Ruchti, 2017).

Needs Analysis – Testing

After completing a needs analysis and establishing key determinants of performance, a suitable test battery can be established to identify the athlete's strengths and weaknesses in comparison to their peers, characteristics of elite performers and/or relevant normative data. Elite performance data can be searched for using Google Scholar and relative normative data can be found in key strength and conditioning textbooks such as *The Essentials of Strength Training and Conditioning*, 4th edition. It is important to identify key benchmarks from normative data outwith the team training data as there is no way to identify if the team scores are a strength or a weakness. For example, an athlete may score the best countermovement jump in comparison with their teammates, which would suggest lower-body leg power is a strength. However, when this is compared with elite data the whole team may score poorly, so in fact it is a weakness and should be a focal point of training. Therefore, creating a testing battery to best suit the needs of your athlete and ensure transfer of training requires appropriate analysis of data post-testing, prior to the creation of a strength and conditioning programme (Read et al., 2016; Brady et al., 2017). Recently Read et al. (2016) published a coherent article on testing specific physical qualities that range across the force–velocity curve – the reader is directed to this article for further knowledge on tests that relate to qualities such as reactive strength index and the stretch-shortening cycle. Finally the testing battery should be periodically revisited to evaluate the training programme and monitor athlete progress. If the planned adaptations have not been reached then the strength and conditioning coach must revisit and evaluate the needs analysis, testing battery and programme design.

The selection of tests to determine fitness qualities can be challenging; generally this is limited by the equipment available. One of the most important factors to consider is the validity and reliability of the test – validity refers to the degree that the test measures what it is intended to measure or claims to measure. Reliability refers to the ability of the test to produce consistent and repeatable results at different time points. For example, if the goal is to assess VO_2max, the running-based activities are carried out in a laboratory with a graded maximal exertion running test completed on a motorized treadmill with full breath-by-breath analysis. In addition, the duration of the test should be between 5 and 8 minutes to maximally stress the aerobic system. For a team of soccer players this would be time-extensive and require access to the specialist equipment that is costly and requires specialized training. The 20-metre shuttle run test has reported a high level relationship with VO_2max r = 0.9 and reliability r = 0.97 and can be deemed a valid and reliable alternative assessment of aerobic capacity compared to a graded maximal exertion VO_2max test (Clarke et al., 2016). The inclusion of this test within the scenario has scientific rationale as well as practical application. Each test should be considered in this manner; is it a valid and reliable test while being applicable and providing useful data?

The collection of test data also needs strategic consideration and planning. To collect accurate data the tests need to be organized with a specific protocol that each athlete adheres to. Vaverka et al. (2016) investigated the countermovement jump with and without arm swing, determining that the use of arms enhanced jump height by 38%. Consequently it is important that test protocols are clearly defined prior to data collection and the athletes have opportunities to familiarize themselves with the test. Confusion with the protocol and different techniques may provide a data set that delivers an inaccurate reflection of physical qualities. This extends beyond technique considerations and should be reflected in the warm-up, activity recommendation 24-hours prior to testing, test order, trials of each test and rest between trials and tests. One of the most important logistical concerns is the order of the test battery as endurance performance can have a detrimental effect on strength (Häkkinen, 2003). Therefore it would be prudent to determine the most exhaustive and fatiguing tests within a test battery and place them towards the end. For example it would be wise to carry out any maximal exertion aerobic testing after lower-body assessments of strength and power, as in the opposite order this is likely to affect results. Finally, where possible the timeframe between tests should be enough to reduce the negative effect of fatigue without losing the positive effects of the warm-up (McGowan *et al.*, 2015). To ensure reliability of results it would be sensible to determine a reliability measure for tests where applicable. The coefficient of variation is easy to determine and provides a valuable insight to the reliability of data; the reader is directed to an article that provides a thorough explanation of excel techniques by Turner *et al.* (2016) called 'Data analysis for strength and conditioning coaches: using Excel to analyze reliability, differences, and relationships'. If sound planning and protocols are not put in place, the validity and reliability of the test data may be reduced, thus decreasing the accuracy of future evaluation.

Needs Analysis – Analyzing And Presenting Data

Upon completion of data collection, appropriate analysis is required. If this is the first time data has been collected, this should be compared with elite or normative values of a similar population to determine the strength and weakness for the athlete, and inform programming. The data obtained can initiate dialogue with both the athlete and technical coach whilst building trust and rapport. Results are important to identify goals and establish physical targets for the athlete, as well as producing integrated physical and performance goals with the technical coach. Analysis, presentation and communication of test data are vital to ensure athlete motivation and unified goals amongst the technical staff (Hoffman, 2012). Advanced methods for analysing and presenting data can be completed on accessible software programmes such as Excel. Total score of athleticism and smallest worthwhile change are two methods that may be of particular interest to the strength and conditioning coach; these methods can provide useful

analysis that informs of strengths and weaknesses whilst evaluating the effectiveness of the strength and conditioning programme (Turner, 2014; Turner *et al.*, 2016). For a full explanation and step-by-step application of these methods in Excel, the reader is directed towards the articles by Turner (2014) and Turner *et al.* (2016).

Testing And Data Analysis – Field Hockey Example

Based on the information provided in this chapter an example test battery, rationale and benchmark scores for female field hockey have been identified in Table 1.1. It should be noted that this example is by no means a comprehensive or complete list of tests that could be included. For example depending on the sport and athlete, further tests that assess physical qualities such as range of motion, flexibility and speed-strength could be included. However, test selection is often dependent on equipment and time available. Table 1.1 has been provided as a guide to illustrate the planning and research that should go into data collection and subsequent data analysis. This will enable coherent determination of athletic strength and weaknesses, thus creating appropriate training goals.

SUMMARY

Designing a strength and conditioning programme to target specific physiological adaptations is a complex process. The strength and conditioning coach must have sufficient knowledge of the basic training principles of overload, specificity and variation. The process of a needs analysis then guides the strength and conditioning coach through a methodical process that considers the fitness qualities typical of elite performers, movements and muscle recruitment within performance and the injuries inherent to the sport. Finally

Test	Rationale	Benchmarks
Skinfold Assessment for body fat percentage.	Monitor body composition and regulation of non-functional mass that may decrease exercise economy. (Thomas et al., 2017a).	Youth elite 18±6.1% and sub-elite 22.9±7% hockey players (Elferink-Gemser et al., 2007). Regional players 24.8±0.7% and club players 27%±0.8% (Keogh et al., 2003).
Countermovement Jump.	Will determine an indication of lower body explosive strength (Read et al., 2016).	Regional players 35±1cm and club players 29±1cm (Keogh et al., 2003).
10-Metre Sprint.	Time motion analysis identifies elite hockey players will on average perform 30 sprints per game with a mean duration of 3 seconds (Spencer et al., 2004).	National players 1.96±0.06s (Rechichi et al., 2013) Regional players 2.01±0.02s and club players 2.16±0.03 (Keogh et al., 2003).
Repeated Sprint Ability (6 x 30-metre sprint ability test).	Time motion analysis identifies elite hockey players will on average perform 4 sprints with a mean recovery time of 15 s (Spencer et al., 2004).	National players total time 29.93±0.92s and percentage decrement 4.8±2.5 (Rechichi et al., 2013).
30-15 Intermittent Fitness Test.	Measure of aerobic capacity for team sports that include intermittent multidirectional movements. Score can be used to estimate VO_2peak (Clarke, 2016; Thomas et al., 2017a).	Australian Women's Hockey squad Vo2peak 55.1±3.49 mL kg-1 min-1 (Bishop et al., 2003). Predicted VO_2peak from multistage fitness test. Regional players 43.7±1.2 mL kg-1 min-1and club players 38.9±1.3 mL kg-1 min-1 (Keogh et al., 2003).
cm = centimetres, s = seconds, mL kg-1 min-1 = millilitres per kilogram per minute and Vo2 = volume of oxygen.		

Table 1.1 Example testing battery, rationale and bench mark scores for field hockey. The tests are also listed in order of the least to most fatiguing.

evaluation of the athlete, determination of a specific testing battery and appropriate analysis of test data compared with elite data or relevant normative values should ensure that the strength and conditioning coach has all the information for programme design. Furthermore intelligent manipulation of the acute programme variables should provide transfer of training and improve performance. The secondary goal of training should be to create a robust, well-balanced athlete that has minimized the potential of injury with an appropriate training intervention. On a final note, the strength and conditioning coach should understand that they are often working as part of a technical support team, where communication is vital and sometimes alterations in programming are required to support and develop the unified goal.

REFERENCES

ACSM (2009) Progression models in resistance training for healthy adults. *Medicine and Science in Sports and Exercise*, 41(3), pp.687–708.

Adams, V.J., Goldufsky, T.M. and Schlaff, R.A. (2016) Perceptions of body weight and nutritional practices among male and female National Collegiate Athletic Association Division II athletes. *Journal of American College Health*, 64(1), pp.19–24.

Appleby, B., Newton, R.U. and Cormie, P. (2012) Changes in strength over a 2-year period in professional rugby union players. *The Journal of Strength and Conditioning Research*, 26(9), pp.2538–2546.

Bird, S.P., Tarpenning, K.M. and Marino, F.E. (2005) Designing resistance training programmes to enhance muscular fitness. *Sports Medicine*, 35(10), pp.841–851.

Bishop, D., Lawrence, S. and Spencer, M. (2003) Predictors of repeated-sprint ability in elite female hockey players. *Journal of Science and Medicine in Sport*, 6(2), pp.199–209.

Brady, C., Comyns, T., Harrison, A. and Warrington, G. (2017) Focus of Attention for Diagnostic Testing of the Force–Velocity Curve. *Strength and Conditioning Journal*, 39(1), pp.57–70.

Buckner, S.L., Mouser, J.G., Dankel, S.J., Jessee, M.B., Mattocks, K.T. and Loenneke, J.P. (2017) The General Adaptation Syndrome: Potential misapplications to resistance exercise. *Journal of Science and Medicine in Sport*. 00: 1–3. [accessed 11 July 2017]

Carfagno, D.G. and Hendrix, J.C. (2014) Overtraining syndrome in the athlete: current clinical practice. *Current Sports Medicine Reports*, 13(1), pp.45–51.

Chiu, L.Z. and Barnes, J.L. (2003) The Fitness-Fatigue Model Revisited: Implications for Planning Short-and Long-Term Training. *Strength and Conditioning Journal*, 25(6), pp.42–51.

Clarke, R., Dobson, A. and Hughes, J. (2016) Metabolic Conditioning: Field Tests to Determine a Training Velocity. *Strength and Conditioning Journal,* 38(1), pp.38–47.

Cormie, P., McCaulley, G.O. and McBride, J.M. (2007) Power versus strength-power jump squat training: influence on the load-power relationship. *Medicine and Science in Sports and Exercise,* 39(6), pp.996–1003.

DiFiori, J.P., Benjamin, H.J., Brenner, J.S., Gregory, A., Jayanthi, N., Landry, G.L. and Luke, A. (2014) Overuse injuries and burnout in youth sports: a position statement from the American Medical Society for Sports Medicine. *British Journal of Sports Medicine,* 48(4), pp.287–288.

Elferink-Gemser, M.T., Visscher, C., Lemmink, K.A. and Mulder, T. (2007) Multidimensional performance characteristics and standard of performance in talented youth field hockey players: A longitudinal study. *Journal of Sports Sciences,* 25(4), pp.481–489.

Fox, A., Spittle, M., Otago, L. and Saunders, N. (2013) Activity profiles of the Australian female netball team players during international competition: Implications for training practice. *Journal of Sports Sciences,* 31(14), pp.1588–1595.

Haff, G.G., Haff, E.E. and Hoffman, J. (2012) 'Training Integration and Periodization' in Hoffman, J. (ed.) *NSCA's Guide to Program Design.* Leeds: Human Kinetics, pp.213–258.

Häkkinen, K., Alen, M., Kraemer, W.J., Gorostiaga, E., Izquierdo, M., Rusko, H., Mikkola, J., Häkkinen, A., Valkeinen, H., Kaarakainen, E. and Romu, S. (2003) Neuromuscular adaptations during concurrent strength and endurance training versus strength training. *European Journal of Applied Physiology,* 89(1), pp.42–52.

Hamill, J., Knutzen, K.M. and Derrick, T.R. (2015) *Biomechanical Basis of Human Movement,* 4th ed., London: Wolters Kluwer.

Herda, T.J. and Cramer, J.T. (2016) 'Bioenergetics of Exercise and Training' in Haff, G.G. and Triplett, N.T. (eds.) *Essentials of Strength Training and Conditioning,* 4th ed., Leeds: Human Kinetics, pp.43–64.

Hetherington, S., King, S., Visentin, D. and Bird, M.L. (2009) A Kinematic and Kinetic Case Study of a Netball Shoulder Pass. *International Journal of Exercise Science,* 2(4).

Hill-Haas, S.V., Dawson, B., Impellizzeri, F.M. and Coutts, A.J. (2011) Physiology of small-sided games training in football. *Sports Medicine,* 41(3), pp.199–220.

Hoffman, R.J. (2012) 'Athlete Testing and Program Evaluation' in Hoffman, J. (ed.) NSCA's *Guide to Program Design.* Leeds: Human Kinetics, pp.213–258.

Howatson, G. and Van Someren, K.A. (2008) The prevention and treatment of exercise-induced muscle damage. *Sports Medicine,* 38(6), pp.483.

Joyner, M.J. and Coyle, E.F. (2008) Endurance exercise performance: the physiology of champions. *The Journal of Physiology,* 586(1), pp.35–44.

Keogh, J.W., Weber, C.L. and Dalton, C.T. (2003) Evaluation of anthropometric, physiological, and skill-related tests for talent identification in female field hockey. *Canadian Journal of Applied Physiology,* 28(3), pp.397–409.

Kraemer, W.J., Comstock, B.A., Clarke, J.E. and Dunn-Lewis, D. (2012) 'Athletes Needs Analysis' in Hoffman, J. (ed.) *NSCA's Guide to Program Design.* Leeds: Human Kinetics, pp.213–258.

Kraemer, W.J., Ratamess, N.A. and French, D.N., 2002. Resistance training for health and performance. *Current Sports Medicine Reports,* 1(3), pp.165–171.

Lloyd, R.S. and Faigenbaum, A.D. (2016) 'Age- and Sex-Related Differences and Their Implications for Resistance Exercise' in Haff, G.G. and Triplett, N.T. (eds.) *Essentials of Strength Training and Conditioning,* 4th ed., Leeds: Human Kinetics, pp.135–154.

Lloyd, R.S. and Oliver, J.L., 2012. The youth physical development model: A new approach to long-term athletic development. *Strength and Conditioning Journal,* 34(3), pp.61–72.

Loturco, I., Pereira, L.A., Kobal, R., Zanetti, V., Kitamura, K., Abad, C.C.C. and Nakamura, F.Y., 2015. Transference effect of vertical and horizontal plyometrics on sprint performance of high-level U-20 soccer players. *Journal of Sports Sciences*, 33(20), pp.2182–2191.

McBride, J.M., Triplett-McBride, T,. Davie, A. and Newton, R.U. (1999) A comparison of strength and power characteristics between power lifters, Olympic lifters, and sprinters. *The Journal of Strength and Conditioning Research*, 13(1), pp.58–66.

McGowan, C.J., Pyne, D.B., Thompson, K.G. and Rattray, B. (2015) Warm-up strategies for sport and exercise: mechanisms and applications. *Sports Medicine*, 45(11), pp.1523–1546.

McMahon, J. and Barker-Ruchti, N., 2017. Assimilating to a boy's body shape for the sake of performance: three female athletes' body experiences in a sporting culture. *Sport, Education and Society*, 22(2), pp.157–174.

Morin, J.B., Edouard, P. and Samozino, P. (2011) Technical ability of force application as a determinant factor of sprint performance. *Medicine and Science in Sports and Exercise*, 43(9), pp.1680–1688.

Myer, G.D., Ford, K.R., Paterno, M.V., Nick, T.G. and Hewett, T.E., 2008. The effects of generalized joint laxity on risk of anterior cruciate ligament injury in young female athletes. *The American Journal of Sports Medicine*, 36(6), pp.1073–1080.

Read, P.J., Bishop, C., Brazier, J. and Turner, A.N., 2016. Performance Modeling: A System-Based Approach to Exercise Selection. *Strength and Conditioning Journal*, 38(4), pp.90–97.

Rechichi, C., Polgaze, T. and Spencer, M. (2012) 'Hockey Players' in Tanner, R. and Gore, C. (eds.) *Physiological Tests for Elite Athletes,* 2nd ed., London: Human Kinetics, pp.331–340.

Reilly, T. and White, C. (2005) Small-sided games as an alternative to interval-training for soccer players. *Science and Football V*, pp.355–358.

Roig, M., O'Brien, K., Kirk, G., Murray, R., McKinnon, P., Shadgan, B. and Reid, W.D. (2009) The effects of eccentric versus concentric resistance training on muscle strength and mass in healthy adults: a systematic review with meta-analysis. *British Journal of Sports Medicine*, 43(8), pp.556–568.

Schoenfeld, B.J. (2010). The mechanisms of muscle hypertrophy and their application to resistance training. *The Journal of Strength and Conditioning Research*, 24(10), pp.2857–2872.

Selye, H. (1956) *The Stress of Life*. London: Longmans Green.

Selye, H. (1950) Stress and the general adaptation syndrome. *British Medical Journal*, 1(4667), p.1383.

Sheppard, J.M. and Triplett, N.T. (2016) 'Programm Design for Resistance Training' in Haff, G.G. and Triplett, N.T. (eds.) *Essentials of Strength Training and Conditioning*, 4th ed., Leeds: Human Kinetics, pp.439–469.

Small, K., McNaughton, L.R., Greig, M., Lohkamp, M. and Lovell, R. (2009) Soccer fatigue, sprinting and hamstring injury risk. *International Journal of Sports Medicine*, 30(08), pp.573–578.

Small, K., McNaughton, L., Greig, M. and Lovell, R. (2010) The effects of multidirectional soccer-specific fatigue on markers of hamstring injury risk. *Journal of Science and Medicine in Sport*, 13(1), pp.120–125.

Spencer, M., Lawrence, S., Rechichi, C., Bishop, D., Dawson, B. and Goodman, C. (2004) Time–motion analysis of elite field hockey, with special reference to repeated-sprint activity. *Journal of Sports Sciences*, 22(9), pp.843–850.

Stone, M.H., Collins, D., Plisk, S., Haff, G. and Stone, M.E. (2000) Training Principles: Evaluation of Modes and Methods of Resistance Training. *Strength and Conditioning Journal*, 22(3), p.65.

Thomas, C., Comfort, P., Jones, P.A. and Dos' Santos, T. (2016) A Comparison of Isometric Mid-Thigh Pull Strength, Vertical Jump, Sprint Speed, and Change of

Direction Speed in Academy Netball Players. *International Journal of Sports Physiology and Performance*, pp.1–20.

Thomas, C., Comfort, P., Jones, P.A. and Dos' Santos, T. (2017a) Strength and Conditioning for Netball: A Needs Analysis and Training Recommendations. *Strength and Conditioning Journal*, 39(4), pp.10-21.

Thomas, C., Ismail, K.T., Simpson, R., Comfort, P., Jones, P.A. and Dos' Santos, T. (2017b) Physical Profiles of Female Academy Netball Players by Position. *The Journal of Strength and Conditioning Research*. 00: 1–15. [accessed 11 July 2017]

Turner, A.N. (2014) Total Score of Athleticism: a strategy for assessing an athlete's athleticism. *Professional Strength and Conditioning*, (33), pp.13–17.

Turner, A., Brazier, J., Bishop, C., Chavda, S., Cree, J. and Read, P. (2015) Data analysis for strength and conditioning coaches: using Excel to analyze reliability, differences, and relationships. *Strength and Conditioning Journal*, 37(1), pp.76–83.

Vaverka, F., Janda ka, D., Zahradník, D., Uchytil, J., Farana, R., Supej, M. and Vodi ar, J. (2016) Effect of an arm swing on countermovement vertical jump performance in elite volleyball players. *Journal of Human Kinetics*, 53(1), pp.41–50.

Vingren, J.L., Kraemer, W.J., Ratamess, N.A., Anderson, J.M., Volek, J.S. and Maresh, C.M. (2010) Testosterone physiology in resistance exercise and training. *Sports Medicine*, 40(12), pp.1037–1053.

Zatsiorsky, V.M. and Kraemer, W.J. (2006) *Science and Practice of Strength Training*, 2nd ed., Leeds: Human Kinetics.

CHAPTER 2
STRENGTH AND POWER

Debby Sargent, MSc, PGDip, ASCC and Richard Clarke, MSc, ASCC
University of Gloucestershire, UK

Power is the product of force and velocity (Stone et al., 2003; Haff and Nimphius, 2012; Newton and Kraemer, 1994) and, for the vast majority of sports, generating high power outputs is suggested to be 'the most important factor in determining success' (Stone et al., 2003). Movements involved in explosive sports such as rapid changes of direction, sprinting, throwing, jumping, kicking and striking are all dependent on maximal power output to achieve a high velocity at release, take off and/or impact. (Newton and Kraemer, 1994; Haff and Nimphius, 2012; Stone et al., 2003).

Cross-sectional comparisons have demonstrated superior power-generating capabilities in athletes with greater strength levels (Stone et al., 2003; Carlock et al., 2004; Peterson et al., 2006; Stone et al., 2016; Secomb et al., 2015; Pallarés et al., 2012), such that these attributes have been shown to successfully differentiate between levels of performer (Carlock et al., 2014; Baker, 2014; Cronin and Hansen 2005; Abdelkrim at al 2010. Platzer et al., 2009; Secomb et al., 2015; Suchomel et al., 2016; Naisidou et al., 2017), with stronger and more powerful athletes more likely to perform at higher levels within their sport (Baker et al., 2014; Granados et al., 2013).

Optimizing strength and power development is therefore an essential training outcome for female athletes. The purpose of this chapter is to firstly provide an overview of the mechanisms that underpin strength and power development, followed by a brief discussion of the relevance and contribution of specific resistance and plyometric training methods to enhance strength and power development. The final section will include recommendations and examples of how to apply these specifically to the needs of the female athlete.

PHYSIOLOGY OF STRENGTH AND POWER

Force–Velocity Relationships

The ability of the muscle to generate force is not only determined by the sarcomere force-length relationship (Herzog et al., 2016), but by the speed and type of muscle contraction (isometric, concentric, and eccentric), with different contraction types demonstrating differences in force behaviour (Kuriki et al., 2012; see Fig. 2.1). An understanding of the force–velocity curve in relation to muscular strength and power production is paramount for the identification of appropriate integration of training methods to optimize sports performance.

When the velocity is zero (no movement occurs), the amount of force produced by the muscle exactly matches the external load – this is known as an isometric contraction. When the external load is less than the isometric strength, the muscle contracts concentrically demonstrating an inverse relationship between force and velocity. In simple terms, this means that as the velocity of contraction increases, the amount of force the muscle can

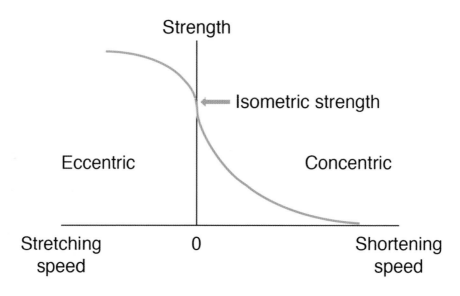

Fig. 2.1 Force-velocity curve for an isolated muscle.

produce decreases, primarily due to the fact that at high velocities of shortening, the number of actin-myosin cross bridges that can attach at any one time is reduced (Cormie et al., 2011a). Negative velocities occur when the muscle is lengthening whilst generating tension (eccentric contraction). The amount of force a muscle can generate is greatest during an eccentric contraction, with the force increasing as the speed of lengthening increases, plateauing around 1.2 times the maximal isometric force (Beltman et al., 2004; Babault et al., 2001). At the very highest rates of lengthening, reflex inhibition may prevent further increases in force generation occurring (Newton, 2011; Beltman et al., 2004; Babault et al., 2001). Various theories have been proposed to explain the greater force outputs demonstrated during eccentric contractions (see review by Nishikawa, 2016; Herzog et al., 2016). Firstly, preferential recruitment of the fast-twitch motor units (MUs) due to a reversal of the size principle is suggested to occur (Hortobágyi et al., 1996; Shepstone et al.,

2005; Nardone et al., 1989), although the evidence to support this is equivocal (Enoka and Duchateau, 1985). Secondly, the stretching of the muscle and the cross bridges themselves are thought to add to the overall tension produced by the muscle, with titin suggested to play a key role (Nishikawa, 2016; Herzog et al., 2016). For most sporting actions, stretch-shortening cycle muscle actions (SSC) are inherent and involve the coupling of eccentric and concentric muscle actions to enhance power output (see plyometric training section).

From an athlete perspective, the optimization of power development requires three key elements (Newton and Kraemer, 1994; Haff and Nimphius, 2012):

- An improvement in overall muscle strength development in order to maximize the force generating capacity of the muscle under all three types of muscle contraction (eccentric, isometric and concentric)
- An increase in the ability to develop large

forces at fast contraction velocities – that is, high rates of force development

- An increase in the capacity to continue producing high forces as the velocity of shortening increases.

Dynamic power can only be generated during the concentric portion of the force–velocity curve (Newton, 2011), with sporting events typically requiring athletes to produce power under loaded conditions. The ability to overcome a heavy resistance is called 'strength-speed' – in sporting situations the resistance may be an athlete's own body weight, an opponent's body weight (grappling and collision sports) or an implement (for example in strongman events). In contrast, the ability to overcome a lighter load (javelin, basketball) and generate high forces at high velocities is called 'speed-strength' (Siff, 2003). Both strength-speed and speed-strength are subsets of power (Baker et al., 2014; Siff, 2003). For most athletes playing their sport, they will need to maximize power over a continuum of loaded conditions, spanning a large portion of the force–velocity curve. For many sports it can be argued that power development over the full concentric range is necessary. Therefore, an athlete's development programme needs to fully reflect this using a diverse range of training modalities to adequately prepare that athlete for the demands of playing the sport.

Adaptations to Strength and Power Training

The main physiological mechanisms underpinning strength and power development are changes in the quantity and structure of the muscle (hypertrophy, pennation angle and fascicle length), together with modifications in the nervous system.

Hypertrophic response

Anatomical and physiological cross-sectional area (CSA) of a muscle is directly proportional to its maximal force-producing capabilities (Cormie et al., 2011a). Whilst this is true for all fibre types, the CSA of Type II MUs is particularly relevant in this chapter because of their superior abilities for power generation per unit CSA (Cormie et al., 2011a). Traditional heavy resistance training stimulates a hypertrophic response (increase in myofibrillar proteins, actin and myosin) (DeFreitas et al., 2011; Coffrey and Hawley, 2007; Phillips et al., 1997; Dreyer et al., 2008), with preferential increases in the Type II MUs (Fry, 2004), reported to occur through a combination of mechanical tension/stretch, increased metabolic stress and muscle damage (Schoenfeld, 2010). CSA increases can occur through the addition of sarcomeres in parallel or in series (increased fascicle length), or through architectural alterations in pennation angle (Stone et al., 2016). Compared to traditional heavy resistance training, eccentric training methods involving supramaximal loads (>100 per cent of 1-Repetition Maximum) have been shown to elicit a greater degree of hypertrophy as well as an increased fascicle length, which produces favourable increases in the velocity of shortening (Cormie et al., 2011a; Aagaard, 2010; Norrbrand et al., 2008; Roig et al., 2009). Hypertrophic responses have also been demonstrated following high-velocity plyometric training (Vissing et al., 2008; Kubo et al., 2007).

Traditionally, skeletal muscle hypertrophy has been deemed to be a relatively slow process, with some authors suggesting that significant increases in whole muscle CSA are only apparent after six to seven weeks of training (Phillips, 2000). However, more recent evidence suggests that this can occur in as little as two to four weeks (Seynnes et al., 2007; Abe et al., 2005; DeFreitas et al., 2011). Acute increases in muscle protein synthesis have been shown to occur within hours of the resistance training session (Dreyer et al., 2008, 2010; MacDougall et al., 1992; Hawley, 2009), with some authors reporting that this can

Olympic Weightlifting World Records

Men

Weight Class (kg)	Snatch (kg)	Clean & Jerk (kg)	Total (kg)	Total/kg BW
56	139	171	310	5.54
62	154	183	337	5.44
69	166	198	364	5.28
77	177	214	391	5.08
85	187	220	407	4.79
94	188	232	420	4.47
105	200	246	446	4.25

Women

Weight Class	Snatch (kg)	Clean & Jerk (kg)	Total (kg)	Total/kg BW
48	98	121	219	4.56
53	103	134	237	4.47
58	112	141	253	4.36
63	117	147	264	4.19
69	128	158	286	4.14
75	135	164	299	3.99
90	130	160	290	3.22

Table 2.1a A comparison of male and female weightlifting world records.

Track and Field World Records

Event	Men	Women	% difference F vs M
100m (secs)	9.58	10.49	9.50
200m (secs)	19.19	21.34	11.20
400m (secs)	43.03	47.6	10.62
High Jump (m)	2.45	2.09	-14.69
Long Jump (m)	8.95	7.52	-15.98
Triple Jump (m)	18.29	15.5	-15.25

Table 2.1b Comparison of male and female track and field world records.

remain elevated for up to 24 (115 per cent) hours in trained individuals, returning to basal levels by 36 hours (MacDougall et al., 1995). In a study comparing male and female responses to high-intensity resistance training (bilateral leg extension), post-exercise muscleprotein synthesis rates increased in both male (52 per cent) and female (47 per cent) physically active subjects and remained elevated for 2 hours. No significant (p<0.05) differences were found between groups (Dreyer et al., 2010). This data supports previous review findings that show that the rate of gain in CSA per day between males and females who have followed the same training programme is similar, with increases of 0.13 per cent and 0.14 per cent respectively (Wernbom et al., 2007; Hunter, 1985).

Although the rate of CSA gain is comparable between the sexes, males are reported to have a 20–30 per cent larger initial CSA than females (Fry, 2004; Dreyer et al., 2010; Hirsch et al., 2015; Maughan et al., 1983; Hunter, 1985; Bishop et al., 1989; Costill et al., 1976; Healy et al., 2014), which means that resistance training-induced absolute gains in CSA is typically greater in males (Fry, 2004; Hirsch et al., 2015; Maughan et al., 1983; Hunter, 1985). These differences in muscle CSA and the subsequent sex differences in force capabilities are evidenced during analysis of strength performances (Peterson et al., 2006; Hirsch et al., 2015; Komi and Karlsson, 1978; Trzaskoma and Trzaskoma, 2006). Table 2.1a shows Olympic weightlifting world records for male and female athletes across the weight classes. Comparisons between athletes competing in the 69kg weight class showed combined totals for the snatch and the clean and jerk, per kg body weight, of 5.28 for males and 4.14 for females (male value 21.6 per cent higher than the female value). Similarly, in Table 2.1b, track and field sprint and jump world records again show female performance values around 10–15 per cent of that for

males. However, it is important to make the point that when adjustments are made for lean muscle mass or body mass, women are reported to be at least as strong as men, at least in the lower body (Stone et al., 2007; Bosco et al., 2002; Hoffman et al., 1979; Miller et al., 1993; Staron et al., 1994; Burger and Burger, 2002).

Sex differences in muscle mass distributions between upper and lower body are a consistent finding reported in the literature (Bishop et al., 1989; Buśko and Gajewski, 2011; Bishop et al., 1987; Miller et al., 1993; Zatsiorsky and Kraemer, 2006; Stone et al., 2007). Generally, females report a significantly lower proportion of lean muscle mass in the upper body, even when adjustments are made for lean muscle mass or body mass (Burger and Burger et al., 2002; Stone et al., 2007). Stone et al. (2007) proposed that females' maximum strength relative to body mass (per kg) and lean body mass (per kg) compared to males' was 60 per cent and 70–75 per cent. For lower body, when compared to males, females' maximal strength relative to body mass (per kg) and lean muscle mass (per kg) is 80–85 per cent and 95–100 per cent.

Acute and chronic endocrine responses to resistance training play a crucial role in the development of muscle strength and power, via the regulation of protein turnover (Cook and Crewther, 2011; French, 2016). Depending on the prescription, resistance training can stimulate acute increases in both anabolic hormones (mainly testosterone and growth hormone) and catabolic hormones (cortisol) and these responses are summarized in Table 2.2 (Crewther et al., 2006; Aizawa et al., 2006). Anabolic hormones stimulate protein synthesis and inhibit protein breakdown, causing an increase in muscle hypertrophy (French, 2016; Crewther et al., 2006), whereas catabolic hormones do the reverse – increase muscle protein breakdown and decrease protein synthesis.

	Strength and Power Training Adaptation			Resting Hormonal Concentrations in athletes* Mean (Standard Deviation)		
Hormone	Strength, Hypertrophy	Strength, Neuronal	Dynamic Power (Explosive/Ballistic)	Male	Female	Training Adaptations Differences (Males vs Females)
Testosterone (TST)	↑↑↑↑	↑↑	↑↑↑↑	M>F (p<0.05) 450.0ng.dl-1 (68.7)	(5-10% of males) 36.0ng.dl-1 (4.8)	M: TST ↑72 % Hyp; 27% N F: ↔
GH	↑↑↑↑↑↑↑	↑	↕	4.6 ng.ml-1(6.9)	14.3ng.ml-1(14.1)	M: ↑ 850 % Hyp; 375% N F: 106% Hyp; nil N M>F regardless of RT programme F >M blood GH levels after RT.
IGF-1	↑↑↑	↑↑↑↑	↕	316.0ng.ml-1 (31.3)	366ng.ml-1 (75.0)	M: ↑ 9% Hyp;12% N M vs F: ↔ Hyp M vs F: M ↑ immediately post-RT; F↑1 hour post-RT
Cortisol	↑↑↑↑↑	↕	↑↑	19.9ug.dl-1 (9.0)	14.5ug.dl-1 (5.1)	M vs F: ↔, when lifting same relative load. M: ↑ 65% Hyp; ↔ N F: ↑125% Hyp; ↔ N

↑ = increase   ↕ = no change

Table 2.2 Summary of research examining the acute anabolic and catabolic hormone responses to hypertrophy, neuronal and dynamic power schemes. (Adapted from Crewther *et al.*, 2006 and Aizawa *et al.*, 2006)

Testosterone

Whilst hormones such as insulin and insulin-like growth factors are known to have anabolic qualities, testosterone and growth hormone are considered the primary anabolic hormones, with resting and acute post-resistance training levels being markedly different between the sexes (Burger *et al.*, 2002; Cardinale and Stone, 2004; Crewther *et al.*, 2006; Vingren *et al.*, 2010; Healey *et al.*, 2014; Kraemer and Ratamess, 2005; Linnamo *et al.*, 2005; Weiss *et al.*, 1983; see Table 2). Females have significantly lower resting testosterone concentrations (~10 per cent of male values) and do not appear to demonstrate acute elevations in testosterone concentrations post-resistance training (Ribeiro *et al.*, 2016; Crewther *et al.*, 2006; see Table 2.2). Chronic adaptations in resting testosterone concentrations are inconsistent or negligible, with some authors suggesting (French, 2016) that changes in resting testosterone over time are more of a reflection of variation in training volume and intensity across an athlete's programme.

The importance of testosterone to strength and power performance is supported by cross-sectional data involving elite track and field and team-based athletes (twenty-two female, forty-eight men). Both male and female athletes demonstrated a positive linear relationship (r=0.61, p<0.001) between testosterone and counter movement jump (CMJ) ability, with women's CMJ scores being 86.3 per cent that of the men (Cardinale and Stone, 2006). In contrast, a significant negative correlation (r=0.94, p<0.001) was found in a group of female athletes (throwers, gymnasts and footballers) between testosterone and relative isokinetic knee extension strength, although correlations were reported between strength measures and dehydroepiandrosterone sulphate (DHEAS). DHEAS is the predominant precursor responsible (r=0.98; p<0.001) for producing 90 per cent of circulating testosterone in females (Aizawa *et al.*, 2006), which suggests that this may be a more relevant marker of adaptation to resistance exercise and trainability of female athletes (Aizawa *et al.*, 2006) than testosterone per se.

Growth Hormone

Growth hormone (GH) is extremely responsive to exercise prescription targeting muscle growth (see Table 2.2) and although relative training-induced increases in GH response is larger in males, absolute values are larger in females (Aiwaza *et al.*, 2006; Healy *et al.*, 2014; Cook and Crewther, 2011; Kraemer and Ratamess, 2005; Linnamo *et al.*, 2005). This may be due to sex differences in GH secretion (Crewther *et al.*, 2006) and/or greater resting concentrations of GH (Aizawa *et al.*, 2006) in females. Longitudinal data does not suggest GH responses adapt chronically to resistance exercise (Cook and Crewther, 2011; French, 2016).

Cortisol

In relation to cortisol, baseline concentrations and training responses are similar between males and females (French, 2016; Crewther *et al.*, 2006; Cook and Crewther, 2011), with cortisol being very sensitive to resistance training aimed at increasing muscle mass (Nunes *et al.*, 2011). For both sexes, the degree of hypertrophy is determined by the balance between anabolic and catabolic factors (Stone *et al.*, 2016). Indeed, testosterone to cortisol ratios (T:C ratio) are commonly used to indicate overall training stress (marker of overtraining and indicator of enhanced tolerance to training) (French, 2016; Kraemer and Ratamess, 2005) and level of preparedness (Stone *et al.*, 2007; Haff *et al.*, 2008). In a study involving elite female weightlifters, moderate to very strong correlations (r=-0.83) were found between the

T:C ratio and volume load, with the authors demonstrating that sustained increases in volume load of more than 30 per cent had significant effects on performance (isometric peak force measures).

Sex differences in resting and training-induced increases in anabolic hormone concentrations are commonly thought to explain the larger increase in muscle mass and subsequent strength differences in men and women. At this point it is worth being reminded that there is no difference in relative strength or per cent increases in muscle mass in response to hypertrophy programmes between the sexes. Furthermore, recent evidence in untrained male subjects has suggested that hypertrophy is not related to circulating hormones post-exercise (Mitchell *et al.*, 2013). There is also considerable between-subject variability in hormone responses. Endocrine profiles measured in female athletes within 2 hours post-competition, found that in a cohort of 239 (across 15 sports), 11 female athletes had testosterone levels greater than 8nmol.l-1, with 3 showing values within the 25 and 35nmol.l.-l range, which is at the upper limit of the male athlete range (Healy *et al.*, 2014). Overall, this suggests that the exact mechanisms responsible for hypertrophy, in particular those relating to gender-specific mechanisms, are yet to be fully understood.

Oestrogen, the Menstrual Cycle and Muscle Mass/Strength

Oestrogen plays a key protective role, stimulating repair and regeneration of the muscle tissue, although a lot of the evidence that support these claims are based on findings from animal studies (Enns and Tiidus, 2010) and not from humans. However, this has led some people to suggest that females may be less prone to muscle damage after a bout of strength training. Radaelli *et al.* (2014) investigated muscle damage responses to a 1-RM unilateral bicep curl exercise in untrained males and females and found that recovery over a 72-hour period was similar between groups, although the men did show significantly greater delayed muscle soreness at 72 hours ($p < 0.05$). In practice the training responses in more athletic groups, following a more realistic strength and conditioning programme (multi-muscle, multi-joint exercises), may provide a different response and will be something to explore in the future.

It is well documented that oestrogen fluctuates across the menstrual cycle (see Chapter 8), so theoretically the proposed effects of oestrogen on muscle mass and muscle strength would suggest that programming of strength and power should complement hormone profiles across the menstrual cycle for optimal training adaptations. In addition, testosterone concentrations also increase very slightly around ovulation, but these effects are minimal (Stone *et al.*, 2007). In reality, the limited available research suggests that strength does not appear to fluctuate across the mesocycle and tailoring strength prescription to the menstrual cycle is not justifiable (Constantini *et al.*, 2005; Xanne and de Jonge, 2003; DiBrezzo *et al.*, 1991; Gür, 1997; de Jonge *et al.*, 2001; Lebrum *et al.*, 1995).

Neuromuscular Response

The maximal amount of strength or power an athlete can generate during a movement is not only determined by the degree of hypertrophy and structure of the muscle, but also by the ability of the nervous system to optimally recruit and activate the relevant motor units. Early phases adaptations to strength training programmes are suggested to occur predominantly through improvements in neural drive (Sale, 1988; Behm, 1995).

Motor Unit Recruitment

The motor unit (MU) consists of the motor neurone and all the muscle fibres it innervates and according to the all-or-none principle once activated, all of the muscle fibres within the MU will contract (Stone *et al.*, 2007). There are generally three types of MUs based on their contractile properties (Type I, Type IIA and Type IIX; see Stone *et al.*, 2007) and these are recruited in an orderly pattern as originally proposed by Henneman *et al.* (1965a,b). It is generally believed that this relationship appears to hold true regardless of the type and speed of muscle contraction (Cormie *et al.*, 2011a; Duchateau and Enoka, 2011), although some authors dispute this (Sale, 1988; Haff and Potteiger, 2001, Hortobágyi *et al.*, 1996; Shepstone *et al.*, 2005; Nardone *et al.*, 1989). Smaller Type I MUs, with lower firing thresholds are recruited at low levels of force, but as the requirement for force or intensity increases, higher threshold, high-force MUs (Type IIA, IIX) are activated (Bompa and Haff, 2009; Stone *et al.*, 2007; Rainoldi and Gazzoni, 2011). For maximal force generation the capacity to fully activate high threshold MUs is paramount (Haff and Potteiger, 2001) and the ability to do this is thought to improve through resistance training (Sale, 1988; Behm, 1995).

Muscle fibre characteristics are genetically determined, with those excelling in endurance sports typically showing a greater percentage of slow twitch (ST) MUs in comparison to strength and power athletes who have a higher percentage of fast twitch (FT) MUs (Costill *et al.*, 1976; Prince *et al.*, 1976).

Whilst the identification of the three major fibre types is useful, in reality this is an oversimplification and there is a much broader spectrum of fibre types in human muscle (see below; Fry, 2004):

I ↔ IC ↔ IIC ↔ IIAC ↔ IIA ↔ IIAX ↔ IIX

(slowest)   (fastest)

Shifts in the profile of MUs can occur as a result of high volumes of heavy resistance training (Stone *et al.*, 2016), typically by a conversion of Type IIX fibres into Type IIA, with the latter suggested to be the preferred fibres for use with this type of training (Fry, 2004). The transition to a 'slower' MU could have detrimental consequences for power generation, but it is thought that the preferential hypertrophy of Type II fibres is able to compensate for this (Cormie *et al.*, 2011a). In addition, fibre type transitions appear to be reversed following a taper (Terzis *et al.*, 2008) or after a period of detraining (Andersen and Aagard, 2000). The literature does not support transitions from Type I to Type II fibre types (Fry, 2004).

Rate coding

Rate coding refers to the frequency of activation of motor units (Bompa and Haff, 2009). An increase in the firing frequency can augment both the magnitude and rate of force development generated by the muscle, without increasing the recruitment of additional MUs (Haff and Potteiger, 2001; Cormie *et al.*, 2011a). 'Explosive strength', or the rate of force development (RFD) is crucial to sports performance as there is usually a

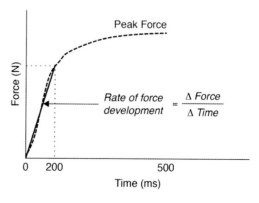

Fig. 2.2 Isometric force-time curve. (Adapted from Haff *et al.*, 1997)

critical timeframe in which force can be generated (Haff and Nimphius, 2012; Stone *et al.*, 2016; Newton and Kraemer, 1994; Maffiuletti *et al.*, 2016). For most powerful muscle actions such as sprinting, jumping and changing direction, 50–250ms is likely (Haff and Nimphius, 2012). Rate of force development can be calculated from the slope of a force-time curve (Haff *et al.*, 1997; see Fig. 2.2):

MU recruitment and rate coding both play an essential role in sporting movements that require large RFDs and can be improved through training. Ballistic contractions are characterized by very high MU firing rates that occur at the onset of contraction, which promptly decline (Maffiuletti *et al.*, 2016; Sale 1998; Duchateau and Enoka, 2011). It is speculated that an increase in the number of doublet discharges (MU firing two consecutive discharges in ≤ 5ms) are thought to contribute to the very high firing rates initially observed (Cormie *et al.*, 2011; Duchateau and Enoka, 2011). In terms of the contribution of MU recruitment to RFD, two things happen. Firstly, the recruitment thresholds of the larger Type II fibres are reduced, which means they are recruited earlier and because they can produce greater force outputs and contract at a faster rate (3–8 times faster than Type 1; Metzger and Moss, 1990), they have a powerful effect on RFD (Maffiuletti *et al.*, 2016). Secondly, synchronization of motor units (several MUs activated simultaneously) is theorized to occur (Cormie *et al.*, 2011a; Bompa and Haff, 2009). Because this will have an additive effect on force output it is logical that this could influence RFD during ballistic contractions although this is not well supported in the literature (Bompa and Haff, 2009; Cormie *et al.*, 2011a). However, a 'pre-movement silent period' (~50ms) has been demonstrated in the agonist muscles before a ballistic action occurs (Behm, 1995). This enables the MUs to complete their refractory periods so that a larger number of MUs can synchronize at the start of the ballistic contraction (Zehr and Sale, 1994). Optimal musculo-tendinous stiffness is another important consideration for movements that require a high RFD (Maffiuletti *et al.*, 2016), but although strength training can positively impact stiffness (Kubo *et al.*, 2006), this will be discussed further in the plyometric section of this chapter.

Power production requires the intricate coordination of multiple muscles, including agonists, antagonists and synergists simultaneously, to produce efficient movement (maximize net force in the required direction) (Newton and Kraemer, 1994; Cormie *et al.*, 2011a). This means that muscles need to be activated at the right time and to the right level to be able to both stabilize joints and generate large forces quickly. For antagonist muscles, although a certain degree of co-activation is necessary for the reasons just described, excessive co-activation would be counterproductive to maximal power generation by the agonist muscles (Cormie *et al.*, 2011a). This can be improved through resistance training, but the degree of movement specificity must be extremely high (Newton and Kraemer, 1994).

Effects of Training on RFD

Explosive type training and traditional heavy resistance training can have positive effects on RFD (Haff and Nimphius, 2012; Newton and Kraemer, 2001; Kawamori and Haff, 2004). In early phase RFD (50–75ms), maximal voluntary activation of the agonist muscles via a decrease in MU activation thresholds (caused by modulation to the nervous system) and, more significantly, an increase in MU firing rates (and the ability to sustain these) at the onset of contraction seem to be the primary factors (Maffiuletti *et al.*, 2016; Cormie *et al.*, 2010). Late phase RFD (50–100ms) is thought to be primarily dependent on intrinsic muscle characteristics (muscle size and fibre type, pennation angle, musculo-tendinous stiffness,

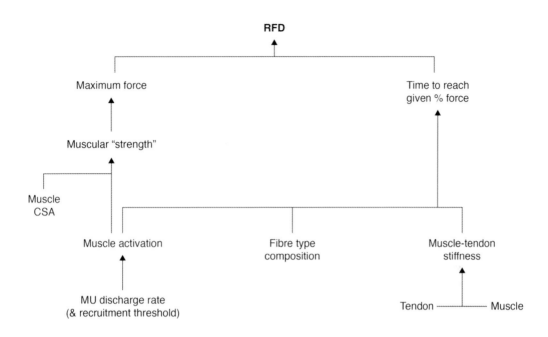

Fig. 2.3 Factors within the neuromuscular system that influence rate of force development. (Adapted from Maffiuletti *et al.*, 2016)

myofibrillar mechanisms) (Maffiuletti *et al.*, 2016). Fig. 2.3 summarizes the trainable neuromuscular factors that impact early and late phase RFD.

MEASURING STRENGTH AND POWER

Maximum strength, or one-repetition maximum (1-RM), is defined as the 'ability to apply maximal levels of force or strength irrespective of time constraints' (Baker, 2014). For a strength and conditioning coach, assessment of an athlete's maximal strength capabilities is useful for two reasons. Firstly, tracking changes in an athlete's absolute or relative (per kg body weight) 1-RM strength typically provides a measure of the degree of adaptation to a strength-training programme.

Secondly, load prescription (training intensity) is traditionally based upon a percentage of an athlete's one-repetition maximum. This requires the coach to either directly (1-RM testing) or indirectly (repetition maximum testing) assess 1-RM values in a number of 'core' lifts. Multiple RM testing involves lifting submaximal loads for a number of specified repetitions and then estimating 1-RM values using established tables (Sheppard and Triplett, 2016; Bompa and Haff, 2009) or prediction equations (Reynolds *et al.*, 2006; Abadie and Wentworth, 2000; Mayhew *et al.*, 1991). For example, according to Sheppard and Triplett (2016) if an athlete can back squat 96kg for 5 repetitions (~87 per cent of 1-RM) they have an estimated 1-RM back squat of 110kg. Whilst there are a number of variables that affect the accuracy of these predictions such as gender, training status, exercise selection (muscle mass and mode) and the assumed relationship between load and repetitions (linear vs. curvilinear) (Sheppard and Triplett, 2016; Bompa and Haff, 2009), it is generally accepted that the accuracy of these predictions increases when the quality of the movement is maintained and the number of repetitions performed is relatively low (≤5 reps, or loads closer to the actual 1-RM value) for core strength and power lifts (for example Olympic lifts, squats, presses) (Reynolds et al., 2006; Shephard and Triplett, 2016).

Strength and power testing should minimally impact normal training and competition performance, but should provide sufficient meaningful data to accurately assess the athlete's response to training (Beckham et al., 2013). Multiple RM and 1-RM testing are both fatiguing and time consuming. In addition, the demands of athlete training schedules and periodization of the sport usually dictate that these traditional methods are often no longer viable (Wang et al., 2016; West et al., 2011; Sheppard and Triplett, 2016; Banyard et al., 2017). Other ways of performing a strength diagnosis (for example linear position transducer and maximal isometric testing) are increasing in popularity and can provide practically viable alternatives for the strength and conditioning coach.

However, if you do not have access to these technologies, estimating 1-RM loads is still a valuable tool. Monitoring of actual repetitions and loads lifted by the athlete allows a consistent estimation of 1-RM strength with no disruption to training. Tracking of 'very heavy' loads will track 1-RM strength for the majority of exercises prescribed in an athlete's programme. Moreover, this can also improve training efficiency because training loads can be predicted to some degree of accuracy as exercise prescription changes (prescribed rep ranges) from one block to another.

Linear Position Transducer

Accurate prediction of the absolute weight (training intensity) that needs to be lifted for a certain repetition range is suggested to be the most important programming variable to achieve specified strength and power adaptations (Bird et al., 2005; Kraemer et al., 2004). This means that an accurate assessment of 1-RM (and percentage 1-RM) is necessary to optimize training. In reality, an athlete's actual 1-RM value can fluctuate on a daily basis. Jovanović and Flanagan (2014) reported that the daily 1-RM could vary as much as ± 15 per cent on a previously reported 1-RM, which they explained by variations in an athlete's 'day-to-day readiness'. For less well-trained athletes, the potential for rapid gains in 1-RM is also greater (Bird et al., 2005), making previously recorded 1-RM values redundant in programming terms.

The inverse relationship between load (percentage 1-RM) and velocity in dynamic muscle actions (see Fig. 2.1) dictates that velocity can be used to estimate load. Indeed, a growing body of literature supports the use of linear position transducers (LPTs) as a valid and reliable device to objectively monitor training load as well as a tool for prescribing 'velocity-based' strength and power training (Harris et al., 2010; Jovanović and Flanagan, 2014). There are a number of different velocity and power measures that an LPT can provide. For traditional, non-aerial, resistance exercises (for example squat, bench press), mean concentric velocity is recommended due to the relatively large amount of time spent decelerating the bar (Jidovtseff et al., 2011). However, both peak (Banyard et al., 2017) and mean concentric velocity (Baker, 2017) have been suggested to be relevant for explosive type exercises (for example jumps, throws). Specific practical applications of velocity-based training include:

1. Power/velocity profiling

Load-velocity and load-power profiles for specific exercises can be achieved by the athlete performing repetitions over a range of pre-determined loads (four to six intensities, ranging from 30–85 per cent of estimated 1-RM, Jovanović and Flanagan, 2014). Within-athlete comparisons will track velocity-specific training adaptations, as well as easily pinpoint the load that elicits the greatest power output in that particular exercise (Harris *et al.*, 2010).

2. Estimating 1-RM

Minimal velocity threshold (MVT) is 'the mean concentric velocity produced on the last successful repetition of a set to failure performed with maximal lifting effort' (Jovanović and Flanagan, 2014). Provided the MVT for an exercise is known (for example ~0.18m.s-1 for bench press, Loturco *et al.*, 2016), 1-RM can be predicted using a regression equation from two to three measures of velocity across increasing loads (Harris *et al.*, 2010). Numerous investigations have reported a strong linear relationship between mean concentric velocity in traditional strength exercises (for example bench press) and the relative load as a per cent 1-RM, with r values commonly reported as being at or greater than 0.95 (González-Badillo and Sánchez-Medina, 2010; Harris *et al.*, 2010; Jovanović and Flanagan, 2014; Sánchez-Medina *et al.*, 2013; Loturco *et al.*, 2016). This relationship means that for a strength and conditioning coach, monitoring velocity during warm-up sets will not only provide the coach and the athlete with an accurate assessment of daily 1-RM (daily readiness), but can provide an accurate estimate of the per cent 1-RM for any absolute load, allowing the coach to adjust training loads accordingly to optimize training.

3. Other benefits of velocity-based training

There are other additional benefits of embracing velocity-based training, which are beyond the scope of this chapter. They include: a) Prescribing loading (repetitions and sets) based on velocity or power output, as either velocity/power stops or velocity/power bands (Jovanović and Flanagan, 2014; Harris *et al.*, 2010). For example, a velocity/power stop would mean that when the athlete's ability to maintain a certain movement velocity or power output drops below a predetermined value, repetitions cease. This aids to maintain 'quality' of training as well as provide a degree of control over fatigue (Morán-Navarro *et al.*, 2017; Sánchez-Medina and González-Badillo, 2011); and b) Provide the athlete with real-time feedback (visual and auditory) on their performance. This can have positive effects on motivation, increasing engagement and concentration of effort during sessions.

Isometric Mid-Thigh Pull

On the basis that peak force and peak rate of force development are fundamental performance variables in a range of sports (Haff *et al.*, 2005), the isometric mid-thigh pull is acknowledged to be a valuable tool for assessing strength and power (James *et al.*, 2015; Haff *et al.*, 2005) in athletes. Tests can be carried out relatively quickly (~5–8 minutes per athlete; Stone *et al.*, 2016) with minimal disruption to normal training. Plus, the skill requirements to perform the test correctly are low in comparison to traditional 1-RM testing methods, carrying a lower level of injury risk as well as being applicable across a broader range of performance levels (de Witt *et al.*, 2016).

The IMTP position is standardized to reflect the 'power position' or second pull in weightlifting (trunk upright, knee bend 130–140 degrees) where the largest force and power outputs are registered (Haff *et al.*, 1997; DeWeese *et al.*, 2013). Isometric peak force and rate of force development measures have been significantly correlated with sprinting (West *et al.*, 2011; Wang *et al.*, 2016) jumping

(West *et al.*, 2011; Beckham *et al.*, 2013; Kawamori *et al.*, 2006), weightlifting (Wang *et al.*, 2016;Witt *et al.*, 2016; Beckham *et al.*, 2013; Haff *et al.*, 2005; Kawamori *et al.*, 2006; McGuigan *et al.*, 2006), change of direction (Wang *et al.*, 2016; Thomas *et al.*, 2015), cycling (Stone *et al.*, 2004) and throwing (Stone *et al.*, 2003). With respect to the analysis of the force-time curves produced from IMTP testing it is recommended that strength and conditioning coaches use predetermined time zone bands such as 0–30, 0–50, 0–90, 0–100, 0–150, 0–200 and 0–250ms as these produce the highest degree of reliability (Haff *et al.*, 2015).

It has been suggested that the closer the similarity between the IMTP position and the dynamic test (Haff *et al.*, 2005; Stone *et al.*, 2007), the more significant the relationship is likely to be. For example, in a group of elite women weightlifters isometric peak force was found to be strongly correlated with an athlete's snatch (r=0.93), clean and jerk (r=0.64) and combined total (r=0.80) (Haff *et al.*, 2005). Other researchers have also suggested that the isometric force-time correlations are strongest with dynamic tests that involve heavy external loads, decreasing as the loads get lighter (Haff *et al.*, 1997; Murphy *et al.*, 1994; Kawamori *et al.*, 2006). In a study of elite male weightlifters (Kawamori *et al.*, 2006) investigating the relationship between isometric (IMTP) PF and dynamic PF during clean pulls (from mid-thigh) across a range of intensities (30–120 per cent of their 1-RM power clean) strong to very strong correlations were found (r=0.51–0.82) across all intensities. However, lower, non-significant correlations were reported at lighter loads (30 and 60 per cent 1-RM power clean), compared to heavy loaded conditions, where correlations were statistically significant (p<0.05).

More recent investigations into the use the IMTP testing, using a dual force-plate system, to assess force-time characteristics between dominant and non-dominant limbs (Dos' Santos *et al.*, 2016) have provided evidence to suggest that unilateral stance IMTP may also be a useful tool for the strength and conditioning coach. Specifically it has the potential to measure muscle strength asymmetry, which has implications for injury risk (Hewit *et al.*, 2012b; Knapik *et al.*, 1991) and performance in sports involving unilateral movements.

The ability for both LPT devices and the IMTP test to provide a richer amount of information about an athlete's development beyond 1-RM strength is important. A within-athlete comparison may not necessarily reveal improvements in 1-RM strength, but velocity/power specific adaptations to submaximal loads may be evident. An understanding of what parts of the load-velocity or load-power spectrum are being affected by different exercise prescriptions will allow the coach to be able to tailor training more effectively to strength and power qualities identified in the needs analysis. Between-athlete comparisons are also relevant. Two athletes who possess the same 1-RM values can show very different load-velocity or load-power profiles (Harris *et al.*, 2010). For both the coach and the athlete this will enhance their understanding of what differentiates 'winners' and 'losers' (between sports and positional differences) and may help coaches make better prescription decisions to aid transfer into actual sports performance.

TRAINING STRENGTH AND POWER

The primary goal of periodization is to maximize an athlete's performance capabilities at predetermined time points, or over a season, sustain elevated performances for an extended period of time (Haff, 2016). Because of the importance of power to success, optimizing power output is a primary goal for coaches and athletes, who strive to rationally and systematically structure a variety of different training methods to achieve the required physiological outcome. This 'mixed methods approach' (Haff and Nimphius, 2012; Newton and Kraemer, 1994; Kawamori and Haff, 2004), that requires an athlete to produce force (strength) over a diverse range of contraction velocities ('surf' the curve), has been suggested to: a) produce superior gains in maximum power output and b) allow for a better transfer of training effect (Haff and Nimphius, 2012). Fig. 2.4 illustrates how various training interventions can impact the force–velocity curve, with the overall aim being to shift the concentric portion of the force–velocity curve up and to the right (shift the power line; Brewer, 2017). What this means for the athlete is that they will be able to apply a given force at a higher velocity and/or demonstrate increased strength for the same velocity (Brewer, 2017). The use of maximum strength training, weightlifting and ballistic training to improve power development will be discussed in more detail.

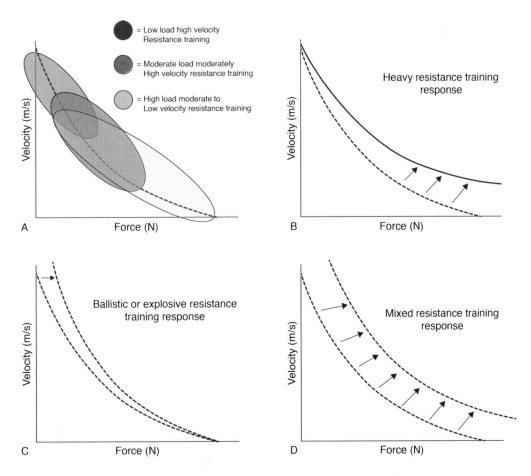

Fig. 2.4 Potential training interventions which impact the force-velocity curve.
(Adapted from Haff & Nimphius, 2012)

Maximal Strength Training

Traditional resistance training exercises such as the deadlift, squat and bench press are programmed predominantly to increase an athlete's maximal force (maximal strength) generating capacities. Based on the fact that the time taken to generate maximal forces can be in excess of 300ms (Aagaard et al., 2002; Aagaard, 2003) and that a large proportion of the lifting time is spent decelerating the load towards the end of range of movement (23 per cent of time to complete a 1-RM bench press; Elliott et al., 1989), the importance of maximal strength to power development is often undervalued (Cormie et al., 2011b).

Despite this apparent lack of task specificity to sporting actions, there is a wealth of evidence (at least in males) supporting the notion that maximal strength is a key fundamental quality, essential for power development (see Table 2.3; adapted from Suchomel et al., 2016). In a recent extensive review, Suchomel et al. (2016) demonstrated that muscular strength shows moderate to large correlations with rate of force development, mechanical power output, generic sports movements (sprinting, jumping and changing direction) as well as the ability to perform sport-specific skills (effective transfer of strength into the sport) (see Table 2.3). Moreover, evidence suggests that when comparing athletes of different strength levels, 'stronger' athletes have a superior capacity to generate RFD, can produce statistically higher external mechanical power outputs, can jump higher, sprint faster and change direction quicker. Additionally, they also appear to show enhanced ability in the actual sports performance compared to their weaker counterparts. What this data shows is that maximal strength can be a major limiting factor to the production of high power outputs, so maximizing strength must be a cornerstone of all athletes' programmes.

Training Considerations

Traditional resistance training (TRT) methods to improve maximal strength, typically involves lifting loads ≥ 80 per cent of the 1-RM (Cormie et al., 2011b; Peterson et al., 2004; Kawamori et al., 2004), which targets the high force, low velocity end of the force–velocity continuum. The increased neural drive associated with the ability of TRT (Cormie et al., 2010; Maffiuletti et al., 2016; Suchomel et al., 2016) to positively affect RFD stems from the theory that the 'intention' to move as explosively as possible is fundamental to achieving the required high velocity-specific adaptations to enhance power (Behm, 1995; Behm and Sale, 1993). Practically, athletes performing strength training will fluctuate intensities of loading across the mesocycle (typically between 80–100 per cent 1-RM) and will inevitably perform 'warm-up' sets in preparation during sessions – logically an athlete who trains 'explosively' has the opportunity to develop power effectively across a range of loads (surfing a greater range of the force–velocity curve) even if the main objective of the training block/session is maximal strength (Haff and Nimphius, 2012).

Post-activation potentiation, or PAP is another factor that can help maximize power development in athletes and refers to the ability to acutely increase strength and power performance as a direct result of a previous muscular activity, usually performed at maximal or near-maximal intensity in order to recruit the maximum number of MUs (known as a conditioning activity) (Evetovich et al., 2015; Seitz and Haff, 2015; Wilson et al., 2013). The pairing up of a conditioning activity with a strength/power exercise (bench press and bench throw) is known as a strength-power-potentiation complex (Seitz and Haff, 2015) (see reviews by Wilson et al., 2013, Seitz and Haff, 2015; Maloney et al., 2014 for more detail) and the mechanism responsible for the PAP response is believed to be enhanced

Relationship to Maximal Strength	Number of studies (no. studies)	Female subjects included	Total number of correlations reported	Correlation data (Moderate, r ≥ 0.3, Large, r ≥ 0.5)	
				No. studies (%) showing moderate correlations	No. studies (%) showing large correlations
Rate Force Development	13	4	59	57 (97%)	44 (75%)
Peak Power	20	4	177	134 (77%)	116 (65%)
Jumping (Height/distance)	29	11	116	91 (78%)	69 (59%)
Sprinting	15	3	67	57 (85%)	44 (66%)
Change of Direction	13	5	45	35 (78%)	27 (60%)
Specific Sport Skill	14	9	107	101 (94%)	89 (83%)
Potentiation Effects	21	6	67	39 (58%)	33 (49%)

Table 2.3 Correlations of maximal strength to power production. (Adapted from Suchomel *et al.*, 2016)

myosin light chain phosphorylation and an increase in Type II motor unit recruitment (Tillin and Bishop, 2009). The use of strength-power-potentiation complexes during maximal strength phases of training is a time-efficient and easy way of incorporating some higher velocity, potentially more sport-specific power work into the session. Complex training and contrast training are two other common strategies used to achieve this (Brewer, 2017). Complex training involves the athlete performing repeated cycles of one set of a maximum strength exercise, followed by one set of a maximal speed exercise or vice versa. Contrast training requires the athlete to perform a number of sets of the strength exercise, followed by multiple sets of the speed exercise or vice versa (Brewer *et al.*, 2017). Stronger athletes have been shown to benefit from PAP effects at an earlier rest interval and to a greater magnitude (Suchomel *et al.*, 2016; see Table 2.3), so some athletes will benefit more from this strategy than others, but for all strength and conditioning coaches, making the most of the limited time you have with athletes is important.

Olympic Lifts

On the basis that weightlifters are probably the most powerful of all athletes (Stone *et al.*, 2006; Hori and Stone, 2005; McBride *et al.*, 1999; Hedrick and Wada, 2008), weightlifting exercises (snatch, clean and jerk) and their derivatives are commonplace in almost all athletes' programmes aimed at developing strength and power. Weightlifting exercises require athletes to perform an explosive 'triple extension' of the hip, knee and ankle, to maximally accelerate the barbell through the entire concentric phase of the lift (no deceleration) (Cormie *et al.*, 2011b). The close degree of similarity between the kinetics and kinematics of the triple extension movement in the weightlifting exercise and that seen in sprinting, jumping and change of direction manoeuvres has led researchers to conclude that these exercises can produce superior gains in performance compared with other power development strategies, with a high potential to transfer positively into a range of sports (Hedrick and Wada, 2008; Suchomel, 2017; Hori *et al.*, 2005; Holmberg, 2013; Suchomel *et al.*, 2015). For the full lifts and for some derivative movements (snatch balance, squat clean from hang, power snatch from hip, and so on), once the athlete has completed a full triple extension they are then required to jump underneath the bar and collect the bar in the 'catch' position by performing a triple flexion movement (Holmberg, 2013; Suchomel *et al.*, 2015). The ability to decelerate a load (absorb force) and maintain appropriate ankle, knee and hip alignment under load (demonstrate good landing mechanics) is an opportunity for female athletes to practice good 'landing mechanics' as well as train deceleration patterns which are important for sports performance (Holmberg, 2013). Weightlifting exercises are also hugely beneficial for females because, depending on the exercise, there is a large emphasis on upper body, as well as lower-body strength. Because of the relatively low upper-body strength levels in females compared to males, weightlifting is an effective way of addressing strength deficits in the female athlete. Elite female weightlifters are capable of pushing loads in excess of two-and-a-half times body weight overhead in some instances (see Table 2.1a) thereby providing evidence of the importance of this type of training in female athlete programmes.

Weightlifting derivatives can be performed from a number of different starting positions (for example start, hang, power, second pull) and can be either snatch-based or clean-based. The starting position of choice has sport-specific application. For example, the 'start' position directly relates to the position a rugby athlete adopts in the scrum and the second pull, or 'power position', to the 'athletic' or 'get ready' position adopted by racquet sport athletes. The second pull (from power position into full triple extension) is particularly relevant to sports performance because it is the portion of the lift that generates the greatest power output (Stone et al., 2006). This phase of the lift occurs within 0.2 seconds (Stone et al., 2006; Souza et al., 2002), which directly correlates to the critical time period (<250ms) for force application during sport-specific movements such as sprinting, jumping and change of direction (Stone et al., 2006; Turner, 2009; Haff and Nimphius, 2012). Athletes may spend a considerable portion of their training time using weightlifting pulling derivatives, which remove the 'catch phase' because it emphasizes, and concentrates the effort, into achieving full completion of the triple extension phase, as well as being less complex to perform (Suchomel et al., 2015). For clean (squat and power), snatch and hang power clean exercises the optimal load for peak power generation is suggested to be between 70–80 per cent 1-RM, but for weightlifting pulling derivatives, higher intensities (90–95 per cent 1-RM) are proposed (Suchomel et al., 2015). This means that pulling-only movements have the potential to more effectively 'overload' the triple extension movement, arguably providing a superior training stimulus to the athlete (Suchomel et al., 2015).

In programming terms, the weightlifting derivatives chosen will reflect the needs analysis of the sport, specific adaptations required from the block of training and the skill

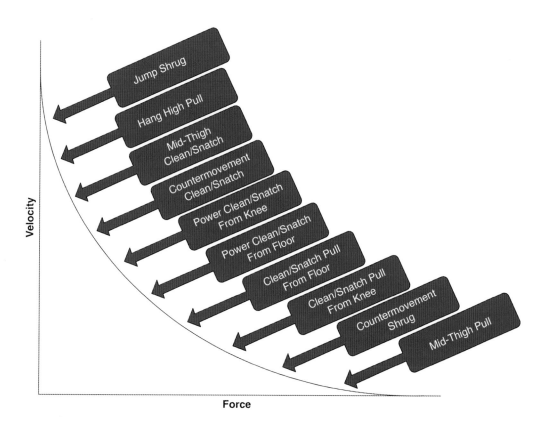

Fig. 2.5a Force-velocity (power) curve with respect to weightlifting derivatives. (Adapted from Suchomel et al., 2017)

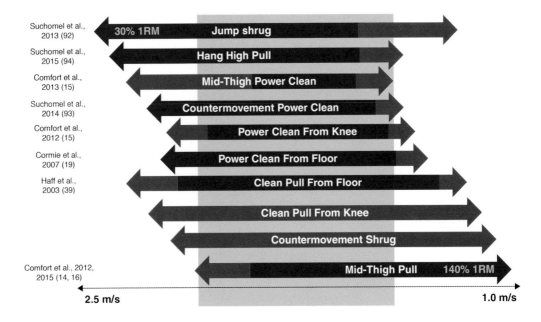

Fig. 2.5b Proposed guidelines for the force-velocity characteristics of weightlifting derivatives with respect to load. Blue = studied loads; red = hypothetical loads; grey area = comparable force-velocity characteristics at given load ranges. (Adapted from Suchomel *et al.*, 2017)

level (technical ability) of the athlete. Clean-based movements can typically be loaded up more than the same snatch-based movement (see Table 2.1a), so tend to affect the strength-speed/high force portion of the force–velocity curve, whereas snatch-based movements sit closer towards the speed-strength/high velocity portion. The huge variation and versatility of weightlifting movements and their derivatives means that they are relevant and appropriate for the majority of athletes and can be tailored to achieving large power outputs across a range of loading conditions (Cormie *et al.*, 2011b). Fig. 2.5a provides an example of how exercise selection can be adapted to feature a different portion of the force–velocity curve (Suchomel *et al.*, 2017). It should be noted that that the same exercise can be prescribed over heavier and lighter loads which will affect its positioning on the

force–velocity continuum. Fig. 2.5b provides further detail demonstrating how load can affect velocity profiles of the lift (Suchomel *et al.*, 2017).

Studies comparing male and female athletes have shown that the peak power output achieved by female athletes in the snatch and clean and jerk is approximately 65 per cent of their male counterparts (Stone *et al.*, 2006). In addition, sex differences have been demonstrated during the clean pull (mid-thigh) exercise across a range of variables (bar displacement, peak power, peak force and impulse (200ms) (Comfort *et al.*, 2015). Overall, males recorded higher values in all measures across loads of 40 per cent, 60 per cent, 80 per cent, 100 per cent, 120 per cent and 140 per cent of 1-RM, except for bar velocity where females demonstrated significantly higher bar velocities at the heaviest loads (120 per cent and 140 per cent 1-RM). Despite these sex differences, peak power and bar velocities were maximal when the load was 40–60 per cent of the 1-RM for both men and women (Comfort *et al.*, 2015).

In summary, the skill complexity (multi-muscle, multi-joint exercises) and high-force (usually 70–85 per cent 1-RM; Stone *et al.*, 2005), high-velocity nature of weightlifting movements, can provide the strength and conditioning coach with an array of exercises that can help maximize strength and power development in athletes. The neuromuscular adaptations hypothesized to achieve this include improved coordination (intra- and inter-muscular) and activation of MUs (increased rate coding, improved recruitment of Type II MUs, muscle fibre adaptations) as well as enhanced neuroendocrine responses to exercise (see review by Hedrick and Wada, 2008 and Cormie *et al.*, 2011b for more detail).

Ballistic Exercise

Ballistic training involves exercises that demand the athlete to maximally exert as much force as possible in very short periods of time, with the primary objective to accelerate a mass (body weight or implement) with maximal velocity into free space (for example jumping, throwing and kicking) – there is no deceleration phase (Cormie *et al.*, 2011b; Kawamori and Haff, 2004). Weightlifting derivatives that include the second pull are examples of ballistic exercises, but this section specifically addresses the use of lighter-load, non-weightlifting movements in the development of power such as loaded and unloaded jump squats and medicine ball throws. Ballistic training has been shown to be effective in targeting improvements in maximal power output and sports performance (Cormie, 2010; Cormie *et al.*, 2011b).

The degree to which training transfers into actual athletic performance is highly dependent on the similarity between the exercises used in training and the competition performance (Gamble, 2006; Reilly *et al.*, 2009). Whilst specificity of training is multifaceted, velocity of training and biomechanical specificity are essential considerations with ballistic exercises. Both the intention to move 'as explosively as possible' and the actual movement velocity are equally important to elicit the necessary adaptations required to enhance performance (Cormie *et al.*, 2011b), with research supporting the concept that training adaptations are velocity dependent (Morrissey *et al.*, 1995; Blazevich *et al.*, 2003; McBride *et al.*, 2002; Gamble, 2006; Harris *et al.*, 2000; Behm, 1995; Hatfield *et al.*, 2006). Therefore, high speed/high power resistance training (ballistic exercises) that typically involve relatively light loads may be particularly relevant for athletes involved in sports that require jumping, throwing, striking, kicking and sprinting. The use of exercises targetting specifically the maximum velocity part of the force–velocity curve are thought to be a superior training stimulus for eliciting increases in RFD, by improving the rate of neural activation, and enhancing coordination abilities (inter- and intra-muscular) during rapid speed movements (Cormie *et al.*, 2011b; Turner, 2009; Behm, 1995).

Biomechanical specificity refers to exercise range of motion, joint angles, planes of motion, limb support (bilateral, unilateral), open/closed kinetic chain and muscle contraction type (isometric, concentric, eccentric) (Gamble, 2006). Exercises that have a high degree of kinematic and kinetic similarity to the actual sporting movement are more likely to have a greater degree of transference into the sport (for example standing medicine overhead throw for a netball player) (Gamble, 2006). Whilst this is an important consideration, it must be remembered that athletes always practice their sport, which is a highly specific activity.

Overloading movements that are too similar to the sport skill(s) may be detrimental to performance as they have the potential to interfere with technique – this is called the 'specificity trap'. For example, weighted sled-towing at loads of 12.6 per cent and 32.2 per cent of an athlete's body mass have been shown to significantly decrease stride frequency and significantly increase the duration of the stance phase, trunk flexion and hip range of motion during a 15m acceleration task (Lockie *et al.*, 2003). The ability of the athlete to display the desired technical model under this degree of load is considerably compromised and in these situations a deviation from the characteristics you are trying to replicate will lessen the effectiveness of the training modality. In summary, ballistic exercise design can be highly creative, allowing the strength and conditioning coach

to programme exercises that are similar to those encountered by the athlete in their sport, exercises that are just not possible with a barbell or a dumbbell. The coach just needs to decide what is an acceptable level of similarity depending on the needs and training experience of the athlete. Athletes with a higher resistance training history and movement competency typically require a greater degree of specificity and variation in their programme (Stone *et al.*, 2007).

Training at the Optimal Load

For any ballistic exercise, the load that produces maximal power is referred to as the 'optimal load' (Haff and Nimphius, 2012; see Fig. 2.6). It is proposed that training at this load, or within ± 10 per cent of this load (Turner, 2009), will provide a potent stimulus

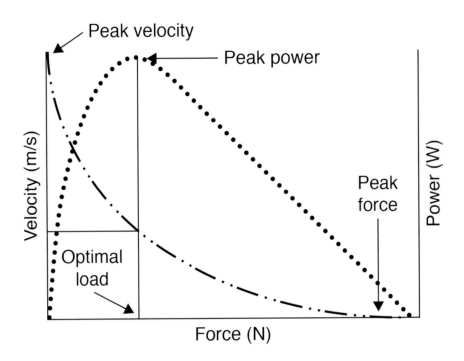

Fig. 2.6 Force-velocity, force-power, velocity-power and optimal load relationship.
(Adapted from Haff & Nimphius, 2012)

for enhancing power output in the belief that it drives specific, positive adaptations in the rate of neural drive (Cormie *et al.* 2011b). In support of this, Newton *et al.* (2006) found that four weeks of optimal load, in-season ballistic training in female volleyball players successfully improved jump performances by 5.3 per cent (p<0.05). Although there is some debate about whether this does provide a superior adaptation to training power (Cormie *et al.*, 2011b; Haff and Nimphius, 2012), this may be more relevant for athletes that require one-off maximal efforts in their performance (shot put for example). For most other athletes, sport-specific requirements will demand that they need to train a variety of loading schemes that accommodate all areas of the force–velocity curve for a greater degree of transference. In practice, when performing ballistic exercises the intention is always to move the resistance (body weight or additional load) with the highest velocity regardless of the absolute load to maximizing power output. Combination loading schemes (using combined RT methods) involving high force/low speed and low force/high speed exercise have been shown to provide superior training adaptations in power output through maximization of both the force and velocity elements of the power calculation (force × velocity) (Harris *et al.*, 2000; Lyttle *et al.*, 1996; Haff and Nimphius, 2012; Cronin *et al.*, 2001; Kawamori and Haff, 2004). In a review paper by Cormie *et al.* (2011b), the optimal loads suggested for use in ballistic and weightlifting exercises to maximize power development were 0 per cent–50 per cent 1-RM and 50 per cent–90 per cent 1-RM respectively.

PROGRAMMING CONSIDERATIONS FOR FEMALE ATHLETES

The evidence clearly shows that in order for an athlete to maximize muscular power development, an overall strong foundation of maximal strength should first be established prior to integrating a range of power-based training strategies within a periodized plan (Haff and Nimphius, 2012). Newton's second law of motion (Force = mass × acceleration; Stone et al., 2002) shows a direct relationship between force and acceleration. From a performance perspective, the greater the force that can be generated (in a defined time period), the greater the acceleration and subsequently the greater the resultant velocity (Suchomel et al., 2016). As discussed earlier, relative increases in strength following a resistance-training programme are similar in males and females, but absolute strength is less, especially in the upper body in females. With this in mind, the key question when working with female athletes is, 'how strong is strong enough' before there should be a shift in training emphasis away from maximal strength?

In a recent review (Haff and Nimphius, 2012), it was recommended that as a minimum requirement for lower-body strength (to realize superior power outputs) athletes should be able to squat twice their body weight. On the basis that a female's lower-body strength is comparable with males when adjusted for body mass or lean body mass, this recommendation is equally valid for both sexes. A theoretical model proposed by Suchomel et al. (2015; see Fig. 2.7), illustrating the association between relative back squat strength and performance, suggested that there are three distinct phases to athletes' developing strength and achieving an optimal performance capacity:

- Strength deficit – increasing the ability to generate force, but not able to fully integrate 'new strength' into actual performance
- Strength association – clear increases in strength with positive impact on performance
- Strength reserve – high levels of strength

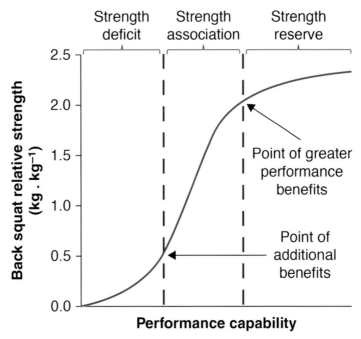

Fig. 2.7 Theoretical relationship between back squat relative strength and performance capability. (Adapted from Suchomel *et al.*, 2016)

already achieved. Gains in strength still possible but the additional benefits to performance become less evident (relates to law of diminishing returns).

Based on previous literature (Keiner *et al.*, 2013, Suchomel *et al.* (2016) deduced that in order to meet the recommended strength level (2 × body weight), this could take up to four to five years of adhering to a structured strength and conditioning plan. With reference to upper body strength, the recommendations are less clear. Needs analysis and testing data will provide you with some guidelines on what level of strength is required in your female athletes to achieve a high level of sports performance. However, if you are in a position where you only have comparative male data, based on the differences previously discussed, females are likely to be able to achieve around

two-thirds the strength levels of their male counterparts in upper body.

In summary, this evidence eludes to the fact that getting 'strong enough' takes a relatively long period of time. Female athletes, through genetic and possibly cultural reasons (depending on sport and athlete perceptions), will often arrive into the strength and conditioning environment with a relatively low resistance training age and level of strength, but large 'window of adaptation' for strength development (Newton and Kraemer, 1994). Considering that all athletes will be getting a significant 'power' stimulus by playing the sport, the biggest impact you are able to have as a strength and conditioning coach to the athletes' performance is by prioritizing strength, provided other aspects of training critical to performance are not being neglected. In support of this statement, it should also be noted that increases in maximal strength will enable the athlete to extend their 'load-power spectrum' (Cormie *et al.*, 2010). What this means is that a stronger athlete will be able to produce greater power over a larger range of absolute loads (Stone *et al.*, 2016), leading to an increase in performance. Development of strength, or aggressive maintenance of strength across the macrocycle, will be a priority on the basis that if strength underpins power performance, a reduction in strength will subsequently result in a reduced power-generating capacity (principle of detraining). A greater percentage of training time should also be dedicated specifically to upper-body strength, particularly for those participating in upper-body dominant sports, such as swimming, throwing and gymnastics. And lastly, exercise selection should also consider the difference in upper- and lower-body strength levels; the intensity of training (load) for combined lifts that involve upper- and lower-body musculature is likely to be limited by the upper body. Whilst combination lifts should not be excluded from training plans, separate exercises that optimally load upper and lower body to develop strength should be featured.

For athletes that do approach what are deemed to be 'high enough' levels of strength, this base level of strength will stimulate further strength and power development through 'phase potentiation' (Stone *et al.*, 1982; Haff and Nimphius, 2012). This refers to the art of sequencing consecutive blocks of training, such that the physiological adaptations from one block will facilitate achievement of training objectives in the next block. For female athletes in terms of strength and power development, this typically refers to shifting the emphasis of training from maximum strength through to strength-speed (greater use of weightlifting techniques) and finally speed-strength (combination loads and ballistic exercises).

STRENGTH AND INJURY PREVENTION

Strength and power training do not just influence performance capabilities for female athletes, but are also important to minimize the risk of injury, with stronger athletes less likely to become injured (Suchomel, 2015; Holmberg, 2013; Lauersen *et al.*, 2014). This is achieved in a number of ways:

- Strength training induces structural changes to muscles, but also has a positive impact on all the other tissues that have been simultaneously stressed, such as bone, ligaments and tendons (Suchomel, 2015; Holmberg, 2013; Lauersen *et al.*, 2014).

- Strength and power asymmetry between dominant and non-dominant sides is recognized as a risk factor for injury (Fort-Vanmeerhaeghe *et al.*, 2015; Maly *et al.*, 2015; Bailey *et al.*, 2015; Bell *et al.*, 2014). Female athletes (volleyball and basketball) have been shown to display a high inter-limb asymmetry index (ASI) (Fort-Vanmeerhaeghe *et al.*, 2015; Hewit *et al.*, 2012) and have also demonstrated (Division I, collegiate athletes) a greater propensity to produce forces asymmetrically compared with males during weight distribution testing and jumping tasks (Bailey *et al.*, 2015). Some authors have suggested that absolute strength may play a bigger role in influencing the extent of asymmetry rather than sex (Bell *et al.*, 2014; Bailey *et al.*, 2015). Therefore, 'strong' females are less likely to experience the adverse effects of asymmetry on performance and injury.

- Strength training induces favourable changes in body composition (increase lean muscle mass, decreased fat mass) (Chiu and Schilling, 2005; Stone *et al.*, 2006; Hedrick and Wada, 2008), as evidenced by weightlifting populations that display high lean body mass and a relatively low percentage of body fat. Data comparing elite male and female weightlifters reported values of around 13 per cent and 20 per cent respectively for percentage of fat, with decreases in fat percentage typically seen in higher-level athletes (Stone et al., 2006). According to Newton's second law, an athlete can become more powerful without getting stronger, by decreasing mass, in particular fat mass, which cannot contribute to force generation. Whilst optimizing 'power-to-weight ratio' provides immediate performance benefits (for example jump higher; MacDonald et al., 2013), it will also reduce impact loads for athletes that perform aerial-based movements (for example track and field athletes, gymnasts, team-sport players), reducing the likelihood of injury through accumulated repetitive loadings or 'bad landings' because of less time in the air (Sands et al., 2000).

Strength training produces a more robust athlete, but RFD is also an important point to consider. Prioritizing strength in female athletes does not mean that other more velocity-dependent types of training are excluded from the programme; in fact, they are necessary. The greater risk of ACL injury in female athletes is a feature across this publication. A hamstring/quadriceps (H/Q) strength ratio, usually based on a maximal voluntary contraction (MVC), has been used to explain the potential for knee stabilization (Zebis et al., 2011). However, the time frame for ACL injury after initial ground contact time is thought to be between 17–50ms (Krosshaug et al., 2007). This is outside of the time frame for achieving a MVC, therefore some power-based activities to stabilize the knee on landing should be included (see plyometric section). Consistent inclusion of unilateral exercises, particularly in lower body is important for female athletes, based on the high risk of ACL injury, relevance of unilateral movement patterns to the needs analysis and common asymmetries found between dominant and non-dominant limbs. In fact, evidence exists to suggest that unilateral exercises can be equally as effective in improving strength as bilateral patterns (Speirs et al., 2016; McCurdy et al., 2005).

PLYOMETRIC TRAINING IN FEMALE ATHLETES

Definition and Classifications

Plyometric exercises are typically categorized by the use of the stretch shortening cycle (SSC) and include high-velocity jumping or rebound exercises (Kyröläinen et al., 2004; Markovic and Mikulic, 2010; McBride, McCaulley, and Cormie, 2008; Spurrs, Murphy, and Watsford, 2003). The SSC is characterized by an eccentric contraction and an amortization phase (the time between eccentric and concentric phases) that is immediately followed by a concentric contraction (Bobbert, Gerritsen, Litjens, and Van Soest, 1996). The SSC enhances the ability of the neural and musculo-tendon system to produce maximal force in the shortest amount of time via pre-activation and elastic energy (EE) return (Bobbert et al., 1996). Schmidtbleicher (1992) categorized SSC expression into either fast or slow; characterized by small or large angular displacements in the hip, knee and ankle joints and a ground contact time (GCT) below or above 250ms respectively.

Hill (1938) identified a mechanical model of muscle, consisting of a series elastic component (SEC), largely composed of the tendon, titin and the intrinsic elasticity of the myofilaments (Siff, 2003); the contractile component (CC), associated with actin and myosin cross-bridge formations; and the parallel elastic component (PEC), consisting of the sarcolemma and other passive tissue structures. Each component of this model is reported to have a key role and in combination make up the properties of the musculo-tendon unit (MTU). The SEC is currently recognized as the primary site for the storage of EE and is key for optimal SSC utilization (Kubo, Kawakami, and Fukunaga, 1999; Kubo et al., 2007; Lichtwark and Wilson, 2007). The role of the CC is to produce force via cross-bridge formation, aiding in all phases of the movement but directly contributing to force output during the concentric phase, while finally the PEC passively exerts force upon muscle stretch (Komi, 1992). Lichtwark and Wilson (2007) suggest that recoil of the SEC is responsible for both increasing concentric power output and conserving energy during locomotion. Komi (1986) suggests that a 'stiff' MTU is optimal for performance of SSC activities as it allows for a rapid and more efficient transmission of muscle force and EE to the skeleton and consequently, higher rates of force development. Stiffness is described as the relationship between the deformation of a body and a given force and can be described from the level of a single muscle fibre, to modelling the entire body as a mass and a spring (Butler, Crowell, and Davis, 2003).

MECHANISMS DURING SSC EXPRESSION

Zatsiorsky and Kraemer (1995) and Ingen Schenau et al. (1997) reported that the mechanisms contributing to the enhanced performance of SSC utilization include more time for force development, storage and utilization of EE, potentiation of contractile structures and stretch reflex contributions. However, as has been mentioned, Schmidtbleicher (1992) categorized SSC expression into either fast or slow actions (less than or greater than 250ms GCT respectively). Understandably, this results in a slight

variation in the relative contribution of these mechanisms in different SSC tasks. For example, during fast SSC performance, Komi, (1992) suggests that higher stiffness levels increase the amount of stored and reused EE. This has been reported to be due to the distribution of the stored energy (EE should be transferred to the SEC as efficiently as possible, as contractile muscle tissue is not efficient for energy storage and return), which is dependent on the level of deformation or stiffness at each tissue (Zatsiorsky and Kraemer, 1995). During active movement the stiffness of the muscle tissue is variable due to the active forces exerted but should be able to exceed the stiffness of the tendon due to its stiffness levels being constant (Turner and Jeffreys, 2010; Zatsiorsky and Kraemer, 1995). Farley, Houdijk, Van Strien, and Louie (1998) report that leg stiffness is influenced by agonist muscle activation, as well as the magnitude of antagonistic co-activation immediately prior to and post ground contact, known as a co-contraction. Supporting this theory, many authors suggest that during a fast SSC, the CC, while not lengthening or shortening is in fact undergoing an isometric action (Fukunaga et al., 2001; Kubo et al., 2000; Wilson and Flanagan, 2008) and co-contractions are taking place to aid stability. An isometric contraction at the muscle may be of benefit as it allows for a greater transition of EE to the SEC due to greater CC stiffness levels (Zatsiorsky and Kraemer, 1995). Supporting this, during gait Ishikawa, Pakaslahti, and Komi (2007) found no significant change in fascicle length during the first half of plantar flexion, whereas there was a rapid lengthening of the tendon. During the second half of plantar flexion both the tendon and muscle rapidly shortened. Therefore, in order to develop efficient fast SSC function, training should be designed to transfer the potential energy of a pre-stretch towards the tendon structure via high force and potentially isometric muscle contractions (Turner and Jeffreys, 2010). In contrast, when the magnitude of force exceeds the stiffness capability of the MTU, more joint compliance and a longer GCT will be seen, resulting in a 'slow' SSC. This also results in the CC of the muscle generating less active stiffness, resulting in less EE being transferred to the SEC. While some EE is stored through the PEC and the cross bridge structure, these structures have less EE storage and returning capabilities (Turner and Jeffreys, 2010; Zatsiorsky and Kraemer, 1995). Subsequently, it is generally found that the increased performance observed during the concentric action of a slow SSC has a lower relative contribution of EE return and is due to other mechanisms such as an increased time to produce force, contractile element potentiation and the stretch reflex (Wilson and Flanagan, 2008). It should be noted that although stored EE may increase with a rise in eccentric force absorption (Zatsiorsky and Kraemer, 1995) there is an individual limit where once the eccentric loading reaches a critical threshold, the subsequent concentric contraction and EE return may actually decrease (Wilson, Murphy, and Pryor, 1994). This may be associated with the amortization phase taking too long as the time span for cross bridge maintenance has been estimated to be in the region of 15–120 milliseconds, therefore the amortization period needs to be minimal to augment energy return from the SEC structures (Siff, 2003) as energy is lost at the instance of cross bridge detachment and eccentric muscle actions (Fleck and Kraemer, 2014).

Furthermore, during plyometric activity, mechanoreceptors are active in order to help return energy through the stretch reflex and provide the MTU protection from excessive tension build-up (Chen, Hippenmeyer, Arber, and Frank, 2003; Jami, 1992). For example, when the MTU stretch reaches a critical length the muscle spindle activates a contraction of the agonist, supporting force output (Komi and Gollhofer, 1997). However, sudden high muscular tension may cause the Golgi tendon organ (GTO) to simultaneously inhibit the agonist's neural drive in order to avoid the potential for injury (Leukel, Taube, Gruber, Hodapp, and Gollhofer, 2008). Swanik et al. (2002) theorized that the positive adaptations of plyometric training could be attributed to increased sensitivity of the muscle spindle and a decrease in GTO sensitivity, allowing the athlete to withstand higher landing forces without a decrease in exerted muscular force. However, it may be postulated that during slow SSC expression, the potential for GTO inhibition may be reduced compared to a fast SSC as the eccentric muscle action inherently reduces tension due to cross bridge detachment (Fleck and Kraemer, 2014), whereas during fast SSC useage the isometric muscle action maintains tension and stiffness in order to increase EE storage (Fukunaga et al., 2001). Therefore, in order to benefit from these neuromuscular adaptations of plyometric training, a gradual increase in muscle tension (via increased exercise intensity and fast SSC tasks) should be developed over time.

TRAINING ADAPTATIONS

Research shows that plyometric training can improve jump height (Faigenbaum et al., 2007; Meylan and Malatesta, 2009), running velocity (Kotzamanidis, 2006), running economy (Saunders et al., 2006; Turner, Owings and Schwane, 2003), and acceleration (Markovic and Mikulic, 2010). When striving for a specific performance outcome, it is important that a plyometric training intervention is designed to eventually have a level of specificity to the GCTs and movements of desired improvements (Markovic and Mikulic, 2010). At the onset of plyometric training, programmes should be designed in order to create the desired mechanistic adaptations; for example, reduced GTO sensitivity and increased pre-activation ability.

Therefore when comparing the types and magnitudes of performance enhancement found within the literature, the specific details of the training protocols and exercises are extremely important. However, this may be challenging as even if a training programme has reported the exercise names and doses, this may be insufficient to determine the GCT and SSC utilized throughout training.

In a study by Paavolainen, Häkkinen, Hämäläinen, Nummela, and Rusko (1999), participants improved running economy after a period of plyometric training, which, along with an increased muscle power, resulted in a 3.1 per cent relative improvement in a 5km running performance. Markovic and Mikulic (2010) also reported increases in sprint performance over 10 and 50m with the greatest improvement over 10m (2.2 per cent vs. 1.5 per cent respectively), which represents the acceleration phase, indicative of slow-SSC ability and knee-joint stiffness (Kuitunen, Komi, and Kyrolainen, 2002). These improvements may have simply been due to the velocity of muscle action and GCT used in training, as slow SSC exercise is associated with enhanced 10m-acceleration and fast SSC is associated with enhanced running economy and maximal velocity (Kotzamanidis, 2006; Saunders et al., 2006; Turner, Owings and Schwane, 2003). Supporting this specificity, it is also commonly reported that plyometric training programmes produce an increase in countermovement jump height, but not necessarily squat jump height due to the absence of the SSC in squat jump performance (Bosco, Viitasalo, Komi and Luhtanen, 1982).

In order to optimize training and specific performance outcomes, an understanding of the specific adaptations that are likely to occur is important. For example, Kubo et al. (2007) reported an increase of 63.4 per cent in overall ankle joint stiffness assessed during drop jumps after a plyometric training intervention. An increase in Achilles tendon elongation was reported but no significant change in tendon stiffness was found. It may be postulated that ankle joint stiffness increased from a rise in muscle stiffness, which subsequently allowed greater transfer of EE to the tendon, resulting in improved EE re-utilization. In contrast, Burgess Connick and Graham-Smith (2007), found increases in jump performance while also reporting a rise in Achilles tendon stiffness after six weeks of plyometric training. It may again be that the different results shown throughout the research are caused by varied training prescription and athlete characteristics. However, this can only be speculated as some researchers failed to report the exact training prescription.

Overall, plyometric training has been shown to improve SSC function via the following mechanisms:

- A muscle's maximal shortening velocity (Malisoux, Francaux, Nielens and Theisen, 2006)
- Inter-muscular coordination and co-contraction ability (Markovic and Mikulic, 2010)
- Pre-activation prior to landing (Kuitunen et al., 2002)
- Elastic energy storage and return (Kubo et al., 2007; Lichtwark and Wilson, 2007)
- Maximum tendon elongation (Kubo et al., 2007)
- The stretch reflex mechanism (Adams, O'Shea, O'Shea, and Climstein, 1992)
- Dampening of GTO sensitivity (Hutton and Atwater, 1992)
- Motor unit recruitment and neural firing frequency (Adams et al., 1992; Kyröläinen et al., 2005)
- Rate of force development (Komi, 1986).

Testing for Plyometric Ability

In order to correctly identify athletes who are in need of plyometric development, it is important to quantify the individual's plyometric ability. The Reactive Strength Index

(RSI) was developed in order to quantify an athlete's reactive strength capability (Young, 1995). RSI is described as jump height (mm)/GCT (ms) (Young, 1995). This measure can be attained through a drop jump protocol (McClymont, 2003), a five-jump protocol (Lloyd, Oliver, Hughes and Williams, 2009) or through a ten-jump protocol (Harper, 2011). The drop jump procedure should be performed from a standardized drop height, typically of 30cm, while the five- and ten-jump protocol require the athlete to perform continuous rebound jumps of a self-selected height with minimal GCT. The RSI is calculated as an average of four jumps or the best five jumps in the five-jump and ten-jump protocols respectively.

Recent research has indicated that different test protocols measure different expressions of the SSC (Lloyd, Oliver, Hughes and Williams, 2011). For example, leg stiffness can be measured via a sub-maximal hopping protocol and represents a more isolated physical quality than that measured during the RSI (Lloyd et al., 2011). Lloyd et al., (2011) concluded that the sub-maximal hopping protocol may more validly measure fast SSC function with the RSI and CMJ representing intermediate and slow SSC respectively. However, it has also previously been reported that a countermovement jump does not provide an adequate model of SSC behaviour or stretch reflex potentiation (Komi and Gollhoffer, 1997). Therefore it may be that in order to validly quantify SSC function, the RSI may be a suitable and convenient test to implement. Although, if the athlete's performance requires a more specific SSC function such as that expressed in leg stiffness or a CMJ, these tests may then be considered.

Training Intensity

In order to elicit the desired training adaptations from plyometrics, intensity needs to be controlled and progressed. However, our traditional view of plyometric intensity via exercise names and styles may be insufficient due to the impact of exercise variables and participant characteristics (Bobbert et al., 1996). More recently, plyometric intensity has been defined via the eccentric rate of force development (first peak force/time to peak force from landing) (Jensen and Ebben, 2007). In exercises when the eccentric rate of force development loading is high (dropping from a height, landing on the forefoot with a fast ground contact), the need for high-intensity muscle contraction (muscle stiffness) is increased to ensure that energy is transferred to the SEC where passive EE return can be exploited (Zatsiorsky and Kraemer, 1995). However, while this mechanical view of intensity may be suitable for fast rebound-type plyometric exercises, slow rebound type exercises may require a more neuromuscular quantification of intensity such as surface electromyography (sEMG) (Jarvis, Graham-Smith, and Comfort, 2016). During slower SSC performance, the sEMG measures are greater due to the reliance of concentric muscle force compared to that from passive force enhancement in a fast SSC action. Cappa and Behm (2013) reported longer GCTs were associated with higher rectus femoris sEMG (47 per cent) compared with shorter GCT associated with higher RFD (45 per cent). Therefore, although mechanical stress reduces, muscular stress increases with potentially greater motor unit recruitment (Ebben, Simenz, and Jensen, 2008). However, in contrast to this, Jarvis et al. (2016) reported muscular intensity to be more homogenous between rebound and ballistic exercises and that mechanical intensity has a greater ability to distinguish between exercises. It is hypothesized that this may be related to ensuring a maximal intent on all tasks. Jarvis et al. (2016) conclude that three mechanical factors should be considered to quantify plyometric intensity; impulse, peak force and peak eccentric power, quantifying the overall mechanical stress through the movement, the peak stress associated with yielding and the rate of this yielding application respectively.

In order to manipulate these variables within training it is important to consider the details of the exercise selection and how a plyometric movement performed by an athlete may vary in intensity (Fig. 2.8). Firstly, individual athlete characteristics will decrease or increase the mechanical loading experienced during the exercise. For example, increased intensity will be experienced by athletes who have a) an increased body mass, b) a greater reactive strength capability and c)

optimum kinematics allowing a stiff landing strategy (Jarvis et al., 2016). Importantly, the coach must be mostly aware of the athlete's kinematics, as these are able to be acutely manipulated. The exercise set-up can also increase the experienced mechanical loading and intensity via a) a decreased GCT (increased rate) from an appropriate moderate desired jump height, b) an increase in the velocity at which the COM hits the ground (increased 'ECC force'), manipulated by drop height and linear velocity, and c) the available musculature to deal with the stress upon landing (relative force to tissue contribution),

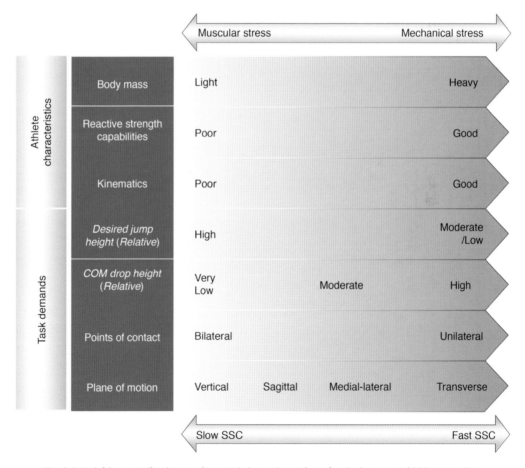

Fig. 2.8 Variables contributing to plyometric intensity and mechanical stress and SSC expression.

manipulated via the number of points of contact (bilateral or unilateral) or the plane of motion (sagittal, frontal, transverse) (Radcliffe and Farentinos, 2015).

An athlete's exercise kinematics are a primary area of development as poor kinematics reduce an athlete's ability to utilize a fast SSC expression. From then the desired GCT should be achieved via manipulating the desired jump height and the velocity at which the COM hits the ground, while intent for minimal GCT remains constant. For example, a very low COM velocity with a moderate to high jumping target, such as that in a CMJ, will not allow for enough potential energy to be stored or for sufficient pre-activation to take place in order for a fast SSC to be utilized. A moderate COM velocity with the same jumping target may allow a fast SSC to be expressed, due to sufficient SEC energy transfer and time for pre-activation. However, if COM velocity increases above an individual's relative capability (associated with their RSI) to store EE and deal with muscular tension, the GTO may reduce neural drive and likely remove the effectiveness of the exercise. This continuum of execution results in a low-magnitude 'inverted u' shape relationship between COM velocity at ground contact and GCT. It must also be understood that although COM velocity may be one key in determining the SSC utilized, this will be secondary to the desired jump height. For example, during tasks with consistent landing velocity, intent for maximal jump height is likely to produce a longer GCT to allow a greater contribution of

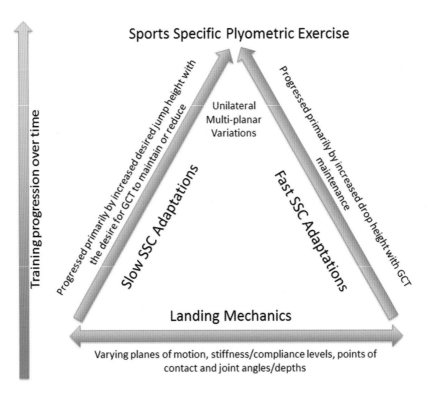

Fig. 2.9 Proposed plyometric training progression for the development of sports specific SSC function.

concentric force production and more time to generate force, while a lower desired jump height will allow a faster SSC expression (Fig. 2.8).

While GCT is important to manipulate, due to its effect on training adaptations and sports specificity, its relationship with task intensity (which must also be controlled) is poor. For example, once a task with moderate COM velocity and jump height (allowing a fast SSC execution) has been designed, there is a window where further increase in COM velocity may increase force at ground contact, but have very little effect on GCT (Walsh, Arampatzis, Schade and Bruggemann, 2004). During this scenario, it is also possible that an increase in desired jump height may result in an increased GCT but also be associated with an increased level of mechanical loading. However, these intricacies are currently not understood well, and it is recommended that a coach considers all contributing intensity variables when designing training progressions (Fig. 2.9).

If the end goal of the training programme is to improve fast/intermediate SSC function, starting a training programme only with low intensity exercises that utilise a slow SSC, such as bilateral in place jumping with minimal eccentric loading may be sub-optimal due to the discrepancy in mechanisms that contribute to fast SSC performance (Fig. 2.9). For example, a slow SSC CMJ (low COM drop height and high desired jump height) may be utilized to minimize mechanical stress, but this may be programmed alongside a pogo hop (a low COM drop height and a low desired jump height), which allows for fast SSC utilization to be developed while still limiting mechanical loading. As a programme progresses, slow SSC expression may then be progressed via a decreased GCT or a maintained GCT but with a greater drop and jump height, while fast SSC exercise could then be progressed via a maintained GCT with increased drop and jump height.

TRAINING RECOMMENDATIONS FOR FEMALE ATHLETES

When planning a female athlete plyometric training programme, there are both general and specific gender considerations that must be made. The obvious differences between males and females are anthropometrical measurements such as body fat percentage, muscle cross sectional area and lower limb biomechanics (Lloyd and Faigenbaum, 2016; Ryan et al., 2009; Sugimoto, Myer, Foss, and Hewett, 2015). However, when considering the jumping and landing activities involved in plyometrics, females demonstrate different neuromuscular strategies than male athletes (Myer, Ford, and Hewett, 2005; Rozzi, Lephart, Gear, and Fu, 1999). For example, females show deficits in dynamic neuromuscular control of joint stability in all three axes of motion through the lower-body kinetic chain, which contributes to a four- to six-fold higher incidence of ACL injury rate compared to males (Hewett et al., 2005). Females also display a longer latency period (electro mechanical delay) between preparatory and reactive muscle activation (Winter and Brookes, 1991) potentially due to a lower level of tendon stiffness (Kubo et al., 2007). Therefore training should focus on plyometric exercises, which subject the joint to rapid loads and can activate pre-activation mechanisms (approx. 100ms prior to ground contact) and enhance motor control during landing.

In general, to benefit from the adaptations of plyometric training, exercises must involve a level of landing stress to increase the rate of eccentric force development (COM fall height) and eventually increase stiffness and reactive strength. However, landing is also a highly likely site for injury during performance (Sugimoto et al., 2015) and the biomechanical positions associated with landing should be the focus of training adaptations for all novice athletes. This becomes more imperative for female athletes who present more at-risk lower limb biomechanics (Sugimoto et al., 2015). In order to land effectively in a range of sporting scenarios, the athlete needs to be able to both land in a stable joint position with stiffness via effective co-contraction and also have the ability to dissipate force through compliance and eccentric muscle actions. This means that the athlete must be able to land in a biomechanically effective position and be able to regulate their stiffness and GCT to control their COM to meet the task demands. It may also be beneficial to ensure that the athlete is able to land with the desired stiffness or compliance at varied muscle lengths, joint angles, points of contact and planes of motion. For example, incorporating lateral or medial jump and landing tasks may help to balance the lateral and medial hamstring and quadriceps contribution ratios (Myer et al., 2005; Rozzi et al., 1999) and improve neuromuscular control of knee valgus collapse. These skills and physical capacities should be developed at the onset of all training programmes before any further increase in intensity is warranted. The development of these abilities should also be accomplished concurrently with strength training to allow necessary MTU adaptations to occur and reduce injury risk (Solomonow and Krogsgaard, 2001; Turner and Jeffreys, 2010). This approach should be considered for a substantial period of time depending on the athlete's baseline training status, which commonly in female athletes is very low. While some practitioners may be keen to move to increased intensity in order to improve reactive strength, the ability to improve reactive strength and performance via being in a more advantageous position with greater stability, improved pre-activation and reduced electromechanical delay at landing should not be overlooked. For example, improvements in pre-activation strategies can enhance performance via greater cross-bridge formation, co-contraction force at ground contact and increased joint and muscle stiffness (Moritani, Oddsson, and Thorstensson, 1991).

Once effective and robust landing skills have been developed, training programmes can be progressed via increases in plyometric exercise intensity with a consideration of the desired adaptations (Fig. 2.9). If adaptations in SSC function are to be realized, the load experienced within the eccentric phase should be within the limits of the athlete's CC force production and the amortization phase should be as rapid as possible without increasing eccentric loading rate so much that the GTO inhibits the muscular contraction (Turner and Jeffreys, 2010). However, the stress and loading during the eccentric phase should be increased and the athlete should be challenged over time. It is important within the training process that maximal intention (minimal GCT possible with desired jump height) is ensured during all repetitions. If a slower GCT is required, this should be completed via manipulating the task (COM drop height and/or desired jump height), while a faster GCT may be achieved via both task manipulation and improving an athlete's jumping kinematics (Fig. 2.8). It may also be desirable to train the mechanisms of both slow and fast SSC function, as slow SSC exercises allow for some intensity to be utilized during training while limiting the mechanical stress, but fast SSC exercises may have more specific adaptations for improving reactive strength and stiffness capabilities.

Upper-Body Plyometrics

Plyometric training is typically referred to within the lower body, although it may be expected that the theory underpinning plyometric training applies to any muscle group including those in the upper body and that a number of sports may benefit from improved SSC performance in the upper extremities (Bosco and Komi, 1979; Heiderscheit, McLean, and Davies, 1996). However, while there has been limited research into upper-body plyometric training, current evidence does not suggest the same level of performance enhancement as that which can be expected in lower-limb plyometric programmes (Heiderscheit et al., 1996; Schulte-Edelmann, Davies, Kernozek, and Gerberding, 2005). Heiderscheit et al. (1996) compared the effects of isokinetic vs. plyometric training of the shoulder internal rotators and reported no significant improvements in isokinetic performance in the plyometric group. Similarly, plyometric training resulted in no improvement in isokinetic performance in the posterior shoulder (Schulte-Edelmann et al., 2005). However, Wilson, Murphy, and Giorgi (1996) compared the effects of weight vs. plyometric training on force production for both the lower and upper extremities. Their results showed improvement in the rate of force development of the lower extremities but not the upper extremities. Interestingly, Fletcher and Hartwell (2004) reported improved golf drive performance after a combined resistance and plyometric training programme, although it is unclear if improvements came from plyometric training or resistance exercise, and the subjects used were of a very low training age which may mean that adaptations were not hard to come by. It may also support that much more research is needed into upper-body plyometric training at both the shoulder and the trunk.

CONCLUSION

When utilizing plyometrics in female athletes, it is important that suitable co-contraction and landing ability is developed prior to and early on during the programme. These skills should be developed and challenged in different planes of motion and with different landing strategies (stiff or compliant) to ensure injury risk is reduced and the body is prepared for the increased intensity of the later stages of the programme. It is also recommended that a period of strength training is used to increase strength of the connective tissues. From thereafter, a plyometric programme must be developed to improve the sports-specific SSC ability with progressive increases in intensity and concurrent slow and fast SSC development.

Case Study Example: The case study shown in Table 2.4 provides guidelines for speed and power development for a female athlete participating in a multidirectional land-based sport.

Programme Level	General Introductory	Basic	Intermediate
Mesocycle Objectives	• Introduce key movement patterns • Address asymmetries and imbalances • Improve whole-body maximum strength & stimulate tissue adaption –hypertrophy. • Increase work capacity	• Increase force generating capacity (maximum strength) • Continue to increase hypertrophy in key areas (e.g., upper body) • Introduce high force-low velocity RFD • Improve/ maintain posture under load. • Increase ability to absorb force.	• Increase skill complexity of lifts/plyometrics • Improve maximum & RFD (slight shift towards higher velocity than basic) • Higher degree of sport specificity
Exercise Selection	BB BN Shoulder Press	BB BN Push Press	BB Split Jerk
	Back Squat	**Clean Pull from Thigh, Concentric Box Jump	Squat clean from thigh
	Bilateral Stiff-Legged Deadlift	Front Squat	Clean first pull (3 second hold in hang)
	Horizontal Row	BB Bent Over Row	Chin Ups
	DB Split Squat	*BB BN FWD lunge, SL hop and stick for distance.	* BB Lateral lunge, multi directional hopping drill.
	Press up to Side Plank	Tricep Dips	*Palloff rotations, MB Side Toss
Suggested Prescription	3-5 sets, 5-8 repetitions, 3-5 minutes between sets.	3-5 sets, 5-8 repetitions, 3-5 minutes between sets.	3-5 sets, 3-5 repetitions, 3-5 minutes rest

Table 2.4 Strength and power development (gym-based case study example).

BB= Barbell; BN=Behind the neck; MB=Medicine Ball; * Complex training; **= Contrast Training; RFD=Rate of Force Development.

REFERENCES

Aagaard, P., Simonsen, E. B., Andersen, J. L., Magnusson, P., and Dyhre-Poulsen, P. (2002) Increased rate of force development and neural drive of human skeletal muscle following resistance training. *Journal of Applied Physiology*, 93(4), 1318–1326.

Aagaard, P. (2003) Training-induced changes in neural function. *Exercise and Sport Sciences Reviews*, 31(2), 61–67.

Aagaard, P. (2010) The use of eccentric strength training to enhance maximal muscle strength, explosive force (RDF) and muscular power-consequences for athletic performance. *The Open Sports Sciences Journal*, 3(5).

Abadie, B.R. and Wentworth, M.C. (2000) Prediction of one repetition maximum strength from a 5–10 repetition submaximal strength test in college-aged females. *Journal of Exercise Physiology Online*, 3(3).

Abe, T., Yasuda, T., Midorikawa, T., Sato, Y., Inoue, K., Koizumi, K. and Ishii, N. (2005) Skeletal muscle size and circulating IGF-1 are increased after two weeks of twice daily 'KAATSU' resistance training. *International Journal of KAATSU Training Research*, 1(1), 6–12.

Adams, K., O'Shea, J.P., O'Shea, K.L. and Climstein, M. (1992) The Effect of Six Weeks of Squat, Plyometric and Squat-Plyometric Training on Power Production. *Journal of Applied Sports Science Research*, 6(1), 36–41.

Abdelkrim, N.B., Chaouachi, A., Chamari, K., Chtara, M. and Castagna, C. (2010) Positional role and competitive-level differences in elite-level men's basketball players. *The Journal of Strength and Conditioning Research*, 24(5), 1346–1355.

Aizawa, K., Hayashi, K. and Mesaki, N. (2006) Relationship of muscle strength with dehydroepiandrosterone sulfate (DHEAS), testosterone and insulin-like growth factor-I in male and female athletes. *Advances in Exercise and Sports Physiology*, 12(1), 29–34.

Andersen, J.L. and Aagaard, P. (2000) Myosin heavy chain IIX overshoot in human skeletal muscle. *Muscle and Nerve*, 23(7), 1095–1104.

Babault, N., Pousson, M., Ballay, Y. and Van Hoecke, J. (2001) Activation of human quadriceps femoris during isometric, concentric, and eccentric contractions. *Journal of Applied Physiology*, 91(6), 2628–2634.

Bailey, C.A., Sato, K., Burnett, A. and Stone, M.H. (2015). Force-production asymmetry in male and female athletes of differing strength levels. International Journal of Sports *Physiology and Performance*, 10(4), 504–508.

Baker, D. (2014) Using strength platforms for explosive performance. In: Joyce, D. and Lewindon, D. (eds.). (2014). *High-Performance Training for Sports. Human Kinetics*, pp.127–144

Baker, D. (2017) Using velocity measures to improve resistance training programming and coaching. *UKSCA 13th Annual Conference, UK*.

Banyard, H.G., Nosaka, K. and Haff, G.G. (2017) Reliability and Validity of the Load–Velocity Relationship to Predict the 1-RM Back Squat. *The Journal of Strength and Conditioning Research*, 31(7), 1897–1904.

Bazuelo-Ruiz, B., Padial, P., García-Ramos, A., Morales-Artacho, A.J., Miranda, M.T. and Feriche, B. (2015) Predicting maximal dynamic strength from the load-velocity relationship in squat exercise. *The Journal of Strength and Conditioning Research*, 29(7), 1999–2005.

Beckham, G., Mizuguchi, S., Carter, C., Sato, K., Ramsey, M., Lamont, H. ... and Stone, M. (2013) Relationships of isometric mid-thigh pull variables to weightlifting performance. *Journal of Sports Medicine and Physical Fitness*, 53(5), 573–581.

Beckham, G.K., Suchomel, T.J., Bailey, C.A., Sole, C.J. and Grazer, J.L. (2014, October) The relationship of the reactive strength index-modified and measures of force development in the isometric mid-thigh pull. In *ISBS-Conference Proceedings Archive*.

Behm, D.G. and Sale, D.G. (1993) Intended

rather than actual movement velocity determines velocity-specific training response. *Journal of Applied Physiology*, 74(1), 359–368.

Behm, D.G. (1995) Neuromuscular implications and applications of resistance training. *Journal of Strength and Conditioning Research*, 9, 264–274.

Bell, D.R., Sanfilippo, J.L., Binkley, N. and Heiderscheit, B.C. (2014) Lean mass asymmetry influences force and power asymmetry during jumping in collegiate athletes. *Journal of Strength and Conditioning Research/National Strength and Conditioning Association*, 28(4), 884.

Beltman, J.G.M., Sargeant, A.J., Van Mechelen, W. and De Haan, A. (2004) Voluntary activation level and muscle fibre recruitment of human quadriceps during lengthening contractions. *Journal of Applied Physiology*, 97(2), 619–626.

Bird, S.P., Tarpenning, K.M. and Marino, F.E. (2005) Designing resistance training programmes to enhance muscular fitness. *Sports Medicine*, 35(10), 841–851.

Bishop, P., Cureton, K. and Collins, M. (1987) Sex difference in muscular strength in equally trained men and women. *Ergonomics*, 30(4), 675–687.

Bishop, P., Cureton, K., Conerly, M. and Collins, M. (1989) Sex difference in muscle cross-sectional area of athletes and non-athletes. *Journal of Sports Sciences*, 7(1), 31–39.

Blazevich, A.J. and Jenkins, D.G. (2002) Effect of the movement speed of resistance training exercises on sprint and strength performance in concurrently training elite junior sprinters. *Journal of Sports Sciences*, 20(12), 981–990.

Bobbert, M.F., Gerritsen, K.G., Litjens, M.C. and Van Soest, A.J. (1996) Why is countermovement jump height greater than squat jump height? *Medicine and Science in Sports and Exercise*, 28, 1402–1412.

Bompa, T.O. and Haff, G.G. (2009) Periodization: *Theory and Methodology of Training*. Human Kinetics Publishers.

Bosco, C. and Komi, P.V. (1979) Potentiation of the mechanical behavior of the human skeletal muscle through prestretching. *Acta Physiologica Scandinavica*, 106(4), 467–472.

Bosco, C., Viitasalo, J.T., Komi, P.V. and Luhtanen, P. (1982) Combined effect of elastic energy and myoelectrical potentiation during stretch-shortening cycle exercise. *Acta Physiologica Scandinavica*, 114(4), 557–565.

Bosco, C., Tsarpela, O., Foti, C., Cardinale, M., Tihanyi, J., Bonifazi, M. ... and Viru, A. (2002) Mechanical behaviour of leg extensor muscles in male and female sprinters. *Biology of Sport*, 19(3), 189–202.

Brewer, C. (2017) *Athletic Movement Skills: Training for Sports Performance*. Human Kinetics.

Burger, M.E. and Burger, T.A. (2002) Neuromuscular and Hormonal Adaptations to Resistance Training: Implications for Strength Development in Female Athletes. *Strength and Conditioning Journal*, 24(3), 51–59.

Burgess, K.E., Connick, M.J., Graham-Smith, P. and Pearson, S.J. (2007) Plyometric vs. isometric training influences on tendon properties and muscle output. *Journal of Strength and Condititong Research*, 21(3), 986–989.

Busko, K. and Gajewski, J. (2011) Muscle strength and power of elite female and male swimmers. *Baltic Journal of Health and Physical Activity*, 3(1), 13.

Butler, R.J., Crowell, H.P. and Davis, I.M. (2003) Lower extremity stiffness: implications for performance and injury. *Clinical Biomechanics* (Bristol, Avon), 18(6), 511–517.

Cappa, D.F. and Behm, D.G. (2013). Neuromuscular characteristics of drop and hurdle jumps with different types of landings. *Journal of Strength and Conditioning Research*, 27(11), 3011–3020.

Cardinale, M. and Stone, M.H. (2006). Is testosterone influencing explosive performance? *Journal of Strength and Conditioning Research*, 20(1), 103.

Carlock, J.M., Smith, S.L., Hartman, M.J., Morris, R.T., Ciroslan, D.A., Pierce, K.C., ...

and Stone, M.H. (2004) The relationship between vertical jump power estimates and weightlifting ability: a field-test approach. *The Journal of Strength and Conditioning Research*, 18(3), 534–539.

Chen, H.H., Hippenmeyer, S., Arber, S. and F rank, E. (2003) Development of the monosynaptic stretch reflex circuit. *Current Opinion in Neurobiology*, 13(1), 96–102.

Chiu, L.Z. and Schilling, B.K. (2005) A primer on weightlifting: From sport to sports training. *Strength and Conditioning Journal*, 27(1), 42.

Coffey, V.G. and Hawley, J.A. (2007) The molecular bases of training adaptation. *Sports Medicine*, 37(9), 737–763.

Comfort, P., Jones, P.A. and Udall, R. (2015) The effect of load and sex on kinematic and kinetic variables during the mid-thigh clean pull. *Sports Biomechanics*, 14(2), 139–156.

Constantini, N.W., Dubnov, G. and Lebrun, C.M. (2005) The menstrual cycle and sport performance. *Clinics in Sports Medicine*, 24(2), e51–e82.

Cook, C. and Crewther, B. (2011) Biochemical markers and resistance training. In: Cardinale, M., Newton, R. and Nosaka, K. (eds.). *Strength and Conditioning: Biological principles and practical applications* (pp.155–164). John Wiley and Sons.

Cormie, P., McGuigan, M.R. and Newton, R.U. (2010a) Influence of Strength on the Magnitude and Mechanisms of Adaptation to Power Training. *Medicine and Science in Sports and Exercise*, 42(8), 1566–1581.

Cormie, P., Mcguigan, M.R. and Newton, R.U. (2010b) Adaptations in athletic performance after ballistic power versus strength training. *Medicine and Science in Sports and Exercise*, 42(8), 1582–1598.

Cormie, P., McGuigan, M.R. and Newton, R.U. (2011a) Developing maximal neuromuscular power. *Sports Medicine*, 41(1), 17–38.

Cormie, P., McGuigan, M.R. and Newton, R.U. (2011b) Developing maximal neuromuscular power. *Sports Medicine*, 41(1), 17–38.

Costill, D.L., Daniels, J., Evans, W., Fink, W., Krahenbuhl, G. and Saltin, B. (1976) Skeletal muscle enzymes and fiber composition in male and female track athletes. Journal of *Applied Physiology*, 40(2), 149–154.

Crewther, B., Keogh, J., Cronin, J. and Cook, C. (2006) Possible stimuli for strength and power adaptation. *Sports Medicine*, 36(3), 215–238.

Cronin, J., McNair, P.J. and Marshall, R.N. (2001) Velocity specificity, combination training and sport specific tasks. *Journal of Science and Medicine in Sport*, 4(2), 168–178.

Cronin, J. and Sleivert, G. (2005) Challenges in understanding the influence of maximal power training on improving athletic performance. *Sports Medicine*, 35(3), 213–234.

Cronin, J. and Hansen, K.T. (2006) Resisted sprint training for the acceleration phase of sprinting. *Strength and Conditioning Journal*, 28(4), 42.

DeFreitas, J.M., Beck, T.W., Stock, M.S., Dillon, M.A. and Kasishke, P.R. (2011) An examination of the time course of training-induced skeletal muscle hypertrophy. *European Journal of Applied Physiology*, 111(11), 2785–2790.

de Jonge, X.A.J. (2003) Effects of the menstrual cycle on exercise performance. *Sports Medicine*, 33(11), 833–851.

DeWeese, B.H., Serrano, A.J., Scruggs, S.K. and Burton, J.D. (2013) The midthigh pull: proper application and progressions of a weightlifting movement derivative. *Strength and Conditioning Journal*, 35(6), 54–58.

De Witt, J.K., English, K.L., Crowell, J.B., Kalogera, K.L., Guilliams, M.E., Nieschwitz, B.E. ... and Ploutz-Snyder, L.L. (2016) Isometric Mid-thigh Pull Reliability and Relationship to Deadlift 1-RM. *Journal of Strength and Conditioning Research*.

DiBrezzo, R., Fort, I.L. and Brown, B. (1991) Relationships among strength, endurance, weight and body fat during three phases of the menstrual cycle. *The Journal of Sports Medicine and Physical Fitness*, 31(1), 89–94.

Dos' Santos, T., Thomas, C., Jones, P.A. and Comfort, P. (2016) Assessing muscle strength asymmetry via a unilateral stance isometric mid-thigh pull. *International Journal of Sports Physiology and Performance*, 1–24.

Dreyer, H.C., Drummond, M.J., Pennings, B., Fujita, S., Glynn, E.L., Chinkes, D.L. ... and Rasmussen, B.B. (2008) Leucine-enriched essential amino acid and carbohydrate ingestion following resistance exercise enhances mTOR signaling and protein synthesis in human muscle. *American Journal of Physiology-Endocrinology and Metabolism*, 294(2), E392–E400.

Dreyer, H.C., Fujita, S., Glynn, E.L., Drummond, M.J., Volpi, E. and Rasmussen, B.B. (2010) Resistance exercise increases leg muscle protein synthesis and mTOR signalling independent of sex. *Acta Physiologica*, 199(1), 71–81.

Duchateau, J. and Enoka, R.M. (2011) Human motor unit recordings: origins and insight into the integrated motor system. *Brain Research*, 1409, 42–61.

Ebben, W.P., Simenz, C. and Jensen, R.L. (2008) Evaluation of plyometric intensity using electromyography. *Journal of Strength and Conditioning Research*, 22(3), 861–868.

Elliott, B.C., Wilson, G.J. and Kerr, G.K. (1989) A biomechanical analysis of the sticking region in the bench press. *Medicine and Science in Sports and Exercise*, 21(4), 450–462.

Enns, D.L. and Tiidus, P.M. (2010) The influence of estrogen on skeletal muscle. *Sports Medicine*, 40(1), 41–58.

Enoka, R.M. (1996) Eccentric contractions require unique activation strategies by the nervous system. *Journal of Applied Physiology*, 81(6), 2339–2346.

Evetovich, T.K., Conley, D.S. and McCawley, P.F. (2015) Postactivation potentiation enhances upper- and lower-body athletic performance in collegiate male and female athletes. *Journal of Strength and Conditioning Research*, 29(2), 336–342.

Faigenbaum, A.D., McFarland, J.E., Keiper, F.B., Tevlin, W., Ratamess, N.A., Kang, J. and Hoffman, J.R. (2007) Effects of a short-term plyometric and resistance training

program on fitness performance in boys age 12 to 15 years. *Journal of Sports Science and Medicine*, 6(4), 519–525.

Farley, C.T., Houdijk, H.H., Van Strien, C. and Louie, M. (1998) Mechanism of leg stiffness adjustment for hopping on surfaces of different stiffnesses. *Journal of Applied Physiology*, (1985), 85(3), 1044–1055.

Fleck, S.J. and Kraemer, W. (2014) *Designing Resistance Training Programs* (4th ed.): Human Kinetics.

Fletcher, I.M. and Hartwell, M. (2004) Effect of an 8-week combined weights and plyometrics training program on golf drive performance. *Journal of Strength and Conditioning Research*, 18(1), 59–62.

Fort-Vanmeerhaeghe, A., Gual, G., Romero-Rodriguez, D. and Unnitha, V. (2016) Lower Limb Neuromuscular Asymmetry in Volleyball and Basketball Players. *Journal of Human Kinetics*, 50(1), 135–143.

Franchi, M.V., Reeves, N.D. and Narici, M.V. (2017) Skeletal muscle remodeling in response to eccentric vs. concentric loading: morphological, molecular, and metabolic adaptations. *Frontiers in Physiology*, 8.

French, D. (2016) The endocrine responses to training. In: Jeffreys, I. and Moody, J. (eds.). *Strength and Conditioning for Sports Performance*, (pp.118–142). Routledge.

Fridén, C., Hirschberg, A.L. and Saartok, T. (2003) Muscle strength and endurance do not significantly vary across 3 phases of the menstrual cycle in moderately active premenopausal women. *Clinical Journal of Sport Medicine*, 13(4), 238–241.

Fry, A.C. (2004) The role of resistance exercise intensity on muscle fibre adaptations. *Sports Medicine*, 34(10), 663–679.

Fukunaga, T., Kubo, K., Kawakami, Y., Fukashiro, S., Kanehisa, H. and Maganaris, C.N. (2001). In vivo behaviour of human muscle tendon during walking. *Proceedings: Biological Sciences*, 268(1464), 229–233.

Gamble, P. (2006) Implications and applications of training specificity for coaches and athletes. *Strength and Conditioning Journal*, 28(3), 54.

González-Badillo, J.J. and Sánchez-Medina, L. (2010) Movement velocity as a measure of loading intensity in resistance training. *International Journal of Sports Medicine*, 31(05), 347–352.

Granados, C., Izquierdo, M., Ibáñez, J., Ruesta, M. and Gorostiaga, E.M. (2013) Are there any differences in physical fitness and throwing velocity between national and international elite female handball players? *The Journal of Strength and Conditioning Research*, 27(3), 723–732.

Gür, H. (1997) Concentric and eccentric isokinetic measurements in knee muscles during the menstrual cycle: a special reference to reciprocal moment ratios. *Archives of Physical Medicine and Rehabilitation*, 78(5), 501–505.

Haff, G.G., Stone, M.H., O'Bryant, H.S., Harman, E., Dinan, C.N., Johnson, R. and Han, K.H. (1997). Force-time dependent characteristics of dynamic and isometric muscle actions. *Journal of Strength and Conditioning Research*, 11(4), 269–272.

Haff, G.G., Whitley, A. and Potteiger, J.A. (2001) A Brief Review: Explosive Exercises and Sports Performance. *Strength and Conditioning Journal*, 23(3), 13.

Haff, G.G., Carlock, J.M., Hartman, M.J. and Kilgore, J.L. (2005) Force-time curve characteristics of dynamic and isometric muscle actions of elite women Olympic weightlifters. *Journal of Strength and Conditioning Research*, 19(4), 741.

Haff, G.G., Jackson, J.R., Kawamori, N., Carlock, J.M., Hartman, M.J., Kilgore, J.L. ... and Stone, M.H. (2008) Force-time curve characteristics and hormonal alterations during an eleven-week training period in elite women weightlifters. The *Journal of Strength and Conditioning Research*, 22(2), 433–446.

Haff, G.G. and Nimphius, S. (2012) Training principles for power. *Strength and Conditioning Journal*, 34(6), 2–12.

Haff, G.G., Ruben, R.P., Lider, J., Twine, C. and Cormie, P. (2015) A comparison of methods for determining the rate of force development during isometric midthigh clean pulls. *The Journal of Strength and Conditioning Research*, 29(2), 386–395.

Haff, G.G. (2016) The essentials of periodisation. In: Jeffreys, I., and Moody, J. (eds.) *Strength and Conditioning for Sports Performance*, (pp.404–448). Routledge.

Harper, D. (2011) *The 10 to 5 repeated jump test. A new test for evaluating reactive strength*. Paper presented at the British Association of Sports and Exercises Sciences Student Conference, Chester, UK.

Harris, G.R., Stone, M.H., O'Bryant, H.S., Proulx, C.M. and Johnson, R.L. (2000) Short-Term Performance Effects of High Power, High Force, or Combined Weight-Training Methods. *The Journal of Strength and Conditioning Research*, 14(1), 14–20.

Harris, N.K., Cronin, J., Taylor, K.L., Boris, J. and Sheppard, J. (2010) Understanding position transducer technology for strength and conditioning practitioners. *Strength and Conditioning Journal*, 32(4), 66–79.

Hatfield, D.L., Kraemer, W.J., Spiering, B.A. and Häkkinen, K. (2006) The impact of velocity of movement on performance factors in resistance exercise. *Journal of Strength and Conditioning Research*, 20(4), 760.

Hawley, J.A. (2009) Molecular responses to strength and endurance training: Are they incompatible? This paper article is one of a selection of papers published in this Special Issue, entitled 14th International Biochemistry of Exercise Conference – Muscles as Molecular and Metabolic Machines, and has undergone the Journal's usual peer review process. *Applied Physiology, Nutrition, and Metabolism*, 34(3), 355–361.

Healy, M.L., Gibney, J., Pentecost, C., Wheeler, M.J. and Sonksen, P.H. (2014) Endocrine profiles in 693 elite athletes in the post-competition setting. *Clinical Endocrinology*, 81(2), 294–305.

Hedrick, A. and Wada, H. (2008) Weightlifting movements: do the benefits outweigh the risks? *Strength and Conditioning Journal*, 30(6), 26–35.

Heiderscheit, B.C., McLean, K.P. and Davies, G.J. (1996) The effects of isokinetic vs. plyometric training on the shoulder internal rotators. *Journal of Orthopaedic and Sports Physical Therapy*, 23(2), 125–133.

Henneman, E., Somjen, G. and Carpenter, D.O. (1965a) Functional significance of cell size in spinal motoneurons. *Journal of Neurophysiology*, 28(3), 560–580.

Henneman, E., Somjen, G. and Carpenter, D.O. (1965b) Excitability and inhibitability of motoneurons of different sizes. *Journal of Neurophysiology*, 28(3), 599–620.

Herzog, W., Schappacher, G., DuVall, M., Leonard, T.R. and Herzog, J.A. (2016) Residual force enhancement following eccentric contractions: a new mechanism involving titin. *Physiology*, 31(4), 300–312.

Hewett, T.E., Myer, G.D., Ford, K.R., Heidt, R.S., Colosimo, A.J., McLean, S.G. ... Succop, P. (2005) Biomechanical measures of neuromuscular control and valgus loading of the knee predict anterior cruciate ligament injury risk in female athletes: a prospective study. *American Journal of Sports Medicine*, 33(4), 492–501.

Hewit, J.K., Cronin, J.B. and Hume, P.A. (2012a). Asymmetry in multi-directional jumping tasks. *Physical Therapy in Sport*, 13(4), 238–242.

Hewit, J., Cronin, J. and Hume, P. (2012b) Multidirectional leg asymmetry assessment in sport. *Strength and Conditioning Journal*, 34(1), 82–86.

Hill, A. (1938) The heat of shortening and the dynamic constants of muscle. Proceedings of the Royal Society of London. *Series B, Biological Sciences*, 126(843), 136–195.

Hirsch, K.R., Smith-Ryan, A.E., Trexler, E.T. and Roelofs, E.J. (2016) Body Composition and Muscle Characteristics of Division I Track and Field Athletes. *Journal of Strength and Conditioning Research/National Strength and Conditioning Association*, 30(5), 1231.

Hoffman, T., Stauffer, R.W. and Jackson, A.S. (1979) Sex difference in strength. *The American Journal of Sports Medicine*, 7(4), 265–267.

Holmberg, P.M. (2013) Weightlifting to improve volleyball performance. *Strength and Conditioning Journal*, 35(2), 79–88.

Hori, N., Newton, R.U., Nosaka, K. and Stone, M.H. (2005) Weightlifting exercises enhance athletic performance that requires high-load speed strength. *Strength and Conditioning Journal*, 24(4), 50.

Hortobagyi, T.I.B.O.R., Hill, J.P., Houmard, J.A., Fraser, D.D., Lambert, N.J. and Israel, R.G. (1996) Adaptive responses to muscle lengthening and shortening in humans. *Journal of Applied Physiology*, 80(3), 765–772.

Hubal, M.J., Gordish-Dressman, H.E.A.T.H.E.R., Thompson, P.D., Price, T.B., Hoffman, E.P., Angelopoulos, T.J. ... and Zoeller, R.F. (2005) Variability in muscle size and strength gain after unilateral resistance training. *Medicine and Science in Sports and Exercise*, 37(6), 964–972.

Hunter, G.R. (1985) Changes in body composition, body build and performance associated with different weight training frequencies in males and females. *Strength and Conditioning Journal*, 7(1), 26–28.

Hutton, R.S. and Atwater, S.W. (1992) Acute and chronic adaptations of muscle proprioceptors in response to increased use. *Sports Medicine*, 14(6), 406–421.

Ingen Schenau, G.V., Bobbert, M. and Haan, A.D. (1997) Mechanics and energetics of the stretch-shortening cycle: a stimulating discussion.

Ishikawa, M., Pakaslahti, J. and Komi, P.V. (2007) Medial gastrocnemius muscle behavior during human running and walking. *Gait Posture*, 25(3), 380–384.

James, L.P., Roberts, L.A., Haff, G.G., Kelly, V.G. and Beckman, E.M. (2017) Validity and Reliability of a Portable Isometric Mid-Thigh Clean Pull. *The Journal of Strength and Conditioning Research*, 31(5), 1378–1386.

Jami, L. (1992) Golgi tendon organs in mammalian skeletal muscle: functional properties and central actions. *Physiological Reviews*, 72(3), 623–666.

Jarvis, M.M., Graham-Smith, P. and Comfort, P. (2016) A Methodological Approach to Quantifying Plyometric Intensity. *Journal of Strength and Conditioning Research*, 30(9), 2522–2532.

Jensen, R.L. and Ebben, W.P. (2007)

Quantifying plyometric intensity via rate of force development, knee joint, and ground reaction forces. *Journal of Strength and Conditioning Research*, 21(3), 763–767.

Jidovtseff, B., Croisier, J.L., Lhermerout, C., Serre, L., Sac, D. and Crielaard, J.M. (2006) The concept of iso-inertial assessment: reproducibility analysis and descriptive data. *Isokinetics and Exercise Science,* 14(1), 53–62.

Jidovtseff, B., Harris, N.K., Crielaard, J.M. and Cronin, J.B. (2011) Using the load-velocity relationship for 1RM prediction. *The Journal of Strength and Conditioning Research*, 25(1), 267–270.

Jones, E.J., Bishop, P.A., Woods, A.K. and Green, J.M. (2008) Cross-sectional area and muscular strength. *Sports Medicine*, 38(12), 987–994.

Jonge, X.A.K., Boot, C.R.L., Thom, J.M., Ruell, P.A. and Thompson, M.W. (2001) The influence of menstrual cycle phase on skeletal muscle contractile characteristics in humans. *The Journal of Physiology*, 530(1), 161–166.

Jovanović, M. and Flanagan, E.P. (2014) Researched applications of velocity based strength training. *Journal of Australian Strength and Conditioning*, 22(2), 58–69.

Kawamori, N. and Haff, G.G. (2004). The optimal training load for the development of muscular power. *The Journal of Strength and Conditioning Research*, 18(3), 675–684.

Kawamori, N., Rossi, S.J., Justice, B.D. and Haff, E.E. (2006) Peak force and rate of force development during isometric and dynamic mid-thigh clean pulls performed at various intensities. *Journal of Strength and Conditioning Research,* 20(3), 483.

Keiner, M., Sander, A., Wirth, K., Caruso, O., Immesberger, P. and Zawieja, M. (2013) Strength performance in youth: trainability of adolescents and children in the back and front squats. *The Journal of Strength and Conditioning Research*, 27(2), 357–362.

Knapik, J.J., Bauman, C.L., Jones, B.H., Harris, J.M. and Vaughan, L. (1991) Preseason strength and flexibility imbalances associated with athletic injuries in female collegiate athletes. *The American Journal of*

Sports Medicine, 19(1), 76–81.

Komi, P.V. and Karlsson, J. (1978) Skeletal muscle fibre types, enzyme activities and physical performance in young males and females. *Acta Physiologica*, 103(2), 210–218.

Komi, P.V. (1992) Strength and Power in Sport: Blackwell Scientific Publications, Oxford.

Komi, P.V. and Gollhoffer, A. (1997) Stretch reflex can have an important role in force enhancement during SSC-exercise. *Journal of Applied Biomechanics*, 33, 1197–1206.

Komi, P.V. (1986). Training of muscle strength and power: interaction of neuromotoric, hypertrophic, and mechanical factors. *International Journal of Sports Medicine*, 7 Suppl 1, 10–15.

Kotzamanidis, C. (2006) Effect of plyometric t raining on running performance and vertical jumping in prepubertal boys. *Journal of Strength and Conditioning Research*, 20(2), 441–445.

Kraemer, W.J. and Ratamess, N.A. (2004) Fundamentals of resistance training: progression and exercise prescription. *Medicine and Science in Sports and Exercise*, 36(4), 674–688.

Kraemer, W.J. and Ratamess, N.A. (2005) Hormonal responses and adaptations to resistance exercise and training. *Sports Medicine*, 35(4), 339–361.

Krosshaug, T., Nakamae, A., Boden, B.P., Engebretsen, L., Smith, G., Slauterbeck, J.R. ... and Bahr, R. (2007) Mechanisms of anterior cruciate ligament injury in basketball. *The American Journal of Sports Medicine*, 35(3), 359–367.

Kubo, K., Kanehisa, H., Takeshita, D., Kawakami, Y., Fukashiro, S. and Fukunaga, T. (2000) In vivo dynamics of human medial gastrocnemius muscle-tendon complex during stretch-shortening cycle exercise. *Acta Physiologica Scandinavica*, 170(2), 127–135.

Kubo, K., Kawakami, Y. and Fukunaga, T. (1999) Influence of elastic properties of tendon structures on jump performance in humans. *Journal of Applied Physiology*, (1985), 87(6), 2090–2096.

Kubo, K., Yata, H., Kanehisa, H. and Fukunaga,

T. (2006) Effects of isometric squat training on the tendon stiffness and jump performance. *European Journal of Applied Physiology*, 96(3), 305–314.

Kubo, K., Morimoto, M., Komuro, T., Yata, H., Tsunoda, N., Kanehisa, H. and Fukunaga, T. (2007) Effects of plyometric and weight training on muscle-tendon complex and jump performance. *Medicine and Science in Sports and Exercise*, 39(10), 1801–1810.

Kuitunen, S., Komi, P.V. and Kyrolainen, H. (2002) Knee and ankle joint stiffness in sprint running. *Medicine and Science in Sports and Exercise*, 34(1), 166–173.

Kuriki, H.U., De Azevedo, F.M., Takahashi, L.S.O., Mello, E.M., de Faria Negrão Filho, R. and Alves, N. (2012) The relationship between electromyography and muscle force. In EMG Methods for evaluating muscle and nerve function. *InTech*.

Kyröläinen, H., Avela, J., McBride, J.M., Koskinen, S., Andersen, J.L., Sipilä, S., ... Komi, P.V. (2004) Effects of power training on mechanical efficiency in jumping. *European Journal of Applied Physiology*, 91(2–3), 155–159.

Kyröläinen, H., Avela, J., McBride, J.M., Koskinen, S., Andersen, J.L., Sipilä, S., ... Komi, P.V. (2005). Effects of power training on muscle structure and neuromuscular performance. Scandinavian *Journal of Medicine and Science in Sports*, 15(1), 58–64.

Lauersen, J.B., Bertelsen, D.M. and Andersen, L.B. (2014) The effectiveness of exercise interventions to prevent sports injuries: a systematic review and meta-analysis of randomised controlled trials. *British Journal of Sports Medicine*, 48(11), 871–877.

Lebrun, C.M., McKenzie, D.C., Prior, J.C. and Taunton, J.E. (1995) Effects of menstrual cycle phase on athletic performance. *Medicine and Science in Sports and Exercise*, 27(3), 437–444.

Leukel, C., Taube, W., Gruber, M., Hodapp, M. and Gollhofer, A. (2008) Influence of falling height on the excitability of the soleus H-reflex during drop-jumps. *Acta Physiologica* (Oxford), 192(4), 569–576.

Lichtwark, G.A. and Wilson, A.M. (2007) Is Achilles tendon compliance optimised for maximum muscle efficiency during locomotion? *Journal of Biomechanics*, 40(8), 1768–1775.

Linnamo, V., Pakarinen, A., Komi, P.V., Kraemer, W.J. and Häkkinen, K. (2005) Acute hormonal responses to submaximal and maximal heavy resistance and explosive exercises in men and women. *Journal of Strength and Conditioning Research*, 19(3), 566.

Lloyd, Oliver, J.L., Hughes, M.G. and Williams, C.A. (2009) Reliability and validity of field-based measures of leg stiffness and reactive strength index in youths. *Journal of Sports Science*, 27(14), 1565–1573.

Lloyd, R., Oliver, J., Hughes, M. and Williams, C. (2011) Specificity of test selection for the appropriate assessment of different measures of stretch-shortening cycle function in children. *Journal of Sports Medicine and Physical Fitness*, 51(4), 595–602.

Lloyd, R.S. and Faigenbaum, A.D. (2016) Age- and Sex-Related Differences and Their Implications for Resistance Exercise. In G.G. Haff and N.T. Triplett, (eds.), *Essentials of Strength Training and Conditioning*, (4th ed., pp.135–154). Leeds: Human Kinetics.

Lockie, R.G., Murphy, A.J. and Spinks, C.D. (2003) Effects of resisted sled towing on sprint kinematics in field-sport athletes. *The Journal of Strength and Conditioning Research*, 17(4), 760–767.

Loturco, I., Kobal, R., Moraes, J.E., Kitamura, K., Abad, C.C.C., Pereira, L.A. and Nakamura, F.Y. (2017) Predicting the Maximum Dynamic Strength in Bench Press: The High Precision of the Bar Velocity Approach. *The Journal of Strength and Conditioning Research*, 31(4), 1127–1131.

Lyttle, A.D., Wilson, G.J. and Ostrowski, K.J. (1996) Enhancing performance: Maximal power versus combined weights and plyometrics training. *Journal of Strength and Conditioning Research*, 10, 173–179.

MacDonald, C.J., Israetel, M.A., Dabbs, N.C., Chander, H., Allen, C.R., Lamont, H.S. and Garner, J.C. (2013) Influence of body composition on selected jump performance measures in collegiate female athletes. *Journal of Trainology*, 2(2), 33–37.

MacDougall, J.D., Tarnopolsky, M.A., Chesley, A. and Atkinson, S.A. (1992) Changes in muscle protein synthesis following heavy resistance exercise in humans: a pilot study. *Acta Physiologica*, 146(3), 403–404.

MacDougall, J.D., Gibala, M.J., Tarnopolsky, M.A., MacDonald, J.R., Interisano, S.A. and Yarasheski, K.E. (1995) The time course for elevated muscle protein synthesis following heavy resistance exercise. *Canadian Journal of Applied Physiology*, 20(4), 480–486.

Maffiuletti, N.A., Aagaard, P., Blazevich, A.J., Folland, J., Tillin, N. and Duchateau, J. (2016) Rate of force development: physiological and methodological considerations. *European Journal of Applied Physiology*, 116(6), 1091–1116.

Malisoux, L., Francaux, M., Nielens, H. and Theisen, D. (2006) Stretch-shortening cycle exercises: an effective training paradigm to enhance power output of human single muscle fibers. *Journal of Applied Physiology* (1985), 100(3), 771–779.

Maloney, S.J., Turner, A.N. and Fletcher, I.M. (2014) Ballistic exercise as a pre-activation stimulus: a review of the literature and practical applications. *Sports Medicine*, 44(10), 1347–1359.

Maly, T., Zahalka, F., Bonacin, D., Mala, L. and Bujnovsky, D. (2015) Muscular strength and strength asymmetries of high elite female soccer players. *Sport Science*, 8(Suppl 1), 7–14.

Markovic, G. and Mikulic, P. (2010) Neuro-musculoskeletal and performance adaptations to lower-extremity plyometric training. *Sports Medicine*, 40(10), 859–895.

Maughan, R.J., Watson, J.S. and Weir, J. (1983) Strength and cross–sectional area of human skeletal muscle. *The Journal of Physiology*, 338(1), 37–49.

Mayhew, J.L., Ball, T.E., Arnold, M.D. and Bowen, J.C. (1992) Relative Muscular Endurance Performance as a Predictor of Bench Press Strength in College Men and Women. *The Journal of Strength and Conditioning Research*, 6(4), 200–206.

McBride, J.M., Triplett-McBride, T., Davie, A. and Newton, R.U. (1999) A comparison of strength and power characteristics between power lifters, Olympic lifters, and sprinters. *The Journal of Strength and Conditioning Research*, 13(1), 58–66.

McBride, J.M., Triplett-McBride, T., Davie, A. and Newton, R.U. (2002) The effect of heavy-vs. light-load jump squats on the development of strength, power, and speed. *The Journal of Strength and Conditioning Research,* 16(1), 75–82.

McBride, J.M., McCaulley, G.O. and Cormie, P. (2008) Influence of preactivity and eccentric muscle activity on concentric performance during vertical jumping. *Journal of Strength and Conditioning Research*, 22(3), 750–757.

McClymont, D. (2003) *Use of the reactive strength index (RSI) as an indicator of plyometric training conditions*. Paper presented at the *Science and Football V: The proceedings of the fifth World Congress on Sports Science and Football*, Lisbon, Portugal.

McCurdy, K.W., Langford, G.A., Doscher, M.W., Wiley, L.P. and Mallard, K.G. (2005) The effects of short-term unilateral and bilateral lower-body resistance training on measures of strength and power. *Journal of Strength and Conditioning Research*, 19(1), 9.

McGuigan, M.R., Winchester, J.B. and Erickson, T. (2006) The importance of isometric maximum strength in college wrestlers. *Journal of Sports Science and Medicine*, 5(CSSI), 108.

Metzger, J.M. and Moss, R.L. (1990) Calcium-sensitive cross-bridge transitions in mammalian fast and slow skeletal muscle fibers. *Science*, 247(4946), 1088–1091.

Meylan, C. and Malatesta, D. (2009) Effects of in-season plyometric training within soccer practice on explosive actions of young players. *Journal of Strength and Conditioning Research*, 23(9), 2605–2613.

Mike, J., Kerksick, C.M. and Kravitz, L. (2015) How to incorporate eccentric training into a resistance training program. *Strength and*

Conditioning Journal, 37(1), 5–17.

Miller, A.E.J., MacDougall, J.D., Tarnopolsky, M.A. and Sale, D.G. (1993) Gender differences in strength and muscle fiber characteristics. European Journal of Applied Physiology and Occupational Physiology, 66(3), 254–262.

Mitchell, C.J., Churchward-Venne, T.A., Bellamy, L., Parise, G., Baker, S.K. and Phillips, S.M. (2013) Muscular and systemic correlates of resistance training-induced muscle hypertrophy. PloS One, 8(10), e78636.

Morán-Navarro, R., Martínez-Cava, A., Sánchez-Medina, L., Mora-Rodríguez, R., González-Badillo, J.J. and Pallarés, J.G. (2017) Movement velocity as a measure of level of effort during resistance exercise. The Journal of Strength and Conditioning Research.

Moritani, T., Oddsson, L. and Thorstensson, A. (1991). Activation patterns of the soleus and gastrocnemius muscles during different motor tasks. J Electromyogr Kinesiol, 1(2), 81–88.

Morrissey, M.C., Harman, E.A. and Johnson, M.J. (1995). Resistance training modes: Specificity and effectiveness. Medicine and Science in Sports and Exercise, 27(5), 648–660.

Murphy, A.J., Wilson, G.J. and Pryor, J.F. (1994) Use of the iso-inertial force mass relationship in the prediction of dynamic human performance. European Journal of Applied Physiology and Occupational Physiology, 69(3), 250–257.

Myer, G.D., Ford, K.R. and Hewett, T.E. (2005) The effects of gender on quadriceps muscle activation strategies during a maneuver that mimics a high ACL injury risk position. J Electromyogr Kinesiol, 15(2), 181–189.

Naisidou, S., Kepesidou, M., Kontostergiou, M. and Zapartidis, I. (2017) Differences of physical abilities between successful and less successful young female athletes. Journal of Physical Education and Sport, 17(1), 294.

Nardone, A., Romano, C. and Schieppati, M. (1989) Selective recruitment of high–threshold human motor units during voluntary isotonic lengthening of active muscles. The Journal of Physiology, 409(1), 451–471.

Newton, R.U. and Kraemer, W.J. (1994) Developing Explosive Muscular Power: Implications for a Mixed Methods Training Strategy. Strength and Conditioning Journal, 16(5), 20–31.

Newton, R.U., Rogers, R.A., Volek, J.S., Häkkinen, K. and Kraemer, W.J. (2006) Four weeks of optimal load ballistic resistance training at the end of season attenuates declining jump performance of women volleyball players. Journal of Strength and Conditioning Research, 20(4), 955.

Newton, R.U. (2011) Strength and conditioning biomechanics. In: Cardinale, M., Newton, R. and Nosaka, K. (eds.) Strength and conditioning: biological principles and practical applications (pp.89–101). John Wiley and Sons.

Nishikawa, K. (2016) Eccentric contraction: unraveling mechanisms of force enhancement and energy conservation. Journal of Experimental Biology, 219(2), 189–196.

Norrbrand, L., Fluckey, J.D., Pozzo, M. and Tesch, P.A. (2008) Resistance training using eccentric overload induces early adaptations in skeletal muscle size. European Journal of Applied Physiology, 102(3), 271–281.

Nunes, J.A., Crewther, B.T., Ugrinowitsch, C., Tricoli, V., Viveiros, L., de Rose Jr, D. and Aoki, M.S. (2011) Salivary hormone and immune responses to three resistance exercise schemes in elite female athletes. The Journal of Strength and Conditioning Research, 25(8), 2322–2327.

Paavolainen, L., Häkkinen, K., Hämäläinen, I., Nummela, A. and Rusko, H. (1999) Explosive-strength training improves 5-km running time by improving running economy and muscle power. Journal of Applied Physiology (1985), 86(5), 1527–1533.

Pallarés, J.G., López-Gullón, J.M., Torres-Bonete, M.D. and Izquierdo, M. (2012) Physical fitness factors to predict female

Olympic wrestling performance and sex differences. *The Journal of Strength and Conditioning Research*, 26(3), 794–803.

Pereira, M.I. and Gomes, P.S. (2003) Movement velocity in resistance training. *Sports Medicine*, 33(6), 427–438.

Peterson, M.D., Rhea, M.R. and Alvar, B.A. (2004) Maximizing strength development in athletes: a meta-analysis to determine the dose-response relationship. *The Journal of Strength and Conditioning Research*, 18(2), 377–382.

Peterson, M.D., Alvar, B.A. and Rhea, M.R. (2006) The contribution of maximal force production to explosive movement among young collegiate athletes. *The Journal of Strength and Conditioning Research*, 20(4), 867.

Phillips, S.M., Tipton, K.D., Aarsland, A., Wolf, S.E. and Wolfe, R.R. (1997) Mixed muscle protein synthesis and breakdown after resistance exercise in humans. *American Journal of Physiology-Endocrinology and Metabolism*, 273(1), E99–E107.

Phillips, S.M. (2000) Short-term training: when do repeated bouts of resistance exercise become training? *Canadian Journal of Applied Physiology*, 25(3), 185–193.

Picerno, P., Iannetta, D., Comotto, S., Donati, M., Pecoraro, F., Zok, M. ... and Patrizio, F. (2016) 1-RM prediction: a novel methodology based on the force–velocity and load–velocity relationships. *European Journal of Applied Physiology*, 116(10), 2035–2043.

Platzer, H.P., Raschner, C., Patterson, C. and Lembert, S. (2009) Comparison of physical characteristics and performance among elite snowboarders. *The Journal of Strength and Conditioning Research*, 23(5), 1427–1432.

Prince, F.P., Hikida, R.S. and Hagerman, F.C. (1976) Human muscle fiber types in power lifters, distance runners and untrained subjects. *Pflügers Archiv*, 363(1), 19–26.

Radaelli, R., Bottaro, M., Wagner, D.R., Wilhelm, E.N., Pompermayer, M.G. and Pinto, R.S. (2014) Men and women experience similar muscle damage after traditional resistance training protocol. *Isokinetics and Exercise Science*, 22(1), 47–54.

Radcliffe, J. and Farentinos, R. (2015) High Powered Plyometrics (2nd ed.): Human Kinetics.

Rainoldi, A. and Gazzoni, M. (2011). Neuromuscular physiology. In: Cardinale, M., Newton, R. and Nosaka, K. (eds.) *Strength and conditioning: Biological principles and practical applications* (pp.17–27). John Wiley and Sons.

Reilly, T., Morris, T. and Whyte, G. (2009) The specificity of training prescription and physiological assessment: A review. *Journal of Sports Sciences*, 27(6), 575–589.

Reynolds, J.M., Gordon, T.J. and Roberts, R.A. (2006) Prediction of one repetition maximum strength from multiple repetition maximum testing and anthropometry. *Journal of Strength and Conditioning Research*, 20(3), 584.

Ribeiro, A.S., Schoenfeld, B.J., Fleck, S.J., Pina, F.L., Nascimento, M.A. and Cyrino, E.S. (2017) Effects of traditional and pyramidal resistance training systems on muscular strength, muscle mass, and hormonal responses in older women: a randomized crossover trial. *The Journal of Strength and Conditioning Research,* 31(7), 1888–1896.

Rozzi, S.L., Lephart, S.M., Gear, W.S. and Fu, F.H. (1999) Knee joint laxity and neuromuscular characteristics of male and female soccer and basketball players. *American Journal of Sports Medicine,* 27(3), 312–319.

Ryan, E.D., Herda, T.J., Costa, P.B., Defreitas, J.M., Beck, T.W., Stout, J.R. and Cramer, J.T. (2009) Passive properties of the muscle-tendon unit: the influence of muscle cross-sectional area. *Muscle Nerve*, 39(2), 227–229.

Sale, D.G. (1988) Neural adaptation to resistance training. *Medicine and Science in Sports and Exercise*, 20(5 Suppl), S135–45.

Sanchez-Medina, L. and González-Badillo, J.J. (2011) Velocity loss as an indicator of neuromuscular fatigue during resistance training. *Medicine and Science in Sports and Exercise*, 43(9), 1725–1734.

Sánchez-Medina, L., Gonzalez-Badillo, J.J., Perez, C.E. and Pallarés, J.G. (2014) Velocity-and power-load relationships of the bench pull vs. bench press exercises. *International Journal of Sports Medicine*, 35(03), 209–216.

Sands, W.A. (2000) Injury prevention in women's gymnastics. *Sports Medicine*, 30(5), 359–373.

Sapega, A.A. and Drillings, G. (1983) The definition and assessment of muscular power. *Journal of Orthopaedic and Sports Physical Therapy*, 5(1), 7–9.

Saunders, P.U., Telford, R.D., Pyne, D.B., Peltola, E.M., Cunningham, R.B., Gore, C.J. and Hawley, J.A. (2006) Short-term plyometric training improves running economy in highly trained middle and long distance runners. *Journal of Strength and Conditioning Research*, 20(4), 947–954.

Schmidtbleicher, D. (1992) Training for power events. In P. Komi (Ed.), *Strength and Power in Sport* (Vol. 1, pp.381–395) Oxford, England: Blackwell Scientific Publications.

Schulte-Edelmann, J.A., Davies, G.J., Kernozek, T.W. and Gerberding, E.D. (2005) The effects of plyometric training of the posterior shoulder and elbow. *Journal of Strength and Conditioning Research*, 19(1), 129–134.

Schoenfeld, B.J. (2010) The mechanisms of muscle hypertrophy and their application to resistance training. *The Journal of Strength and Conditioning Research*, 24(10), 2857–2872.

Schoenfeld, B.J., Ogborn, D., Vigotsky, A.D., Franchi, M. and Krieger, J.W. (2017) Hypertrophic effects of concentric versus eccentric muscle actions: A systematic review and meta-analysis. *The Journal of Strength and Conditioning Research*.

Secomb, J.L., Farley, O.R., Lundgren, L., Tran, T.T., King, A., Nimphius, S. and Sheppard, J.M. (2015) Associations between the performance of scoring manoeuvres and lower-body strength and power in elite surfers. *International Journal of Sports Science and Coaching*, 10(5), 911–918.

Seitz, L.B. and Haff, G.G. (2016) Factors modulating post-activation potentiation of jump, sprint, throw, and upper-body ballistic performances: A systematic review with meta-analysis. *Sports Medicine*, 46(2), 231–240.

Seynnes, O.R., de Boer, M. and Narici, M.V. (2007) Early skeletal muscle hypertrophy and architectural changes in response to high-intensity resistance training. *Journal of Applied Physiology*, 102(1), 368–373.

Sheppard, J.M. and Triplett, N.T. (2016) Program design for resistance training. In: Haff, G.G. and Triplett, N.T. (eds.) (2016) *Essentials of Strength Training and Conditioning*, 4th ed., Human Kinetics, pp. 439–470.

Shepstone, T.N., Tang, J.E., Dallaire, S., Schuenke, M.D., Staron, R.S. and Phillips, S.M. (2005) Short-term high-vs. low-velocity isokinetic lengthening training results in greater hypertrophy of the elbow flexors in young men. *Journal of Applied Physiology*, 98(5), 1768–1776.

Siff, M.C. (2003) *Supertraining*: Supertraining Institute.

Solomonow, M. and Krogsgaard, M. (2001) Sensorimotor control of knee stability. A review. *Scandinavian Journal of Medicine and Science in Sports*, 11(2), 64–80.

Souza, A.L., Shimada, S.D. and Koontz, A. (2002) Ground reaction forces during the power clean. *The Journal of Strength and Conditioning Research*, 16(3), 423–427.

Speirs, D.E., Bennett, M.A., Finn, C.V. and Turner, A.P. (2016) Unilateral vs. Bilateral Squat Training for Strength, Sprints, and Agility in Academy Rugby Players. *The Journal of Strength and Conditioning Research*, 30(2), 386–392.

Spurrs, R.W., Murphy, A.J. and Watsford, M.L. (2003) The effect of plyometric training on distance running performance. *European Journal of Applied Physiology*, 89(1), 1–7.

Staron, R.S., Karapondo, D.L., Kraemer, W.J., Fry, A.C., Gordon, S.E., Falkel, J.E. ... and Hikida, R.S. (1994) Skeletal muscle adaptations during early phase of heavy-resistance training in men and women. *Journal of Applied Physiology*, 76(3), 1247–1255.

Stone, M.H., O'Bryant, H., Garhammer, J.,

McMillan, J. and Rozenek, R. (1982) A Theoretical Model of Strength Training. *Strength and Conditioning Journal*, 4(4), 36–39.

Stone, M.H., Moir, G., Glaister, M. and Sanders, R. (2002) How much strength is necessary? *Physical Therapy in Sport*, 3(2), 88–96.

Stone, M.H., Sanborn, K.I.M., O'Bryant, H.S., Hartman, M., Stone, M.E., Proulx, C. ... and Hruby, J. (2003) Maximum strength-power-performance relationships in collegiate throwers. *The Journal of Strength and Conditioning Research*, 17(4), 739–745.

Stone, M.H., Sands, W.A., Carlock, J.O.N., Callan, S.A.M., Dickie, D.E.S., Daigle, K. ... and Hartman, M. (2004) The importance of isometric maximum strength and peak rate-of-force development in sprint cycling. *The Journal of Strength and Conditioning Research*, 18(4), 878–884.

Stone, M.H., Pierce, K.C., Sands, W.A. and Stone, M.E. (2006a) Weightlifting: A brief overview. *Strength and Conditioning Journal*, 28(1), 50.

Stone, M.H., Sands, W.A. and Stone, M.E. (2006b) Weightlifting: program design. *Strength and Conditioning Journal*, 28(2), 10.

Stone, M.H., Stone, M. and Sands, W.A. (2007) *Principles and practice of resistance training*. Human Kinetics.

Stone, M.H., Cormie, P. and Stone, M. (2016) Developing strength and power. In: Jeffreys, I., and Moody, J. (eds.) *Strength and Conditioning for Sports Performance* (pp.230–260). Routledge.

Suchomel, T.J., Comfort, P. and Stone, M.H. (2015) Weightlifting pulling derivatives: Rationale for implementation and application. *Sports Medicine*, 45(6), 823–839.

Suchomel, T.J., Nimphius, S. and Stone, M.H. (2016) The importance of muscular strength in athletic performance. *Sports Medicine*, 46(10), 1419–1449.

Suchomel, T.J., Comfort, P. and Lake, J.P. (2017) Enhancing the Force–Velocity Profile of Athletes Using Weightlifting Derivatives. *Strength and Conditioning Journal*, 39(1), 10–20.

Sugimoto, D., Myer, G.D., Foss, K.D. and Hewett, T.E. (2015) Specific exercise effects of preventive neuromuscular training intervention on anterior cruciate ligament injury risk reduction in young females: meta-analysis and subgroup analysis. *British Journal of Sports Medicine*, 49(5), 282–289.

Swanik, K.A., Lephart, S.M., Swanik, C.B., Lephart, S.P., Stone, D.A. and Fu, F.H. (2002) The effects of shoulder plyometric training on proprioception and selected muscle performance characteristics. *Journal of Shoulder and Elbow Surgery*, 11(6), 579–586.

Terzis, G., Stratakos, G., Manta, P. and Georgiadis, G. (2008) Throwing performance after resistance training and detraining. *The Journal of Strength and Conditioning Research*, 22(4), 1198–1204.

Thomas, C., Comfort, P., Chiang, C.Y. and Jones, P.A. (2015) Relationship between isometric mid-thigh pull variables and sprint and change of direction performance in collegiate athletes. *Journal of Trainology*, 4(1), 6–10.

Tillin, N.A. and Bishop, D. (2009) Factors modulating post-activation potentiation and its effect on performance of subsequent explosive activities. *Sports Medicine*, 39(2), 147–166.

Trzaskoma, Z. and Trzaskoma, L. (2006) Structure of maximal muscle strength of lower extremities in highly experienced athletes. *Wychowanie Fizyczne I Sport*, 50(3), 169.

Turner, A. (2009) Training for power: principles and practice. *Professional Strength and Conditioning*, 14, 20–32.

Turner, A. and Jeffreys, I. (2010) The Stretch-Shortening Cycle: Proposed Mechanisms and Methods for Enhancement. *Strength and Conditioning Journal*, 32(4), 87–99.

Turner, A.M., Owings, M. and Schwane, J.A. (2003) Improvement in running economy after 6 weeks of plyometric training. *Journal of Strength and Conditioning Research*, 17(1), 60–67.

Vingren, J.L., Kraemer, W.J., Ratamess, N.A.,

Anderson, J.M., Volek, J.S. and Maresh, C.M. (2010) Testosterone physiology in resistance exercise and training. *Sports Medicine,* 40(12), 1037–1053.

Vissing, K., Brink, M., Lønbro, S., Sørensen, H., Overgaard, K., Danborg, K. … and Andersen, J.L. (2008) Muscle adaptations to plyometric vs. resistance training in untrained young men. *The Journal of Strength and Conditioning Research*, 22(6), 1799–1810.

Wang, R., Hoffman, J.R., Tanigawa, S., Miramonti, A.A., La Monica, M.B., Beyer, K.S. … and Stout, J.R. (2016) Isometric Mid-Thigh Pull Correlates With Strength, Sprint, and Agility Performance in Collegiate Rugby Union Players. *The Journal of Strength and Conditioning Research*, 30(11), 3051–3056.

Weiss, L.W., Cureton, K.J. and Thompson, F.N. (1983) Comparison of serum testosterone and androstenedione responses to weight lifting in men and women. E*uropean Journal of Applied Physiology and Occupational Physiology*, 50(3), 413–419.

Wernbom, M., Augustsson, J. and Thomeé, R. (2007) The influence of frequency, intensity, volume and mode of strength training on whole muscle cross-sectional area in humans. *Sports Medicine,* 37(3), 225–264.

West, D.J., Owen, N.J., Jones, M.R., Bracken, R.M., Cook, C.J., Cunningham, D.J. … and Kilduff, L.P. (2011) Relationships between force–time characteristics of the isometric midthigh pull and dynamic performance in professional rugby league players. *The Journal of Strength and Conditioning Research*, 25(11), 3070–3075.

Wilson, G.J., Murphy, A.J. and Giorgi, A. (1996) Weight and plyometric training: effects on eccentric and concentric force production. *Canadian Journal of Applied Physiology*, 21(4), 301–315.

Wilson, G.J., Murphy, A.J. and Pryor, J.F. (1994) Musculotendinous stiffness: its relationship to eccentric, isometric, and concentric performance. *Journal of Applied Physiology (1985)*, 76(6), 2714–2719.

Wilson, J.M. and Flanagan, E.P. (2008) The role of elastic energy in activities with high force and power requirements: a brief review. *Journal of Strength and Conditioning Research*, 22(5), 1705–1715.

Wilson, J.M., Duncan, N.M., Marin, P.J., Brown, L.E., Loenneke, J.P., Wilson, S.M. … and Ugrinowitsch, C. (2013) Meta-analysis of postactivation potentiation and power: effects of conditioning activity, volume, gender, rest periods, and training status. *The Journal of Strength and Conditioning Research*, 27(3), 854–859.

Winter, E.M. and Brookes, F.B. (1991) Electromechanical response times and muscle elasticity in men and women. *European Journal of Applied Physiology and Occupational Physiology*, 63(2), 124–128.

Young, W. (1995) Laboratory strength assessment of athletes. *New Studies in Athletics*, 10, 89–89.

Zatsiorsky, V.M. and Kraemer, W.J. (1995) *Science and Practice of Strength Training*: Human Kinetics, Champaign.

Zatsiorsky, V.M. and Kraemer, W.J. (2006) *Science and Practice of Strength Training*: Human Kinetics, Champaign.

Zebis, M.K. Andersen, L.L., Ellingsgaard, H. and Aagaard, P. (2011) Rapid hamstring/quadriceps force capacity in male vs. female elite soccer players. *The Journal of Strength and Conditioning Research,* 25(7), 1989–1993.

Zehr, E.P. and Sale, D.G. (1994) Ballistic movement: muscle activation and neuromuscular adaptation. *Canadian Journal of Applied Physiology*, 19(4), 363–378.

CHAPTER 3
SPEED AND AGILITY DEVELOPMENT FOR FEMALE ATHLETES

Keith Barker MSc, ASCC

The abilities to run at high velocity and/or accelerate, decelerate and change direction effectively are key performance determinants in many sports, so are precious commodities in female athletes. In most sports, the athletes who demonstrate greatest speed or agility tend to dominate their opponents. Although genetics clearly play a major role in an athlete's potential to run and move quickly, there are several trainable elements that can positively impact upon speed and agility performance. The role of strength and conditioning interventions in this area should normally focus upon the development of relevant physical qualities alongside improving fundamental movement mechanics that can then be applied in sport-specific contexts, rather than attempting to copy and overload specific actions from the sport. These outcomes are best achieved through a combination of training modalities and stimuli whether they are undertaken on the track, field, court or in the gym.

Linear sprinting may be considered in two distinct phases of acceleration and maximal velocity running, with a gradual transition between the two being optimal for performance. Starting from a variety of different positions, stopping and changing direction activities within sports require different skills, techniques and physical attributes than linear running. 'Agility' as defined by Sheppard and Young (2006) refers to 'a rapid whole-body movement with change of velocity or direction in response to a stimulus.' Agility therefore requires the effective response to a stimulus that may be very specific to the sport, is extremely context-specific and highly variable. Without an intimate knowledge of the sport that an athlete is preparing for, it is likely that 'sport-specific' strength and conditioning exercises will not accurately recreate sports scenarios and may actually result in a negative transfer into sports performance. For female athletes it is essential that any multi-directional running activities are strategically prescribed considering the whole training process and the strength and stability qualities of the athlete in order to moderate injury risk and maximize positive adaptation.

For athletes who are required to perform maximal velocity sprinting within their sport, then high-speed running activities should form a significant portion of the training programme. The initial priority of strength and conditioning activities related to speed and/or agility performance must be the development and subsequent maintenance of underpinning strength qualities along with excellent movement mechanics and technical performance. For female athletes undertaking multi-directional running there should be a focus upon eccentric strength, mechanical proficiency, dynamic stabilization and knee alignment throughout high-intensity movements.

There is a wide range of popular methods employed by athletes aiming to improve their speed or agility. This chapter will outline underpinning physiological and mechanical considerations for female athletes undertaking speed or agility training, before providing a framework that may be effectively employed in order to improve speed or agility performance, with example interventions to illustrate how principles may be effectively applied in specific contexts.

PHYSIOLOGICAL AND MECHANICAL OVERVIEW

The energy requirements of brief maximal intensity movements exceed the capabilities of the oxidative system, which is the body's normal method for providing energy. The majority of energy production for maximal speed-agility tasks is initially provided by stores of intra-muscular adenosine triphosphate (ATP) lasting for approximately 2 seconds and the resynthesis of ATP from creatine phosphate (CP) until its depletion from the muscle in approximately 4–6 seconds. In total the anaerobic ATP-CP energy pathway can fuel up to approximately 8 seconds of maximal activity, although this does vary between individuals. When training to improve speed or agility performance it is therefore essential that the ATP-CP pathway is appropriately challenged in order to develop the energy production capability of this pathway.

Through the application of a relevant training stimulus, female athletes can improve the production and utilization of the energy provided by the ATP-CP pathway, in turn improving explosive speed and/or agility. Even well-trained elite athletes who perform maximal sprint efforts require a significant recovery period before their ATP is replenished and they can perform near the level of their previous effort.

Training the ATP-CP system requires very brief periods (10 seconds or less) of very high-intensity effort with plenty of rest (normally 2 minutes or more) between repetitions. Heavy

strength training, explosive medicine ball throws, jumps, short sprints and change of direction or agility drills can all be utilized to challenge this energy system. This chapter is concerned mainly with the running-based modalities of sprinting, change of direction and agility exercises.

Pure sprint athletes rely almost exclusively on the ATP-CP system for the energy production required by their events. Athletes competing in field and court sports such as netball, soccer, tennis and hockey also rely heavily on the ATP-CP system during the explosive maximal efforts in their sports, with the aerobic system facilitating recovery between these explosive activity events. The duration (along with exercise mode and intensity) of recovery between high-intensity efforts is a significant consideration when planning the training of speed or agility performance. Traditional advice regarding recovery between maximal sprint efforts indicates a work:rest ratio of at least 1:12 or 1 minute of recovery time for each 10 metres of maximal sprint running (Francis, C., 1997). The key for each individual athlete is that they are sufficiently recovered prior to each sprint repetition so that intensity and quality remain consistently high.

Greater neuromuscular efficiency can enable improvements in speed-agility performance. In this context, the term 'neuromuscular efficiency' refers to the interaction of the nervous system and muscle firing to produce force. The more efficient the connection, the more force can be rapidly applied in running and change of direction activities. If training is to enhance this connection, the intensity of exercise bouts must be at least near maximal (Ross et al., 2001) with adequate opportunity to recover prior to any further sprint efforts. Within session and more chronic fatigue must therefore be accounted for within prescription, as a tired athlete is unable to achieve the necessary levels of near-maximal intensity running.

Speed and agility training should employ an optimal number of maximal explosive, fast repetitions performed with maximal intent, in sufficient volume and frequency. The 'optimal' training dose will be determined by the individual athlete's characteristics and their response to the stimulus applied. Regular speed training whilst in a fatigued state cannot be effective in the improvement of maximal speed performance as the necessary intensity of stimulus is not attainable in a significantly fatigued state.

The magnitude and direction of the force that an athlete can apply within the time available at ground contact in activities such as running and jumping, is known as impulse (Hunter, Marshall and McNair, 2005). In maximal velocity linear sprinting, ground contact time may be around 0.1 seconds, with slightly longer durations of ground contact (circa 0.15–0.25 seconds) in the early acceleration phase. In deceleration or complex multi-directional tasks, the ground contact time and associated opportunity to apply force is significantly extended and is dependent upon the task and context. Effective agility performance may therefore require both short and long stretch-shortening cycles (SSC and LSSC) demanding either plyometric stiffness or eccentric or concentric muscular force production respectively. Both short and long SSC movements are underpinned heavily by strength characteristics and the development of high levels of strength in relation to the athlete's body mass needs to be a training focus to support high levels of speed and agility in both SSSC and LSSC actions. As force production relative to body mass is a key balance in speed-agility tasks, optimizing athletic body composition and minimizing fat mass can have a positive impact on performance for some female athletes. Nutritional and exercise interventions designed to achieve a modification in body composition should be carefully planned so that the athlete's force production capabilities and running intensities are not compromised in the pursuit of body fat reduction.

Even though in many sports, athletes only rarely have the opportunity to reach peak velocity, there is still great value in an athlete improving their maximum sprinting speed. These infrequent, maximal velocity sprints often occur in events of great significance upon the outcome of the competition, for example sprinting to defend a breakaway attack in hockey. Improved maximal sprinting speed may also have a positive impact upon an athlete's ability to repeat the frequent sub-maximal running efforts required in field-based sports as a sprint of any given velocity becomes easier for the athlete as it is now a lower percentage of a maximum effort than prior to the training intervention.

ASSESSMENT AND MONITORING OF THE SPEED OR AGILITY TRAINING INTERVENTION

With any training intervention, it is essential to have a clear picture of the athlete's current physical state in relation to the intended training outcome. Initial assessments can inform the priority objective(s) and prescription of the programme. Within the programme, frequent assessments integrated into the training schedule can effectively eliminate the practice effect associated with athletes undertaking novel assessments and provide a valid characterization of changes in an athlete's physical qualities.

Field-based measures of speed or agility performance may provide an indication of whether the overall objective of improving sport-specific running or movement capabilities has been achieved. Underpinning the final outcome of improved speed, more isolated measures of relevant physical qualities that have greater reliability and sensitivity provide more precise monitoring of adaptations to the training stimulus being applied. A combined approach of monitoring speed-agility performance within the final task, alongside more isolated measures of physical qualities enables a comprehensive assessment of the athlete's response to the programme.

A standardized drop jump protocol (typically 30cm) with either force plate, switch mat or Optojump analysis of ground contact time and flight time, can provide a measure of reactive strength index (RSI) that is related to the vertical stiffness required during the rapid ground contacts of peak velocity sprinting. An athlete's RSI may show acute variance based upon factors such as fatigue levels or the effectiveness of the preceding warm-up. Impulse for a defined time period (typically 200ms) from either isometric squat, isometric mid-thigh pull or countermovement jump using a force plate, produce a strength measure associated with the ability to effectively apply force during the acceleration phase of running. Measurement of countermovement jump height either simply using a wall-mounted tape measure or other device may also be utilized to monitor characteristics relevant to acceleration, as can barbell velocity in movements such as the clean or barbell counter movement jump. Drop landings onto a force plate may be used

Speed Quality	Physical Ability	Example Assessments
Acceleration	ATP-PC system output, Max Strength, Rate of concentric force production, Acceleration technique.	5m, 10m, 20m, 30m times from stationary start, Counter Movement Jump, Isometric Squat, Isometric Pull from mid-thigh.
Peak Velocity	Peak sprint velocity, vertical ground reaction forces, reduced ground contact time.	GPS competition data, flying 30 metres with 20m-30m prior acceleration, 'Optojump' ground contact time whilst sprinting, Drop Jump Reactive Strength Index.
Deceleration	Application of braking forces (eccentric strength).	Bilateral and unilateral altitude landings onto force plate to assess rate and magnitude of force production.
Change of Direction	Multi-directional manipulation of momentum.	Sport-specific CoD or agility assessments supported by simple video analysis of posture, foot strike, joint angles, centre of mass vs base of support against technical models and/or mechanical principles.

Table 3.1 Outline of possible speed-agility assessments.

to provide information relating to the eccentric strength and braking forces required in the performance of decelerations in sport.

The assessment of linear sprinting speed by timing (preferably using timing gates) the athlete over an appropriate distance including split times at relevant points provides a measure of velocity. Either accelerations from a static start or flying sprints with a rolling start of at least 20 metres using timing gates can measure the athlete's ability to accelerate or reach their peak velocity respectively. GPS data either from an assessment event or competition performance can also be used to quantify an athlete's linear sprinting velocity. Athletes with access to systems such as Optojump can also gather supplementary data regarding ground contact times or time to a pre-determined number of steps.

Table 3.1 provides a brief outline of assessment protocol that may provide valuable information regarding an athlete's physical qualities in relation to speed-agility and monitor adaptations to a training intervention.

There are several traditionally accepted time-based assessment protocols for change of direction ability that are readily available for coaches and athletes to access and apply, for example T-Test, 505, Illinois agility and L-Run. For athletes training to improve specific speed-agility capabilities in order to perform better in their sport, these well-established protocols may not be relevant, as the movement patterns and key qualities required for successful test performance may be different to those being targeted by training or required in the sport. An example of this is the 505 test, which is often used to assess 'agility' when in fact it is a self-paced sprint drill that is more closely related to peak linear sprint velocity than agility (Nimphius et al., 2016). For female athletes competing in sports requiring effective agility performance, it is best practice to develop bespoke protocols that accurately assess characteristics that are important in

their sport. Sport-specific assessment examples from squash and badminton are outlined below:

SQUASH: As shown in Fig. 3.1, the 'Squash-Specific Change of Direction Speed Test' developed by Wilkinson et al. (2009) requires squash athletes to complete a multi-directional course including six lunges to touch the top of small cones. Developed from match-play time-motion data, this test includes very specific movements from the sport and is well correlated with performance level in the sport (Wilkinson et al., 2012). This is an effective example of sport-specific change of direction assessment utilizing pre-planned movements.

Participants are required to move between and around the large cones (denoted by crosses) to reach out and touch the smaller cones (denoted by circles) with either hand, depending on their preference.

BADMINTON: The 'Badcamp' test developed by Loureiro and Barbosa de Freitas (2016) is a badminton-specific agility test designed to assess reactive agility relevant to the sport. The participant begins in the middle of six towers that will act as targets. An LED panel with six arrows corresponding to the targets on the outside of the area indicates the direction the athlete should run. The six arrows light in a random order as the athlete undertakes the test. The athlete touches a switch in the centre of the area to start the test and in between touching each of six targets. This enables split timing for each of the six movements. Although the LED panel utilized does not provide a stimulus similar to that experienced during badminton match-play, the 'Badcamp' test is an excellent example of how a sport-specific assessment of reactive agility rather than pre-planned movements may be developed.

An alternative approach to the assessment of linear running, change of direction or agility performance is to focus upon the technical

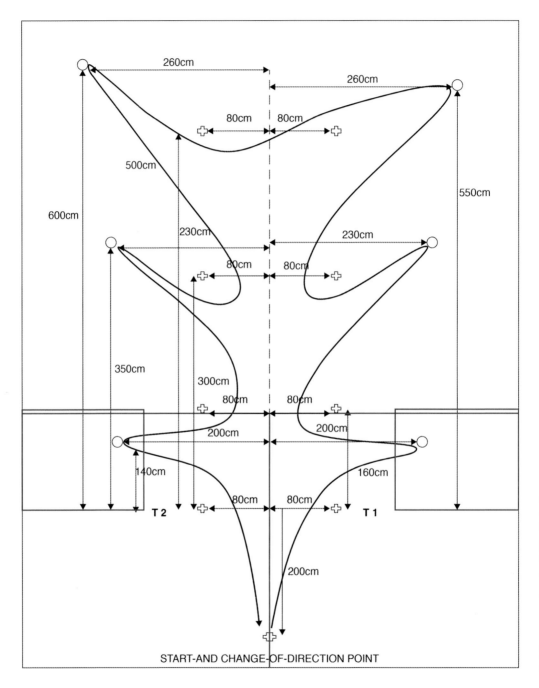

Fig. 3.1 Outline of the set-up for the 'Squash-Specific Test of Change-of-Direction Speed'.
(Wilkinson *et al.*, 2009)

performance of designated speed or agility tasks. The application of a technical model or framework based around key reference points such as joint angles, shin and trunk angles, posture and foot placement may be applied to simple observational or video analysis and coaching. The basis of this approach is that improved technical performance coupled with the development of physical qualities will enable the athlete to maximize improvements in performance.

Screening: Static or isolated movement screening such as the functional movement screen (FMS) (Cook, Burton and Hoogenboom, 2006) is straightforward to administer and may be useful in identifying restrictions in range of movement or stability, but offer little in terms of assessing the athlete's ability to safely and effectively perform speed or agility tasks. Those athletes and coaches with access to force plate analysis may effectively utilize a drop jump protocol to assess reactive strength characteristics. For those without this technology, simple video analysis of jumping and landing, deceleration and standardized change of direction tasks may provide extremely valuable information regarding the athlete's current capabilities, injury risk and movement mechanics. Rehabilitation-based assessments of unilateral dynamic stabilization such as the 'hop and stop' test developed by Juris et al. (2007) can be extremely valuable for both initial needs analysis and the ongoing monitoring of the athlete's movement control and dynamic stabilization throughout the programme. Protocol such as those validated by Imwalle et al. (2009) where the athlete jumps across a line before performing a reactive 45-degree or 90-degree sidestep cutting movement may be used for the initial assessment of generic reactive agility.

PLYOMETRICS, RESISTANCE TRAINING FOR SPEED-AGILITY PERFORMANCE

For many female athletes, improving force production capabilities, the rate of force development in key movements, or more specifically the application of impulse within the time available in ground contacts will improve their ability to manipulate momentum and apply and resist change of direction forces, having a significant impact upon speed, change of direction or agility performance.

Any strength-training programme with the objective of enabling improvement in the athlete's speed performance should predominantly utilize complex, multi-joint/whole body exercises requiring rapid and/or maximal force production from the large muscle groups, for example Olympic weightlifting, squats and lunges. Maximum voluntary effort (intent) to develop force as rapidly as possible is key to improving rate of force development (Young and Bilby, 1993). More isolated strengthening of the gluteal, hamstring and calf complexes may well also support improved speed-agility performance (Seitz et al., 2014).

As detailed in the preceding chapter, plyometric exercises, explosive jumps and medicine ball throws may be effectively utilized to address the explosive strength deficit that may be evident in some female athletes involved in speed-agility activities. Plyometric exercises in particular can be effective in the development of the athlete's ability to create stiffness around the ankle and throughout the whole system. Given that all strength and power training is relatively general and is not specific to running and change of direction activities, these training modalities should supplement the sport-specific elements of the training programme rather than replacing them, in other words if

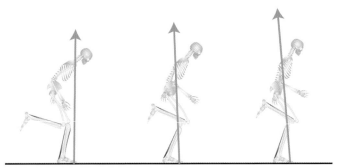

Fig. 3.2 Representation of sprint mechanics in the maximal velocity and acceleration phases of sprinting (Lai *et al.*, 2016).

the goal is to run faster then the training programme should include a significant amount of high-speed running.

DEVELOPING SPRINTING TECHNIQUE

Effective sprinting performance requires the skilful coordination of complex movements involving high forces at high speed. If the training objective is to enable the athlete to run faster, then high speed running with associated supplementary exercises and low-level plyometrics should normally form a significant proportion of the training schedule. Although running is commonly considered a natural action for athletes, many exhibit significant technical errors that limit their sprinting performance. Many female athletes can make initial gains in linear running speed within the first few sessions of a speed-training programme, simply by improving technical proficiency in running technique. It is therefore logical that this set of skills should be practiced and refined within a speed-training programme.

For most athletes who do not specialize in track sprinting, the application of two straightforward technical models provides plenty of opportunity for the improvement of running technique and performance. In sprinting the initial six to eight steps of the acceleration phase (often called 'drive phase') have clear technical markers. As indicated in Fig. 3.2, the athlete should then gradually transition (approximately steps eight to twenty) to maximal velocity sprinting that requires a different set of mechanics.

TECHNICAL POINTS COMMON TO BOTH ACCELERATION AND MAX VELOCITY SPRINTING

There are a number of performance characteristics and technical points that are common to the optimal technical models for both acceleration and maximal velocity sprinting:

- In preparation for ground contact, the athlete should create stiffness around the ankle joint by dorsiflexing the ankle to a neutral position and pre-activating the calf-Achilles complex.
- Broadly speaking, in both acceleration and maximal velocity running, the ball of the foot should strike the ground and be the point where weight is distributed during the stance phase. In acceleration, the forward lean raises the heel, whereas in maximal velocity sprinting the heel will be very close to the ground and may even make contact without any significant force applied through it.
- Stiffness through the stance leg and torso throughout the ground contact enables the effective transmission of ground reaction forces creating effective and efficient displacement and minimizing the

dissipation of energy from the system. In acceleration, the hip and knee extend, ankle plantar flexes during ground contact with greater amplitude than in maximal velocity sprinting. The posture of the athlete's trunk should enable effective force transmission throughout rather than trying to create force through flexion or extension.

• In order to best prepare for the effective application of force at ground contact and maintain effective posture and pelvic and trunk alignment, it is essential that once the foot has left the ground at toe-off (the point when the athlete completes ground contact and leaves the ground), it is recovered into a position in front of the body as early as possible. As the ankle hits level with the knee (shin horizontal) it should have begun travelling forwards. Overall, the athlete should aim to minimize the time the lower limbs spend behind the line of the trunk. This is often termed as either 'minimizing backside

mechanics' or 'positive running'.

ACCELERATION MECHANICS

In acceleration, the athlete should have a significant forward lean of the whole body; the degree of forward lean will vary between athletes based upon strength and the ability to rapidly recover the swing leg. All running involves significant vertical force into the ground (to act against gravity); acceleration also requires the athlete to apply significant horizontal force in order to change momentum (and velocity). Pushing harder into the ground therefore involves greater horizontal and vertical force enabling greater forward lean without falling over. An athlete that can recover their foot underneath their centre of mass more rapidly is also able to lean further forward when accelerating. The shin angle as the foot strikes the ground should match the forward lean of the torso as the foot strikes the ground just behind the hips.

At toe-off the athlete should achieve full

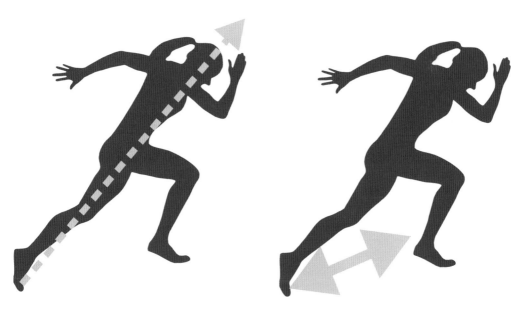

Fig. 3.3 Acceleration toe-off position.

extension at the hip and knee and plantar flexion at the ankle. This is the result of pushing as hard as possible into the ground during ground contact. Explosive concentric force production is a key physical quality in this phase of running. This explosive drive into the ground for the duration of ground contact should be associated with an aggressive arm action of exaggerated amplitude to counterbalance the rotation forces created by the forward lean.

As getting the foot down quickly to push into the ground again (stride frequency) is essential to the change in momentum required in acceleration, the athlete should recover the foot low to the ground between toe-off and the next time the foot strikes the ground, minimizing the time required to recover the leg. This low recovery of the foot and the driving of the foot back and down into the ground mean that the action of the legs in acceleration may be described as piston-like.

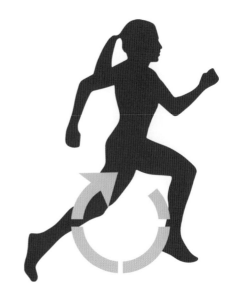

Fig. 3.4 Representation of the 'mid-flight' position in max velocity sprinting.

MAXIMAL VELOCITY SPRINT MECHANICS

In contrast to the acceleration phase, once close to peak velocity, the athlete's torso and associated shin angles should be upright. The forces involved are now predominantly vertical (as velocity is no longer increasing) with the aim of efficiently bouncing along, rebounding rapidly within very brief ground contacts. The shin should also be vertical when the foot strikes the ground underneath the hips, matching the upright posture.

As the ground contact is so brief, the athlete should not now aim for full hip and knee extension or full ankle plantar flexion at the point of toe-off. Muscular stiffness and elasticity are now key qualities. The arm action should be powerful and dynamic counteracting the action of the lower limbs. Shoulders and hands should be relaxed.

At maximum velocity the foot should now be recovered relatively high, crossing the stance leg at or above the knee creating a cycling action of the legs. This is due to the priority now being set up to create greatest vertical velocity and force towards the ground, maximizing vertical ground reaction force.

Table 3.2 summarizes the key technical points for the acceleration and maximal velocity phases of sprinting along with technical points that apply to either phase.

CHANGE OF DIRECTION AND AGILITY TRAINING

As depicted below in the 'Deterministic Model of Agility' presented by Sheppard and Young (2006), 'Agility' may be considered as a combination of change of direction qualities and perceptual and decision-making factors, applied in response to a stimulus within a sport, for example the movement of an opponent, or the movement of the ball.

In most cases, perceptual and decision-

ACCELERATION	V	TOP SPEED
WHOLE BODY LEAN		UPRIGHT
LOW HEEL RECOVERY		HIGH STEPOVER RECOVERY
PISTON ACTION		CYCLIC ACTION
FULL TRIPLE EXTENSION		NOT FULL EXTENSION
	BALL OF FOOT CONTACT	
	STIFF SPRING SYSTEM	
	POSITIVE RUNNING	

Table 3.2 Key characteristics of sprint mechanics (UKSCA, 2016).

making qualities are best developed within sport-specific training led by an expert sport coach. As described by Jeffreys (2011) agility tasks have clear context and situational specificity that vary from one task to the next. Attempts within strength and conditioning exercises to simulate sport-specific stimuli and movement patterns are likely to be incongruent with the environment and task constraints experienced in the sport itself (Young and Farrow, 2013). It is therefore logical that strength and conditioning training prioritizes the ability to start, stop and change direction in a variety of tasks. It is then up to the athlete and their technical sports coach to apply these improved abilities within the performance of the sport.

TECHNICAL PROFICIENCY

Addressing biomechanical errors in key movements and improving the athlete's ability to produce force, transmit force and manage momentum in key change of direction tasks can often have a significant impact upon the speed-agility capabilities of female athletes. Rather than deficits in physical qualities limiting performance, it may be that a lack of technical proficiency is the main limitation.

Maintaining postural integrity and utilizing advantageous joint angles can maximize force production and transmission potential through change of direction movements. As illustrated in Fig. 3.6, within many sports, in this case squash, athletes are required to effectively perform a wide range of multi-directional agility tasks. Although precise technical points may vary between individual athletes based upon anthropometry and other physical characteristics, and vary significantly depending upon the specific sports context, there are fundamental technical principles that should be applied to change of direction and agility tasks for all athletes and those coaching them.

Underpinning Principles for Change of

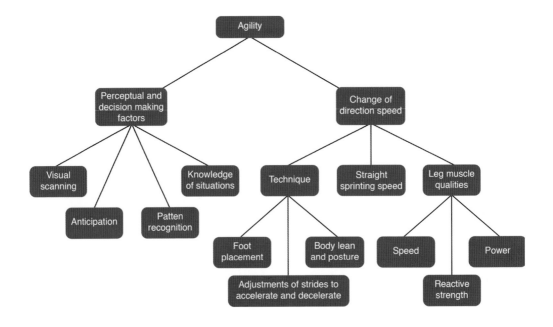

Fig. 3.5 Deterministic model of agility (modified from Sheppard and Young, 2006).

Direction and Agility Performance:

- Starting, stopping and changing direction are predominantly about the management of the base of support and centre of mass whilst setting up joint angles (and possessing the necessary strength) that enable effective application of force in the optimal direction. The relationship between the athlete's centre of mass and base of support is key to effectively manipulating momentum, creating instability to accelerate, or stability for stopping or changing direction.

- The alignment of hip, knee, ankle and trunk are key considerations when the athlete is required to produce, transmit or absorb force (as are strength qualities).

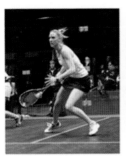 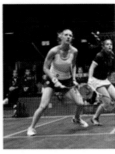 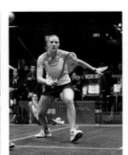 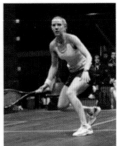

Fig 3.6 Examples of multi-directional agility tasks within squash.

- In change of direction tasks, rotation of the hips should drive the athlete's movement in the new direction. Foot placement must enable the effective loading of the muscles around the hip to re-accelerate in the new direction of travel.
- Trunk angle will vary, a forward lean whilst accelerating and more upright in deceleration. In ready positions and even in decelerations, the shoulders should normally remain slightly in front of the hips to enable rapid reactive acceleration when a new stimulus requires it.
- The athlete must effectively use each foot contact with the ground, not wasting any steps. The athlete should be able to utilize a variety of types of foot contact and be able to apply force in different ways, for example reactive stiffness, concentric explosive force or friction on the ground and flexion of hip, knee and dorsiflexion of the ankle to decelerate.
- The intensity of performance and the athlete's intent in change of direction and agility exercises whilst training must be high if positive neuro-muscular adaptations are to be stimulated.

Effective deceleration and stopping requires a set of technical points that could be considered as a reversal of several of the coaching points for acceleration:

- Rear of foot contact as the athlete lowers centre of mass through the hips to increase stability.
- Hip and knee flex, ankle dorsiflexes through the stance phase.
- The athlete's stride length will shorten as they decelerate but in most cases the athlete should aim to minimize the number of steps required (limited by strength levels) to stop. In most evasive agility sports the stronger athlete who is able to decelerate within the least number of steps will dominate.

- For games players, the shoulders should remain in front of hips throughout, ready to respond to the next stimulus or re-accelerate immediately after completing changes of direction or stopping tasks.

RECOMMENDATIONS FOR SPEED-AGILITY PRESCRIPTION

A thorough warm-up should be completed prior to high-intensity speed, change of direction or agility exercises to moderate injury risk and enable optimal performance. The warm-up should raise heart rate and core temperate and increase blood flow to the muscles that will be most active (around hips, knees and ankles). The hips, knees and ankles should be taken through full ranges of controlled flexion, extension and rotation via dynamic movements that also require activation of the surrounding musculature. Prior to change of direction or agility sessions, multi-planar and multi-directional movement patterns should form a significant portion of the warm-up. Warm-up activity should gradually increase in intensity to prepare the athlete for maximal intensity 'work' repetitions. Skipping and rebounding drills reinforcing ground contact, ankle action, reactive stiffness and key positions can be utilized within the warm-up and can be a valuable tool for conditioning the hamstrings, hip flexors and calf-Achilles complex whilst reinforcing key technical positions through increasingly complex patterns.

Speed and agility training should normally be programmed concurrently alongside traditional strength and power training. An athlete with a solid foundation of movement control and strength should perform their speed work at high intensities. Athletes who are unaccustomed to speed or agility training should begin by integrating a small number of speed or agility exercises into their current programme, on the end of warm-ups or as a lead into weightlifting or conditioning sessions. The development of technical excellence in the performance of basic exercises should be an initial priority before any complex exercises are undertaken.

Progression should be made on a gradual dose-response basis with the response to previous sessions taken into account before increasing either complexity, intensity or volume, so if the athlete feels fine then the volume or complexity may be increased from the last session, if excessive muscle soreness or any joint pain resulted from the previous session, then ease off. Two sessions of approximately 30 minutes speed training per week is normally a reasonable place for beginners to start. As the competence and conditioning of the athlete advances then speed or agility training may be undertaken three to four times per week, providing the athlete is sufficiently recovered in between sessions. Aggressive deceleration and change of direction exercises are not advisable for female athletes with poor movement control and should not be undertaken more than twice each week with any female athlete, particularly if the athlete's competition or event also includes this type of activity.

Intensity and volume are inversely related with each having a significant influence upon the other. When planning phases of training away from competition, volume may be relatively high with the intensity and quality of training being somewhat compromised. As competition approaches, the volume of speed-agility training should be relatively low to enable high quality and intensity. For speed-agility training, the volume of each training session can be calculated to be either the total number of exercise repetitions, accelerations, changes of direction or decelerations. For linear speed work, the total distance covered by high velocity running can be utilized. The intensity of speed-agility training can be manipulated based upon velocity of

movement, change of direction angle or whether movements are planned or in response to an unpredictable stimulus. In order to at least maintain speed qualities, a trained female athlete must experience a high-intensity speed-agility stimulus at least every seven to ten days in order to avoid the detraining of this quality.

Female athletes may generally have lower absolute strength than their male counterparts, which may lead to an elevated injury risk when performing change of direction and agility tasks. When planning linear acceleration and max velocity sprinting training, these gender differences are not a significant consideration, as training age and mechanical competence (skill) are far more important factors. Supplementary strengthening whilst reinforcing the forward lean and piston-like leg actions of acceleration may be undertaken using heavy sled towing or heavy prowler pushing. When designing training programmes to include decelerations and change of direction activity, gender does become a key consideration, as female athletes should be cautious regarding the volume and frequency of high-intensity actions. The heavy eccentric work involved in deceleration and change of direction training is also likely to elicit delayed-onset muscle soreness (DOMS), particularly before the athlete becomes well conditioned to this type of activity. This soreness prohibits a frequency greater than twice a week until the athlete becomes better conditioned and the limiting effects of DOMS are reduced.

For high-level adult athletes, the programme should reflect the competition, for example a track sprinter should focus upon one-off linear acceleration and max velocity exercises, while a netball player should incorporate multi-directional exercises performed for several repetitions. When the objective is the development of linear running acceleration and peak velocity, the training should include a significant volume of high-intensity accelerations and high-speed running. For sprint athletes who are

SPEED TRAINING SESSION PRESCRIPTION FRAMEWORK	
LINEAR SPEED	**CHANGE OF DIRECTION / AGILITY**
• Work time: <6 seconds	• Work time: <6 seconds
• Distance of run: 10m – 60m	• Reps per set: 3–6 reps
• Reps per set: 2 - 4 reps	• Total sets per session: 3–5 (9–30 reps total)
• Total sets per session: 2–4 (6 - 16 reps total)	• Intra-set Work: Rest ratio: 1:6 – 1:10
• Total distance of set: 40m–120m	(e.g. 6sec rep = 36-60sec rest)
• Total distance of session: 160m–600m	• Inter-set Work:Rest ratio: 1:20
• Intra-set recovery: 45–60sec per 10m of	**(e.g. 6sec reps = 120sec rest between sets)**
maximum intensity sprinting	
• Inter-set recovery: 1.5–2x intra-set recovery	

Table 3.3 Speed Training Prescription Framework (UKSCA, 2016).

technically proficient, resisted sprinting using a sled, parachute, weighted vest or slight incline can be integrated into the programme. The aim of this method is to overload the athlete's sprinting and improve explosive force production without compromising running mechanics. The resistance applied should therefore be relatively light. Assisted (over speed) sprinting using partner towing via bungee cord or a shallow decline allows the athlete to experience increased stride frequency. The level of assistance provided should not compromise the running mechanics.

Table 3.3 contains an outline of generic guidelines for the prescription of linear speed and change of direction or agility training. This provides a very general framework that should be manipulated by the coach in order to minimize the athlete's drop-off in speed between repetitions due to fatigue.

Linear speed training can be progressed through a block of training by modulating the emphasis (for example, acceleration or maximal velocity sprinting), frequency (how many sessions each week), complexity of technical drills and volume. The progression of agility training within a session and across a training block may follow one of four themes; closed towards open contexts, simple towards complex movement patterns, single towards multiple chained patterns or moderate to maximal intensity. Table 3.4 outlines examples of how simple agility drills may be progressed to appropriately challenge the athlete.

There can be significant value in even highly competent athletes repeating simple change of direction drills performed with high intensity as they can provide a stimulus for the improvement of relevant strength and stability qualities that may later be applied within more complex tasks. For example, 180-degree turns require sequenced loading of the inside leg to apply braking force and the outside leg to complete the braking and apply accelerative force in the new direction. Task constraints with external focus to support the correct technical performance of agility drills can be an extremely impactful intervention for the improvement of change of direction performance. The use of task constraints with an external focus can refine the loading and/or

EXAMPLE CHANGE OF DIRECTION PROGRESSIONS			
	LEVEL 1	LEVEL 2	LEVEL 3
Closed towards Open	90° turn to accelerate.	Multi-directional partner initiated accelerations.	Small-sided games with large degrees of variation and movement options.
Simple towards Complex patterns	Linear acceleration from a split stance.	Linear accelerations from a 90° and 180° turn.	Multi-directional accelerations from a wide variety of compromised start positions.
Single towards Multiple Patterns	3m lateral shuffle	3m lateral shuffle into 5m linear acceleration	3m lateral shuffle into 5m linear acceleration with a controlled stop in a split stance.
Intensity	Technical practice of outside foot 'power' cut with restricted <5m run-in.	Outside foot 'power' cut with restricted approx.10m run-in.	Combine high velocity sprinting with outside foot 'power' cut patterns.

Table 3.4 Example change of direction progressions.

skill requirements of a drill and address consistent faults in performance. For example, requiring the athlete to touch a cone either on the inside or outside of a 180-degree turn overloads the inside or outside leg respectively. If an athlete is not able to effectively use the inside leg to brake when they perform aggressive cuts or 180-degree turns in their sport, then using the drill with the cone on the inside could trigger performance improvement.

When selecting equipment it is essential to evaluate the effect that its use will have on the performance of an exercise rather than simply using what is popular or fashionable. The over-reliance on novel equipment may negatively impact upon the desired outcome of the exercise. Examples of this negative impact below:

• Successful rapid completion of agility ladder drills reinforces incorrect ground contacts and technical positions for change of direction and agility performance.

• The use of poles for change of direction

drills does not allow the athlete to lean into the change of direction; if a lean into the turn is something you want to promote, marker disks are a better option.
• The use of micro hurdles when training acceleration does not allow the low recovery of the foot that is key to effective performance.

When preparing well-trained, competent female athletes for sports requiring complex agility tasks, the movement patterns utilized within and at least some of their speed or agility training can and should have a high level of variation in movement requirements, neuromuscular demands and sensory input. The rationale for utilizing varied chaotic open drills to improve agility performance is the ability to respond to a variety of stimuli and situations; this should not be the only format used within the agility training programme but should be supplemented with more simple change of direction exercises to enable sufficient consistency of stimulus.

EXAMPLE TRAINING SESSIONS

Table 3.5 outlines three linear speed-training sessions that could be used in order to improve an athlete's maximum velocity, acceleration and early drive phase acceleration respectively.

Table 3.6 provides an example of a change

of direction training session that could be utilized for athletes involved in court sports.

SUMMARY

The development of improved speed-agility performance in female athletes can best be achieved through an intimate understanding of the movement demands of their sport, identification of associated strength qualities and movement competencies, and appropriate assessment of the athlete's current qualities and competencies.

Rather than a simple generic solution to improving the speed and agility of all athletes in all sports situations, a multi-faceted approach to the development of force production, motor control, dynamic stabilization, and sport-specific proficiency should be framed around the demands of the sport and current physical state of the athlete. Traditional resistance training, explosive and plyometric exercises are a valuable part of the training programme for the speed athlete but high-intensity training involving sport-specific actions, for example running, must also form a significant portion of the training.

Generally speaking, when compared to their male counterparts, female athletes tend to have lower strength levels, different neuromuscular recruitment patterns in landing and change of direction tasks, and are subject to acute effects on movement control

	SPEED QUALITY	SETS × REPS × DISTANCE	REST BETWEEN REPS / SETS
Session 1	Max Velocity	3 × 2 × 40m 'flying' sprints (30m acceleration zone)	4 mins / 6 mins
Session 2	Acceleration	3 × 4 × 30m from a 2 point stance	3 mins / 5 mins
Session 3	Early drive phase acceleration	4 × 4 × 10m from a 3 point stance	60 secs / 120 secs

Table 3.5 Linear speed session examples.

Warm-up to include: Line hops, drop squats, drop lunges, stiff legged jumps, multi-directional lunges, accelerations, etc.

Activity	Reps	Rest Between Reps
Set 1) Stiff-legged bound into 3m acceleration	x 4 (2 each leg)	30 Secs
2 Minutes Recovery (light technical practice)		
Set 2) Tuck Jump x5 into 3m acceleration (4 directions)	x 4	30 Secs
2 Minutes Recovery (light technical practice)		
Set 3) Lateral Single Leg Rebounds x6 into 3m acceleration (4 directions)	x 4	30 Secs

Notes:

1. Complete a thorough multi-directional warm-up prior to starting this session.

2. Each repetition of a drill must be done with maximal intensity (as fast as you can).

3. This session can be used as an extended warm-up leading into technical session.

Table 3.6 Example court-based agility session outline.

and joint stability due to their menstrual cycle. Speed and agility training is high-intensity exercise that requires a foundation of strength qualities and movement competence. It is therefore essential that female athletes strategically manage the volume and load provided by change of direction and agility training. Female athletes who are unaccustomed to speed or agility training, or who have not recently undertaken this modality, should introduce speed training gradually into the training regimen, beginning with a low volume of basic linear exercises and progressing from there. The velocity and complexity of change of direction and agility drills combine to create a load that should be managed and progressed in a strategic manner, enabling the athlete to build resilience and capacity and improve performance.

REFERENCES

Bachero-Mena B. and Gonzalez-Badillo J.J. (2014) Effect of resisted sprint training on acceleration with three different loads accounting for 5, 12.5, and 20 per cent of body mass. *Journal of Stress and Conditioning Research*, 28(10), 2954–2960.

Bradley P.S. and Vescovi J.D. (2015) Velocity Thresholds for Women's Soccer Matches: Sex Specificity Dictates High Speed Running and Sprinting Thresholds: Female Athletes in Motion (FAiM). *International Journal of Sports Physiology and Performance*, 10, 112–116.

Brown L.E. and Ferrigno V.A. (2015) *Training for Speed, Agility and Quickness* (3rd ed.). Human Kinetics, Champaign, Ill.

Brughelli M. *et al.* (2008) Understanding Change of Direction ability in Sport: A Review of resistance Training Studies. *Sports Medicine*, 38(12), 1045–1063.

Cook G., Burton L. and Hoogenboom B. (2006) Pre-participation screening: the use of fundamental movements as an assessment of function – part 1. *North American Journal of Sports Physical Therapy*, 1, 62–72.

Cottle, C.A. *et al.* (2014) Effects of sled towing on sprint starts. *Journal of Stress and Conditioning Research*, 28(5), 1241–1245.

Francis, C. (1997) *Training for Speed*. Facciona Speed and Conditioning Consultants.

Francis, C. and Patterson, P. (1986) *The Charlie Francis Training System*. Ottawa, Canada: TBLI Publications Inc.

Gamble, P. (2012) *Training for Sports Speed and Agility: An evidence based approach*. Routledge, New York.

Hewit, J.K., Cronin, J.B. and Hume, P. (2012) Understanding Change of Direction Performance: A Technical Analysis of a 180°Ground-Based Turn and Sprint Task. *Journal of Sports Science and Coaching*, 7(3), 493–501.

Hewit, J.K. *et al.* (2011) Understanding deceleration in sport. *Strength and Conditioning Journal*, 33(1), 47–52.

Holmberg, P.M. (2009) Agility Training for Experienced Athletes: A Dynamical Systems Approach. *Strength and Conditioning Journal*, 31(5), 73–78.

Hunter, J.P., Marshall, R.N. and McNair, P.J. (2005) Relationships Between Ground Reaction Force Impulse and Kinematics of Sprint-Running Acceleration. *Journal of Applied Biomechanics* 21, 31–43.

Jeffreys, I. (2011) A Task-Based Approach to Developing Context-Specific Agility. *Strength and Conditioning Journal*, 33(4), 52–59.

Keiner, M. *et al.* (2014) Long-term strength training effects in change of direction sprint performance. *Journal of Strength and Conditioning Research*, 28(1), 223–231.

Lai, A. *et al.* (2016) Human ankle plantar flexor muscle-tendon mechanics and energetics during maximum acceleration sprinting. *Journal of the Royal Society online* [accessed 28 June 2017]

Loureiro, L.F.B. and Barbosa de Freitas, P. (2016) Development of an Agility Test for Badminton Players and Assessment of its Validity and Test-Retest Reliability. *International Journal of Sports Physiology and Performance*, 11, 305–310.

Marshall, B.M. *et al.* (2014) Biomechanical factors associated with time to complete a change of direction cutting manoeuvre. *Journal of Strength and Conditioning Research*, 28(10), 2845–2851.

Myer, G.D. *et al.* (2006) The effects of plyometric vs. dynamic stabilization and balance training on power, balance, and landing force in female athletes. *Journal of Strength and Conditioning Research*. 20(2), 345–353.

Naoki, K., Kazunori, N. and Newton, R.U. (2013) Relationships between ground reaction impulse and sprint acceleration performance in team sport athletes. *Journal of Strength and Conditioning Research*. 27, 568–573.

Nimphius, S., Callaghan, S.J., Spiteri, T. and Lockie, R.G. (2016) Change of direction deficit: A more isolated measure of change of direction performance than total 505 time. *Journal of Strength and Conditioning*

Research. 30(11), 3024–3032.

Nimphius, S. (2014) in *High Performance Training for Sports.* Human Kinetics. Chapter 13, Increasing agility, 185–198.

Ross, A. *et al.* (2001) Neural influences on sprint running: Training adaptations and acute responses. *Sports Medicine,* 31(6), 409–425.

Schache, A.G. *et al.* (2012) Mechanics of the Human Hamstring Muscles During Sprinting. *Medicine and Science in Sports and Exercise,* 44(4), 647–658.

Seitz, L.B. *et al.* (2014) Increases in lower-body strength transfer positively to sprint performance: a systematic review with meta-analysis. *Sports Medicine,* 44(12), 1693–1702.

Sheppard, J.M. and Young, W.B. (2006) Agility literature review: classifications, training and testing. *Journal of Sports Sciences,* 24(9), 919–932.

Spiteri, T. *et al.* (2014) Contribution of strength characteristics to change of direction and agility performance in female basketball athletes. *Journal of Strength and Conditioning Research,* 28(9), 2415–2423.

Teyhen, D.S. *et al.* (2012) The Functional Movement Screen: A Reliability Study.

Journal of Orthopaedic and Sports Physical Therapy, 42(6), 530–540.

Triplett, N.T. *et al.* (2012) Power associations with running speed. *Stress and Conditioning Journal,* 34(6), 29–33.

UK Strength and Conditioning Association. (2016) *Plyometrics, Agility, Speed Workshop Resource Pack.* UKSCA.

Whelan, N. *et al.* (2014) Resisted sprints do not acutely enhance sprinting performance. *Journal of Strength and Conditioning Research,* 28(7), 1858–1866.

Wilkinson, M., Leedale-Brown, D. and Winter, E.M. (2009) Validity of a squash-specific test of change-of-direction speed. *International Journal of Sport and Physical Performance,* 4, 176–185.

Young, W.B. and Bilby, G.E. (1993) The effect of voluntary effort to influence speed of contraction on strength, muscular power and hypertrophy development. *Journal of Strength and Conditioning Research.* 7(3), 172–178.

Young, W. and Farrow, D. (2013) The importance of a sport-specific stimulus for training agility. *Stress and Conditioning Journal,* 35(2), 39–43.

CHAPTER 4
ENERGY SYSTEM DEVELOPMENT FOR FEMALE ATHLETES

Julian Monk, ASCC, PGDE and Keith Barker, MSc, ASCC

Optimizing sport-specific performance requires the development of both muscular (strength) endurance and energy system output. As described by Gastin (2001), energy production relies upon three interrelated processes:

- ATP–PCr (alactic) system: the splitting of stored phosphagens (adenosine triphosphate [ATP] and phosphocreatine [PCr])
- Glycolytic system: the breakdown of carbohydrate in the absence of oxygen
- Oxidative (aerobic) system: the combustion of carbohydrates and fats in the presence of oxygen.

'Metabolic conditioning' is a commonly used term to describe the training activities utilized to develop the ability of energy systems to maximize power output for the duration of the sports performance. As with any other training activities, it is essential that metabolic conditioning sessions are well matched to the individual athlete's physical state, training age, training phase and developmental needs. Within a comprehensive training programme, an athlete should employ a blend of conditioning activities including sport-specific and non-specific protocol, enabling intensity to be effectively manipulated and a high volume of training completed. Several significant differences in the endurance performance characteristics and responses to metabolic conditioning activities between male and female athletes exist and may

influence the optimal prescription of training. Trends in a range of sports have led to the popular use of 'specific game-related' interval training where competition time-motion data is utilized to create simulated competition intervals of exercise and recovery. Used intelligently around competitive match-play events, this method can form part of an appropriate conditioning regime. Limitations of solely adopting this 'sport-specific' approach to conditioning for sports performance relate to whether it provides appropriate targeted energy system stress in order to elicit positive adaptations to energy system output. Other recently popularized forms of metabolic conditioning such as high-intensity interval training (HITT), CrossFit and maximal aerobic speed (MAS) training may have some value for athletes in certain contexts but should not be the only conditioning formats considered. Many coaches and athletes have largely overlooked long-duration steady state aerobic training activity in favour of shorter, more intense formats but this is probably for reasons of convenience and time efficiency rather than a strategic decision based upon desired adaptations.

This chapter aims to outline the function of the energy systems in the performance of cyclical and acyclical sports activities of wide-ranging duration and intensity. It will also provide an understanding of how the rate of energy production, duration and work:rest ratios of metabolic conditioning activities impact upon resulting adaptations. Examples of how these principles can be developed and applied to specific training activities and sessions within an athlete's training programme will be given.

ANATOMICAL/PHYSIOLOGICAL OVERVIEW

When comparing male and female sporting performances, female athletes are generally around 10 per cent slower compared to the times for males in swimming, speed skating, rowing, cycling, kayaking and marathon running events. This gap however starts to close when it comes to ultra-endurance events, prompting the examination of the key physiological factors that determine success in endurance sports. Consideration needs to be given to a number of specific components including lean muscle mass, VO_2max, size of the heart, movement economy and central drive (the ability of the nervous system to send signals to the muscles to maintain performance over time). Generally, male athletes naturally have advantages in lean muscle mass, VO_2max and the size of the heart, but these can all be changed through

training for both males and females. Potentially the greatest changes in performance for female athletes come through developing central drive and movement economy, which may account for female athletes closing the gap on men in endurance events. A study by Zamparo and Swaine (2012) found that swimmers with a lower VO_2max could perform at the same speeds as those with a higher VO_2max by improving their movement economy.

Other potential factors to consider are fatigability and the ability to derive more energy output from fat stores. Female athletes generally have a higher number of fatigue-resistant muscle fibres in comparison to males, which are utilized during lower-intensity activities (Keller *et al.*, 2011). Due to the increased muscle mass of males the heart works harder as more blood is required to allow male muscle tissue to function. This will also affect fuel utilization because female athletes tend to have less muscle mass and therefore derive more energy from fat stores, which is the primary fuel source for endurance events (Brown, 2017). This pattern of fuel utilization means females may rely more

Female athletes	Male athletes
	More muscle
	Larger heart
	More red blood cells
Increased fat burned at given exercise intensity	
	Increased glycolytic capacity
Less fatigue-able	
Increased number of repetitions at a given % of 1 rep max	
Increased ability to handle higher relative workload	
Strength per unit of muscle is equal	

Table 4.1 Key physiological differences between female and male athletes.

heavily on the aerobic system for the production of energy, giving them a greater ability to tolerate increased workloads and the ability to recover faster.

Sex hormones can explain many of the differences in metabolic characteristics between females and males. Testosterone affects the ability to develop muscle mass, explaining why male athletes tend to have greater muscle mass than females. Females produce greater amounts of oestrogen and research indicates that this could be beneficial to aerobic performance. Muscle sensitivity to oestrogen increases the uptake of glucose, potentially improving metabolic health (Nuckols, 2015).

Table 4.1 summarizes some of the key physiological differences between females and males. Adapted from Nuckols (2015).

When planning a metabolic conditioning programme, an understanding of what it is we are trying to improve or change within the athlete is essential. This requires a clear knowledge of the demands of the sport, the individual needs of the athlete in relation to these demands and how the body adapts to meet this stress. With the development of technology over recent years such as GPS and heart rate monitoring systems it is possible to get a real understanding of the distances covered, the number of high-intensity movements made and the overall intensity of exercise from heart rate data. This provides comprehensive data for both competition and training and the ability to effectively monitor adaptation to training.

Human bodies are complex machines made up of a number of systems working together to maintain the function of the body, or homeostasis (the maintenance of a constant internal environment). Through research, we now understand how these systems interact and adapt to the stresses placed upon them. Research conducted by Hans Selye back in 1936 led to the theory of the general adaptation syndrome (GAS) (Selye, 1984). This

syndrome manifests itself in three stages:
1) Alarm reaction: the reaction when the body is suddenly exposed to a stressor to which it is not adapted. If the imposed stressor does not lead to death, the alarm reaction is followed by adaptation or the stage of resistance;
2) Stage of resistance: complete adaptation with a disappearance of symptoms (super compensation). However, continued application of the stressor can lead to depletion of adaptation resources or the state of exhaustion;
3) State of exhaustion: occurs when adaptation resources are depleted fully (over-training or reaching).

Regardless of the stress imposed, these sequences of events occur. It is important to understand this, as when we undertake any conditioning, whether it is targeted at aerobic or anaerobic development, this is how the body will respond to the stimulus.

Through the training process, we are trying to develop chronic adaptations to our cardiovascular, muscular and energy delivery systems so they are better able to meet the demands of sports performance. These divide into central and peripheral adaptations for both aerobic and anaerobic energy production.

CENTRAL FACTORS

- **Increased systolic volume (cardiac output).** The term used to describe the pumping activity of the heart is cardiac output. Cardiac output is the amount of blood we eject from the heart (stroke volume), each beat multiplied by the heart rate. Expressed mathematically as:

Cardiac Output = Stroke Volume × Heart Rate.

Simply put, stroke volume is the amount of blood that can fit into the left ventricle of the heart and heart rate is the amount of times the heart contracts every minute. From this, we can see that if we want to improve our ability to deliver more blood and oxygen, increasing the size of the heart in particular, the left ventricle is key.

- **Myocardial hypertrophy** and an increase of myocardial ventricular volume. Aerobic endurance training brings about specific changes in cardiac dimension, especially the left ventricle. It has been shown to induce a proportional change in both eccentric (increase in the size of the left ventricle) and concentric (thickness of the left ventricular wall) hypertrophy (Smith and Fernhall, 2011), enabling a greater volume of blood to be pumped out with every heart beat (increased stroke volume).
- **Increase parasympathetic activity** and reduce sympathetic activity within the autonomic nervous system. The autonomic nervous system is not under voluntary control and is responsible for the regulation of bodily functions, in particular heart rate. It consists of two branches: the sympathetic and parasympathetic nervous system. The sympathetic nervous system is often referred to as the fight or flight or the quick-response mobilizing system. It is responsible for increasing heart rate, breathing rate, releasing adrenalin and noradrenaline from the adrenal glands in response to increasing activity. The parasympathetic system is responsible for bringing our bodies back to normal levels by slowing the heart rate, reducing blood pressure and respiration levels. It is often referred to as the rest and digest system. Through conditioning our aerobic system, we improve parasympathetic activity to conserve energy expenditure and improve overall exercise economy.
- **Increased blood volume.** Increased blood volume enables more oxygen and nutrients to be delivered to the working muscles, consequently supporting the increased demands on the working muscles as a result of training.

- **Increased speed and amplitude of cardiac contractions.** This refers to the rate at which the heart is able to contract to force blood out and the strength of the contraction. This improves the response of the sympathetic system.
- **Increasing pulmonary diffusion.** This refers to the increased capacity of the lungs to diffuse oxygen to the red blood cells, enabling more oxygen to reach the working muscles.

Peripheral Factors

Peripheral factors of aerobic energy production involve oxygen utilization within working muscles.

- Increased quantity, size and density of mitochondria: The mitochondria found in the cells throughout our body are responsible for converting oxygen and nutrients into adenosine triphosphate (ATP). Referred to as the powerhouse of the cell.
- Improved elasticity of the blood vessels: A study on aerobic and resistance exercise demonstrated improvement in the elasticity of blood vessels (Lee et al., 2008). Improved elasticity of the blood vessels increases the amount of blood supplied to the working muscles.
- Increased density and quantity of capillaries: Capillaries are the smallest of our blood vessels that supply our working muscles with oxygen, nutrients and remove waste products such as carbon dioxide. With regular training, the density of capillaries in the working muscles may increase as much as 5–20 per cent within 3 months of regular training.
- Increased muscle glycogen stores: Glycogen provides us with our secondary long-term energy source, with the primary source being fats.
- Increased myoglobin content: Myoglobin is an oxygen and iron-binding protein found in our muscle tissue and its primary role is to deliver oxygen to muscle.

ADAPTATIONS FOR ANAEROBIC ENERGY PRODUCTION

Central Factors

Central factors of anaerobic production are dependent upon the function of the central nervous system. Motor units play an important part in controlling the muscles recruited to produce force through the following three ways:

- Increased motor unit firing rate
- Increased motor unit recruitment
- Increased intra- and inter-muscular coordination.

Peripheral Factors

Peripheral factors involve processes of metabolism within muscles listed below:

- Increased glycolytic enzymes
- Increased phosphocreatine levels
- Increased alactic enzymes
- Increased pH buffering capacity.

INCREASED MOVEMENT ECONOMY

An alternative approach to improving endurance performance is to improve an athlete's running or movement economy, reducing the energy cost at a given exercise intensity. By increasing strength (force production) an athlete can reduce the relative force that is needed every stride, reducing overall energy expenditure. The resultant conservation of fuel stores can then be utilized later in the sports performance when called upon. With an increase in strength comes change in rates of force development along with the number of mitochondria and oxidative enzymes. Additionally, there is increased stiffness of the musculotendinous unit, which enhances energy return. As mentioned earlier, this is potentially one of the areas where female athletes can make a significant improvement in their performance, particularly in endurance-based sports.

In summary, desired adaptations may include (Pate and Kiuska, 1984):

- Increase in the size and number of mitochondria
- Increase in oxidative enzymes
- Increased muscle stability leading to less energy expenditure on ground contact
- Increased stiffness of the musculotendinous unit enhancing energy return. Studies have shown that increasing muscle-tendon stiffness can recover up to 60 per cent of mechanical energy, leaving only 40 per cent needing to be restored through metabolic processes (Verkhoshansky, 1966 and Voight *et al.*, 1995).

ENERGY SYSTEMS

Fig. 4.1 shows the key factors that are involved in the production of metabolic energy and how this energy is utilized to produce mechanical work.

The purpose of the body's energy systems is to maintain energy homeostasis by producing adenosine triphosphate (ATP) that sustains cellular function. Metabolic energy systems convert the nutrients we eat from food into fuel to enable muscular work. Homeostasis is maintained when the rate of energy production is equal to the rate of energy expenditure. As exercise intensity increases, the demand for ATP rises, the body responds by increasing the rate of ATP production to match this need for ATP in the working muscles. The ability to use and resynthesize ATP determines performance potential.

To develop the energy systems optimally for sports performance, athletes and coaches need to understand the demands of their

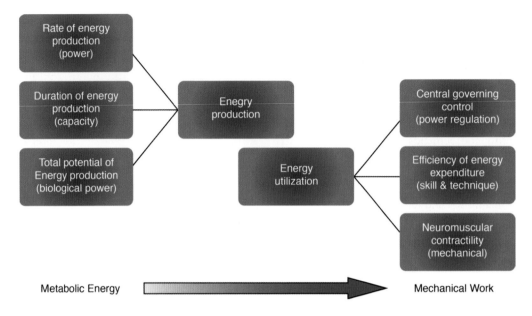

Fig. 4.1 Biological energy transfer (Jamieson, 2009).

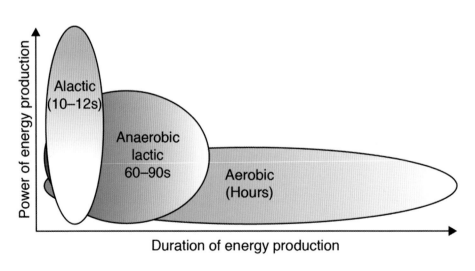

Fig. 4.2 Energy system output comparison (Jamieson, 2009).

sport. This understanding can then be utilized to stress these energy systems with targeted training. For example, when comparing the demands of shot put with those of marathon running, one is over in seconds while the other lasts beyond 2 hours. Both require completely different power output for success, placing different stresses upon the body. In simple terms, the demands placed upon the energy systems by sport can be broken down into the speed of production (intensity), the duration of the event and the work:rest ratios experienced.

Before starting to programme for metabolic conditioning, coaches require an understanding of how the energy systems interact with one another and how female athletes use energy. Females tend to use more fat for energy, having a better distribution of subcutaneous fat as opposed to visceral fat as in males, they have a higher percentage of Type I muscle fibres and are more insulin sensitive. Due to these differences, female athletes use their aerobic systems more efficiently to fuel exercise and recover quicker (Nuckols, 2015).

At the start of the chapter, we have defined the energy systems as:

- ATP – PCr (alactic) system – immediate energy
- Glycolytic system – intermediate energy
- Oxidative (aerobic) system – long-term energy.

Energy systems do not work independently of each other. For example, in the 100m although the aerobic system is working as hard as it can, it just is not able to provide the energy fast enough. Energy systems can be split into a power and an endurance component. Power defined as the rate or speed the system can be switched on to provide ATP, this is dictated by the level of intensity of the activity. Endurance is the total amount of energy that the particular system can provide to support the volume of work being carried out.

ATP-PCr (Anaerobic Alactic System)

This is the immediate energy system and uses creatine phosphate as a source for the resynthesizing of ATP in the absence of oxygen. If you imagine our energy systems as fuel tanks, the ATP-PCr would be the biggest and most powerful. The problem however is that it does not last very long and quickly empties. The athlete is then reliant on how quickly they can resynthesize ATP-PCr to perform again. To replenish this system takes approximately 2–5 minutes recovery, which can also be determined using heart-rate benchmarks before performing the next repetition.

Glycolytic System (Anaerobic Lactic)

This is the intermediate energy system and uses glycogen and glycolysis to resynthesize ATP in the absence of oxygen. The consequence of this process is the production of lactate and hydrogen ions leading to disturbance in homeostasis. Research suggests that the production of lactate does not significantly affect acidosis in the muscle. This is far more likely because of the build-up of hydrogen ions, suggesting that this may be a cause of muscular fatigue.

Lactate, which is often regarded as a cause of fatigue, actually serves as a vital source of energy. It is converted back into pyruvate and oxidized through the aerobic metabolism, allowing it to be used as a source of energy. Lactate accumulation can be used as a marker of aerobic/anaerobic balance. As intensity increases, the body's demand for ATP increases. When the aerobic system cannot provide ATP fast enough we switch to using the anaerobic system, producing and consuming lactate at a faster rate. Eventually the body is working so hard it produces more lactate than the aerobic system can use leading to an accumulation of

Targeted System	Intensity	Duration	Rest between reps	Rest between sets	Reps	No. of Sets
Alactic Anaerobic Power	Maximum	7–10 sec Intervals	2–5 min HR recovery 120	10 minutes	5–6	2
Alactic Anaerobic Capacity	Maximum	7–10 sec Intervals	30seconds-90seconds	5–6 minutes	10–12	2–3
Lactic Anaerobic Power	High or near maximal	20–40 sec Intervals	1–3 minutes	6–10 min	3–4	3–4
Lactic Anaerobic Capacity	High or near maximal	40–90 sec Intervals	1–2 minutes	5–6 min	3–4	3–4
Aerobic Power	Max VO$_2$ HR max 90–100%	30seconds–2 mins Intervals	30seconds–5min HR recovery 120–130 bpm		10–15	1
Threshold Training	HR max 85–90%	3–10mins Intervals	1–5 mins		1	2–5
Cardiac Output	Low-mod <75% HR max 120–150bpm	40–60mins				1
Recovery Stimulation	Low 120–130bpm	20mins				1

Table 4.2 Targeting energy system development.

lactate. This point is referred to as the anaerobic threshold and is when the anaerobic system becomes the primary source of energy and fatigue starts to accumulate.

Aerobic System

This is the long-term energy system using carbohydrates and fats as the primary source for the re-synthesis of ATP in the presence of oxygen. The aerobic system provides ATP at a much slower rate than the anaerobic system. It is capable of sustaining low to moderate intensity for very long periods. However, providing the most ATP per given substrate requires more chemical steps than the anaerobic pathways and takes much longer to generate. Due to this, the aerobic system has a tremendous capacity to produce energy, providing up to 98 per cent in extreme endurance-based events. It also plays a significant role in supporting recovery from high-intensity efforts. This recovery support function is particularly important for sports that require high-intensity efforts to be produced repeatedly over a long period with periods of lower intensity to recover. Females have a distinct advantage in being able to use this system over male athletes, due to their physiological differences in energy utilization.

TRAINING THE ENERGY SYSTEMS

The exercise modality chosen for metabolic conditioning sessions should enable the development of energy systems in relation to neuromuscular fatigue and cardiopulmonary stress. The most direct correspondence from conditioning training to sports performance is with sport-specific actions, enabling both central cardiopulmonary and local neuromuscular adaptations. However, this may not always be possible due to injury or the elevated risk of injury. The use of low-impact, low-risk modalities to build volume of training into the programme, developing central adaptations as opposed to peripheral then become valuable. Whatever the mode used, Table 4.2 outlines the variables to develop the specific energy systems.

AEROBIC SYSTEM

Low-Intensity Aerobic Training (Recovery – Cardiac Output)

Over recent years, it has become increasingly popular to use high-intensity methods for metabolic conditioning rather than lower-intensity aerobic training, with claims that this type of training will lead to making the athlete slower and less powerful. However, as discussed earlier there are key adaptations that occur at these lower intensities. Low-intensity aerobic training plays a key part in the recovery process, especially from high-intensity work. This lower intensity stimulates the adaptive processes of the body to recover both physically and psychologically. To improve cardiac output we have to increase the size of the left ventricle through eccentric hypertrophy. This occurs through continuous training at an intensity of <75 per cent heart rate maximum (HRmax) for 40–60 minutes. Due to the duration of training required to achieve this adaptation, athletes in many sports may be well-advised to utilise non-impact modalities such as cycling and rowing for this type of training. Guided by athlete needs, training phase and competition schedule, this type of training could be undertaken with a frequency of one to three sessions per week.

Improving cardiac output allows the heart to pump out more blood with every beat, making us more efficient at delivering oxygen and nutrients to the working muscles and aiding the resynthesis of ATP, which is crucial for optimizing performance, particularly in team sports that require multiple high-intensity activities performed over a long period.

Threshold Training

The anaerobic threshold is the point at which the body starts to switch from the aerobic system to the anaerobic system. Improving this threshold develops the number of aerobic enzymes and the contractile properties of the aerobic system. By raising this threshold, the athlete relies less on the anaerobic system improving aerobic energy production.

Aerobic Power

Through aerobic power training, specific adaptations to the cardiac muscle tissue can be achieved via higher intensity-based interval work. In particular, as with cardiac output training, the aim is to increase the amount of blood ejected from the left ventricle. However, in this case this is achieved by increasing the contractile strength of the heart (concentric hypertrophy) and number of mitochondria. Improvement in aerobic power is important as it decreases the intensity of stress placed upon the heart at lower activity levels. As the demand for oxygen increases, the strength of the heart then becomes crucial so that it does not fatigue as quickly.

As indicated in Table 4.2, aerobic power training involves exercise intervals ranging from 30 seconds to 2 minutes at an intensity of 90–100 per cent of HRmax. Recovery intervals can be dictated by heart rate recovery to approximately 120–130 bpm. The number of intervals completed can range from ten to fifteen.

Maximal Aerobic Speed Training (MAS)

In recent times, MAS training particularly within team sports has become increasingly popular. MAS is the quickest pace an athlete can maintain while still working aerobically. Research in this area has shown that time spent at or above 100 per cent MAS could be critical in improving aerobic power (Billat and Koralsztein, 1996; Dupont et al., 2002). In particular, at a speed of 120 per cent MAS for short intervals followed by a short rest, for example 15 seconds work followed by 15 seconds rest, repeated for 15 runs.

A simple way to calculate MAS is to run a 5-minute time trial and record the distance covered. Divide the distance by the time resulting in 100 per cent MAS. For example, an athlete runs 1,200m in 300 seconds, their MAS equals 4 metres per second. To determine 120 per cent MAS 4.0 m/s × 120 per cent = 4.8 m/s (Baker, 2011).

ANAEROBIC SYSTEM

In the majority of cases, females have a lower percentage of Type II muscle fibres than males, which has implications when developing speed and power. However, due to their increased percentage of Type I fibres and reliance on the aerobic system, females do not experience the same drop-off in speed and power as males. This has potential implications on recovery time in between intervals and volume of training that can be sustained by female athletes. This information should be used as a guideline; thorough monitoring and knowledge of an individual athlete can be applied to decrease recovery times and increase volume in some cases.

Lactic Anaerobic Power Intervals

The key to the development of anaerobic power is to work at 100 per cent intensity or at the highest possible rate for the duration of the work interval. Intervals can be 20–40 seconds in duration and recovery should be 1–3 minutes between repetitions or if using heart rate, a reduction to 110–130 bpm. The number of repetitions in a set should be 3–4 with at least 6–10 minutes between sets. As mentioned earlier, to develop power the athlete needs to keep the intensity high whilst maintaining quality. In order to do this the athlete requires adequate recovery between repetitions and sets. The aim is to try to avoid fatigue, which prevents high-intensity exercise. This type of training increases the enzymes involved in anaerobic glycolysis developing the muscles' ability to work anaerobically.

Lactic Anaerobic Capacity Intervals

When developing lactic capacity as opposed to lactic power, key differences are evident in the work:rest ratios of the exercise intervals. During lactic power intervals, the body is trying to produce energy as quickly as possible. Lactic capacity intervals are about developing the ability to produce energy for as long as possible. The aim is now to develop the buffering mechanisms involved in allowing anaerobic glycolysis to continue. Exercise intervals now increase to 40–90 seconds with 1–2 minutes between repetitions. Similarly to lactic power training, the athlete should complete 3–4 repetitions per set but with a shorter 5–6 minutes between sets.

When training the above energy systems, specificity of the activities used needs to be considered in relation to the sport being trained for. For example, if the sport involves running then running-based activities can enable peripheral adaptations relevant to sports performance. However if developing these systems as part of the general physical preparation period of training, athletes may choose to add some variety with the use of different modalities. A popular and effective means of creating this variety may be to use circuit training. When performing circuit training, athletes should predominantly utilize exercises that require multi-joint movements and are primarily explosive. For example squat jumps, kettlebell swings, medicine ball throws, tyre flips or sled pushing. Work:rest ratios are as above for developing the specific adaptation you require.

Alactic Anaerobic Power Intervals

As discussed earlier, the alactic system is the body's most powerful and immediate way of producing energy. In most sports, the ability to produce power determines the outcome or the key moments that influence the result. The aim of this type of training is to improve the maximum rate of ATP-PC regeneration through the alactic system by increasing the amount of alactic enzymes involved in its energy production.

When training this system, the intensity of exercise should be maximal for a period of no longer than 7–10 seconds. Rest periods should allow this system to recover fully, ranging from 2–5 minutes, or utilizing heart rate to judge recovery status. A benchmark heart rate value such as 120 beats per minute could be used to indicate that the athlete has recovered sufficiently to begin the next exercise bout. Session volume should be relatively low; for example, 2 sets of 5–6 repetitions. The better the athlete's conditioning becomes, the quicker they will recover between maximal efforts. Any training at lower intensities than this will not stimulate the desired adaptations to alactic anaerobic power.

Quality is the key and this type of training should be performed one to three times per week. This training is particularly taxing on the central nervous system and neuro-muscular system. Regular monitoring of the athlete's neuro-muscular system should be performed before training to assess their readiness. See section on monitoring for ways to assess this system.

Alactic Anaerobic Capacity Intervals

The aim of this type of training is to improve the amount of stored phosphocreatine. Intensity still needs to be 100 per cent and the work intervals are 7–10 seconds. The difference is rest between efforts is now 30–90 seconds and the number of repetitions per set is 10–12 for a total of 2–3 sets with 5–6 minutes between sets. This is more challenging than alactic power training as fatigue will accumulate and focus still needs to be on the quality of repetitions.

A DIFFERENT PERSPECTIVE ON TRAINING TO IMPROVE ANAEROBIC CONDITIONING

Limiting factors to maximal high-intensity exercise are peak power-producing capability and the intensity associated with maximal aerobic capacity (Martin, 2014). Considering this, to train peak power, the athlete should complete high-intensity intervals under 10 seconds in duration combined with high-intensity aerobic intervals of 3–10 minutes. This would completely miss training the glycolytic system (30–60 seconds). Advantages to this approach are physiologically limiting the negative adaptations to the heart through training at high pressures induced by glycolytic training; sessions are tolerable allowing the athlete to train at higher intensities more frequently without feeling nauseous. Psychologically, athletes are able to carry out training without fearing the negative consequences.

This approach fits well with athletes who are involved in team sports, which rely heavily on the alactic and aerobic system due to their multi-sprint activities over 80–90 minutes. It may also suit female athletes better, based on their physiological characteristics.

TRAINING TO IMPROVE MOVEMENT ECONOMY

The development of strength and rate of force production are of particular importance to the conditioning programme of female athletes.

Strength

To develop strength we need to be lifting loads in excess of our 85 per cent of one repetition maximum. Generally in the region of three to five repetitions, however research has shown that females may be able to perform more repetitions with a given percentage of their one repetition maximum than male athletes (Nuckols, 2015). Using compound or multi-joint exercises, for example squats, deadlifts or derivatives of the snatch and clean and jerk, with particular attention given to sets/reps and work/rest ratios, to get the specific adaptations we require. Table 4.3 provides a simple framework to develop a strength-training programme.

Rate of Force Production

Once an athlete has established a strength base (the ability to produce force), the training objective may switch to increasing the rate at which they can produce this force. One of the best ways to achieve this is by using explosive exercises, in particular movements that are

Number of Exercises	Sets	Reps	Rest	Load
3–5	3–5	3–5	3–5 minutes	>85% of 1RM

Table 4.3 Strength training framework.

plyometric in nature. These explosive movements should involve a fast eccentric (lengthening) action immediately and rapidly followed by a concentric (shortening) action. The time between the eccentric and concentric actions is the amortization phase (indicated by ground contact time), which should be as short as possible.

When introducing this type of training into an athlete's programme it is important that this is done gradually, starting with lower-level rebound movements, such as pogos, developing the stiffness of the musculotendinous unit and reducing contact time. Programming needs to take into account the intensity of the exercise, sets, reps and work:rest ratios. The quality and intensity of movement must be prioritized rather than volume, to create the desired training adaptation. For female athletes, it is particularly important that correct landing mechanics are coached throughout plyometric training.

TESTING AND MONITORING

When undertaking any training programme it is important to benchmark the starting point with regards to the current level of conditioning of the athlete. This provides a baseline from which to develop the training programme so that interventions can be targeted appropriately. Ongoing monitoring throughout the training process to assess development of the energy systems and that the athlete is adapting as hoped is also best practice. All the information gathered enables informed decisions about any programme changes that may be required.

When selecting any conditioning test, it should be specific, for example does it measure the physical quality intended? Is it valid (does it measure what it claims)? Is it reliable (can it be used consistently) and objective (does it produce a consistent result if carried out by a different tester)?

The following outlines some tests that can be used to assess the function of the different energy systems.

Aerobic Tests

- Multi-stage fitness test
- Yo-Yo Intermittent Endurance Test
- Cooper run
- MAS 5-minute run.

Anaerobic Tests

Capacity:
- Wingate
- RAST-running-based anaerobic sprint test.

Power:
- Ten-second repeated jump test
- Counter movement jump
- Standing long jump
- Sprint tests, such as 10m acceleration, 40m top speed.

Monitoring

During any training session, it is important to be able to quantify the intensity that the athlete is working at, determining the specific system to be developed. Methods for monitoring training load can be objective (heart rate) or subjective (questionnaires), both can provide reliable information. They also measure internal (heart rate variability, heart rate) and external load (GPS, jump tests). All can produce valuable information, which can inform the training programme.

The ability to quantify the stress placed on the athlete is important in optimizing the dose-response relationship. Greater understanding of the dose-response relationship informs the volume and intensity of training needed plus recovery required for adaptation to occur. Keeping an accurate record of the sets/reps, work:rest ratios allows the modulation of training load on a daily basis; it also enables the planning of different training loads over a micro/meso and macro cycles.

Heart rate (HR) monitoring is an effective tool for quantifying prolonged sub-maximal exercise intensities but is of limited value during maximal or very high-intensity short duration (sprint) exercise intervals. If using heart rate as a guide, it is essential that an individual peak heart rate value used to calculate any percentages of max heart rate (HRmax) as generic estimates of HRmax are likely to be inaccurate for the individual athlete.

In the context of 'all-out' or very high-intensity exercise intervals, rating of perceived exertion (RPE) may be effective for intensity prescription. Following a period of familiarization, athletes are normally able to use RPE as a meaningful method of describing exercise intensity with reasonable consistency regarding how strenuous the exercise feels (Borg, 1998). High-intensity exercise fatigues both the central nervous system (CNS) and the neuro-muscular system. Simple methods to assess neuro-muscular fatigue are the jump test, such as the counter movement jump (CMJ) or standing long jump, carried out daily before training or at the start of the week. If a drop of 10 per cent is observed from their personal best, this is indicating there is some fatigue and the intensity of the subsequent training session should be considered.

The use of questionnaires can be highly effective in monitoring the stress placed on the athlete, not just from training but from daily life. It is often forgotten that external factors to training can not only influence quality of training, but also recovery. You don't have to design your own questionnaire (there are plenty available such as daily analysis of life demands for athletes, DALDA) but simply recording the level of delayed onset muscle soreness (DOMS), hours of sleep and how the athlete feels on the day will help form a picture of the individual's current state of readiness to train.

The above are relatively inexpensive ways of monitoring training load and are available to most people to use. Methods that are more expensive include GPS/accelerometers and heart rate variability, which have become very popular in a range of professional sports contexts. GPS can be used to measure the external load placed on the body through training. It records the total distance covered, number of sprints made and the velocities run at. This gives an objective measure of the load placed on that athlete for the training session. As mentioned, GPS measures external load on the body, it does not measure internal load. For example, there could be two athletes A and B, who have both covered the same distance and number of sprints in a training session. Athlete A has fully recovered the following day, but athlete B has not. Just measuring the external load placed on the athletes does not provide enough information about the readiness of both athletes to train the following day.

Heart rate variability measures the beat-to-beat intervals of the heart. From this information, it is possible to measure the functional state of the autonomic nervous system (ANS). Earlier in this chapter, the role of the ANS in the regulation of the sympathetic and parasympathetic nervous system were outlined. In a fully recovered athlete, you would expect to see these in balance and ready to train, as with athlete A. In athlete B's case we would see the sympathetic system being dominant, indicating they had not fully recovered.

The methods chosen to monitor an athlete's physical state and progress may well depend upon the budget available. It does not matter what method is chosen, it is how the data is used that will impact upon the athlete's progression. The data is there to inform decisions about planning and the readiness of the athlete to train.

PERIODIZATION OF METABOLIC CONDITIONING

When planning for effective energy system development we need to understand the demands of the sport, then the needs of the individual athlete. Developing the energy systems is a continual process running through each stage of the season. Table 4.4 provides an overview of the different phases of a competitive season and outlines the types of conditioning work that are most relevant in each phase of it.

General Physical Preparation

The goal of this phase is about preparing the athlete for the more specific training that will come later in the programme. Depending on the sport, the duration of this period varies; the goal remains the same. The type of activities

FOOTBALL PLAYER

Focus on developing cardiac output 3–4 times per week for 40 mins low intensity. Resistance training 2 times per week focusing on strength development.

utilized may vary as they do not need to replicate movements from the sport, allowing the body to recover. For example if the sport involves weight bearing and the goal is to develop cardiac output, the athlete may want to train on a bike to give their joints a rest. Understanding of the sport will dictate how to approach this phase; is it aerobic, anaerobic dominant or does it require both?

Sport Specific Preparation

The energy systems trained and the movements used are now more specific to the sport. The coach and athlete should now be

General Physical Preparation (GPP) Off Season	Sport Specific Preparation (SSP) Early Preseason	Pre-Competition Late Preseason	Competition In Season
• Aim is to develop a general base the focus being primarily on central adaptations.	• Energy systems trained based on the demands of the sport.	• Increase in specific work capacity in preparation for competition.	• Playing the sport is the main training. • Highly specific to competition.
• Training is not sports specific movements. • A period for the athlete to recover from the competitive season	• Movements become more sport specific. Using same muscle groups.	• Drills from the sport used to condition.	• Training that is non-specific used as accessory work.

Table 4.4 Organization of conditioning around a competition season.

> **FOOTBALL PLAYER**
>
> Moderate to high intensity including threshold training 2 times per week: 4x4mins work/3 mins rest. Alactic power development 2 times per week: 2x5 20m hill sprints.

looking for peripheral adaptations as well as the central adaptations. Work:rest ratios used now are important to replicate the demands that will be placed on the athlete through the sport. The intensity has increased along with the number of sessions per week.

Pre-Competition

This period is increasingly more specific to the sport. Sport-specific drills are the focus for conditioning the energy systems. Work:rest ratios now replicate the demands of the sport. This is to maximize the effect of the energy system development to improve performance.

> **FOOTBALL PLAYER**
>
> Moderate- to high-intensity conditioning training now changes to sport-specific drills and small-sided games.
> Resistance training 2 times per week; focus is now on developing power.

Competition

During this phase, it is about managing the athlete so that they are ready to perform. Conditioning work is through sport-specific training and the frequency depends on the

> **FOOTBALL PLAYER**
>
> Conditioning maintained through small-sided games, frequency dictated by game schedule.
> Resistance training 1–2 times per week, focusing on power and maintaining strength.
> Resistance training 2 times per week focusing on strength development.

number of competitive games. The challenge is finding the right balance to ensure the athlete is ready to compete without fatiguing them.

SUMMARY

Optimizing sporting performance requires an excellent understanding of the demands of the sport being performed. In particular, how the body provides energy and putting together a training plan to develop the different systems to achieve optimal performance. This requires starting with general physical preparation right through to the competitive season. Primary focus in training tends to be on strength/power development. Strength and power do not exist in isolation; to be able to use these qualities effectively the athlete needs to be able to supply the energy to sustain them. Each phase of the training plan should build on the previous, developing the athlete to be able to tolerate greater workloads. Moving from general to sport-specific training enables the athlete to perform at their best.

This chapter has discussed how the body adapts to the stresses placed upon it through training. Creating both central and peripheral adaptations, which are highly specific to the training stimulus (SAID principle; specific adaptations to imposed demands). It is important to understand this in order to plan appropriate training methods to develop the desired energy systems. As has been identified, there are some key physiological differences between female and male athletes. A knowledge of these key differences can enable improved planning and the effective prescription of training programmes. In particular, female athletes use more fat to provide fuel for energy at any given exercise intensity and they are more resistant to fatigue; consequently they may have the ability to tolerate higher relative workloads.

REFERENCES

Baker, D. (2011) Recent trends in high-intensity aerobic training for field sports. *Professional Strength and Conditioning*, 22, 3–8.

Billat, V., and Koralsztein, J.P. (1996) Significance of the velocity at O2max and time to exhaustion at this velocity. *Sports Medicine*, 22, 90–108.

Brown, M. (2017) The Longer the Race, the Stronger we Get. Outside Online. https://www.outsideonline.com/2169856/longer-race-stronger-we-get [accessed April 2017].

Buchheit, M. (2008) The 30–15 Intermittent Fitness Test: Accuracy for individualizing interval training of young intermittent sport players. *Journal of Strength and Conditioning Research*, 22(2), 365–374.

Buchheit, M. and Laursen, P.B. (2013) High intensity interval training, solutions to the programming puzzle. Part I: Cardiopulmonary emphasis. *Sports Medicine,* 43, 313–338.

Buchheit, M., and Laursen, P.B. (2013) High intensity interval training, solutions to the programming puzzle. Part II: Anaerobic energy, neuromuscular load and practical applications. *Sports Medicine*, 43, 927–954.

Clemente, F.M. *et al.* (2014) Developing aerobic and anaerobic fitness using small-sided soccer games: Methodological proposals. *Strength and Conditioning Journal,* 36(3), 76–87.

Copeland, J.L. *et al.* (2002) Hormonal responses to endurance and resistance exercise in females aged 19–69 years. *Journal of Gerontology: Biological Sciences* 57A(4), B158–B165.

Dupont, G. *et al.* (2002) Critical velocity and time spent at a high level of O2 for short intermittent runs at supramaximal velocities. *Canadian Journal of Applied Physiology*, 27, 103–115.

Eliakim, A. *et al.* (2014) Effect of gender on the GH-IGF-T response to anaerobic exercise in young adults. *Journal of Strength and Conditioning Research*, 28(12), 3411–3415.

http://circimaging.ahajournals.org/search?author1=Flavio+D per centE2 per cent80 per cent99Ascenziandsortspec=dateandsubmit=Submit *et al.* (2014) Morphological and Functional Adaptation of Left and Right Atria Induced by Training in Highly Trained Female Athletes. *Circulation: Cardiovascular Imaging*, 7, 222–229.

Gastin, P.B. (2001) Energy system interaction and relative contribution during maximal exercise. *Sports Medicine*, 31(10), 725–741.

Gist, N.H. *et al.* (2014) Sprint interval training effects on aerobic capacity: A systematic review and meta-analysis. *Sports Medicine,* 44(2), 269–279.

Halouani, J. *et al.* (2014) Small-sided games in team sports training: A brief review. *Journal of Strength and Conditioning Research*, 28(12), 3594–3618.

Heavens, K.R. *et al.* (2014) The effects of high intensity short rest resistance exercise on muscle damage markers in men and women. *Journal of Strength and Conditioning Research*, 28(4), 1041–1049.

Jamieson, J. (2009) Ultimate MMA Conditioning. 8WeeksOut Media.

Jamieson J. 8 Weeks Out http://www.8weeksout.com/2011/10/10/ research-review-energy-systems-interval-training-rsa [accessed April 2017]

Keller, M. *et al.* (2011) Supraspinal fatigue is similar in men and women for a low-force fatiguing contraction. *Medicine and Science in Sports and Exercise*, 43(10), 1873–1883.

Laurent, C.M. *et al.* (2014) Sex-specific responses to self-paced high-intensity interval training with variable recovery periods. *Journal of Strength and Conditioning Research*. 28(4), 920–927.

Lee, M.G. *et al.* (2008) Effects of continuous exercise, accumulation of short duration exercise, and resistance exercise on blood pressure, vascular elasticity, and blood variables after exercise. *Korean Journal of Sport Science*. 19, 21–36.

Martin, D. (2014) Chapter 14: Generating Anaerobic Power. *In High Performance Training for Sports*, 4767–5089. Human

Kinetics.

Meckel, Y. et al. (2014) Repeated sprint ability in young soccer players at different game stages. Journal of Strength and Conditioning Research, 28(9), 2578–2584.

Nuckols, G. (2015) Gender Differences in Training and Metabolism. Stronger By Science https://www.strongerbyscience.com/gender-differences-in-training-and-diet/ [accessed April 2017]

Pate, R. and Kiuska, A. (1984). Physiological basis of the sex difference in cardiorespiratory endurance. Sports Medicine, 1, 87–98.

Pettit, R.W. and Clark, E. (2013) High-intensity exercise tolerance: An update on bioenergetics and assessment. Strength and Conditioning Journal, 35(2), 11–16.

Selye, H. (1984) The Stress of Life, revised edition. The McGraw-Hill Companies Inc.

Turner, A.N. and Stewart, P.F. (2013) Repeat sprint ability. Strength and Conditioning Journal, 35(1), 37–46.

Smith, D., and Fernhall, B. (2011) Advanced Cardiovascular Exercise Physiology. Human Kinetics.

Verkhoshansky, Y.U. (1966) Perspectives in the development of speed-strength preparation in the development of jumpers. Track and Field, (9), 11–12.

Voight, M. et al. (1995) The influence of tendon Young's modulus, dimensions and instantaneous moment arms on the efficiency of human movement. Journal of Biomechanics, 28, 281–291.

Zamparo, P. and Swaine, I.L. (2012) Mechanical and propelling efficiency in swimming derived from exercise using a laboratory-based whole-body swimming ergometer. Journal of Applied Physiology, 113, 584–594.

CHAPTER 5
MOBILITY FOR PERFORMANCE IN FEMALE ATHLETES

Debby Sargent, MSc,PGDip, ASCC,
University of Gloucestershire, UK

Flexibility is a measurable quality most commonly defined as the absolute range of motion (ROM) achievable at a joint or series of joints (McNeal and Sands, 2006), which can have static and dynamic components (Jeffreys, 2016, p.320; Siff, 2003, p.182). *The Collins English Dictionary* (2017) defines the word flexible as being 'able to be bent easily without breaking' and some definitions of flexibility make reference to the fact that this joint range of motion is adequate to prevent injury to the surrounding structures (Alter, 2004, p.2) and as such, should be a pain-free range of motion (McNeal and Sands, 2006; Alter; 2004, p.2; Sands *et al.*, 2016a, p.388; Marek *et al.*, 2005).

Despite the fact that sufficient flexibility plays a key role in athletic movement ability and is often a required outcome from a number of different training modalities, it has been suggested that flexibility is a largely inadequately appreciated quality and misunderstood by coaches and researchers (Siff, 2003). Sporting actions involve the optimal amount of neuromuscular coordination, control (motor skill) and interaction of a number of different physical qualities such as flexibility, strength, endurance and speed (Siff, 2003). This concept is expressed in Siff's pyramidal model (see Fig. 5.1, 2003) of musculoskeletal fitness. The central positioning of flexibility at the base of the pyramid highlights both the importance

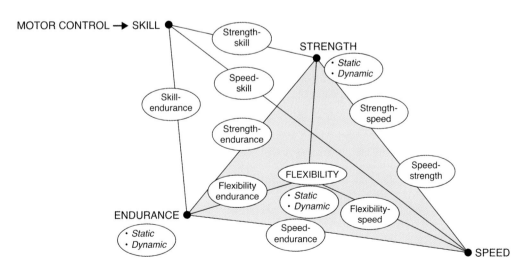

Fig. 5.1 Pyramidal model of the major elements of musculoskeletal fitness. (Adapted from Siff, 2003, p91)

of flexibility and its pivotal role in an athlete's ability to display any of the other major elements of fitness (Siff, 2003, p.91).

The inability of the term 'flexibility' to adequately describe an athlete's ability to move in a more functional sense has seen the introduction of the alternative term, 'mobility', and a deliberate attempt to differentiate between flexibility and mobility. Mobility has been defined by some authors as 'the ability to move joints fluidly through a full range of motion' (Heyward, 1984; Jeffreys, 2007). Others have described it as the 'athlete's ability to function and reach desired positions during activity, being heavily dependent upon stability and proper coordination of multiple joints functioning simultaneously' (Brooks and Cressey, 2013). In athletic populations mobility may be a more important performance goal, rather than pure flexibility (McNeal and Sands, 2016a; Knapp, 2016).

The purpose of this chapter is to first describe the mechanisms underpinning the theorized positive and negative effects of flexibility and/or mobility training on performance and injury outcomes, and second, to explore and evaluate methods currently used for measuring and training range of motion/mobility, addressing specific considerations for female athletes where possible.

FACTORS LIMITING RANGE OF MOTION IN THE FEMALE ATHLETE

All structures located within and over a joint influence the available ROM, including the structure of the joint, extensibility of the musculotendinous unit (MTU), skin, vascular structures, joint capsule and ligaments (Guissard and Duchateau, 2006). Measures of both static and dynamic flexibility are affected by these structures, which also act to resist an imposed stretch to the joints (Siff, 2003; Moir, 2016).

Restructuring the articular surfaces of the joint is generally not regarded as a practical means of increasing ROM (Siff, 2003), although adaptive structural changes to the joint may be a natural consequence of long-term exposure to loaded, full-range, sport-specific movement patterns (Borsa et al., 2007; Crockett et al., 2002; Challoumas et al., 2017). Adolescent club swimmers are reported to accumulate around 40,000m of swim volume per week for an extended 11-month period (Hibberd and Myers, 2013). Given that this does not include weight training and other land-based activity, it should be no surprise that the extreme physiological demands and overhead training load could potentially alter the physical characteristics of the swimmers as the upper extremities adapt to the training demands (Hibberd and Myers, 2013).

Joint Laxity

Joint laxity relates to a lack of stability of a joint, defined as 'abnormal movement of a joint that will not support normal load' (Falsone, 2004, p.61). Whilst joint laxity may confer a competitive advantage in sports that require extreme ranges of movement, increased laxity that is inherited and/or acquired through years of stretching or sport-specific training is associated with an increased injury potential (Gannon and Bird, 1999; Myer et al., 2008). In a study by Gannon and Bird (1999), they not only evidenced a greater laxity of females compared to males, but they also demonstrated a graded increase in laxity when they compared a general sporting group, through novice gymnasts to dancers and then to international gymnasts. Since laxity is more influenced by the ligaments and capsular structures that surround the joint (Nawata et al., 1999), stretching of these structures may destabilize the joint and increase injury risk and should be avoided.

It is generally accepted that the gender differences in ACL injury risk can be partially explained by a greater anterior knee joint laxity in females (Hewett et al., 2007). A systematic review (Hewett et al., 2007), proposed that ACL injury risk was more prevalent during the first half of the menstrual cycle during the time period between menses and ovulation, when oestrogen concentrations are significantly elevated (Hewett et al., 2007). Whilst this is useful information, the large individual variability inherent within the menstrual cycle (Vescovi, 2011) means that accurately determining oestrogen status in female athletes is difficult at best. Moreover, as a coach working with female athletes, unless you are working with elite performers, monitoring of menstrual cycles is not typical and tends to be targeted to those athletes at risk of menstrual cycle abnormalities (for example amenorrhea). There is also further evidence suggesting that an increased knee joint laxity might not necessarily change knee mechanics across the menstrual cycle, so coaching observations within sessions may not indicate periods of increased laxity (Park et al., 2009). Therefore, the priority for female athletes displaying laxity tendencies is firstly, to ensure they have adequate strength to control their ROM; secondly, to continue to provide adequate supervision and coaching to maintain 'good' techniques and lastly to avoid programming exercise that could further increase laxity (such as static and PNF stretching).

Given that adaptations to the skeletal structures of the joint are not an intentional target for improving range of motion in female athletes, in practice this means that attention must be directed elsewhere, typically the extension of the musculotendinous unit (MTU). For the purpose of this chapter, MTU extensibility is defined as the 'ability of a muscle to extend to a predetermined endpoint' (Weppler and Magnusson 2010), which is most often based on athlete sensation. Several mechanical theories (viscoelastic and plastic deformation, neuromuscular relaxation, increased sarcomeres in series) and more recently, a sensory theory, have been proposed to explain observed increases in muscle extensibility following training (Weppler and Magnusson, 2010; Sands and McNeal, 2016a).

Viscoelastic and Plastic Deformation

When stretched slowly, the MTU exhibits time-dependent viscoelasticity. Stress relaxation refers to a decline in the peak resistive force of an MTU when stretched and held at a constant length (McNair et al., 2000; Gadjosik et al., 2006), whereas creep refers to an increase in MTU length in response to a constantly applied force (Ryan et al., 2010; Sobolewski et al., 2014). For example, if an athlete performs a lying straight leg hamstring stretch they will flex at the hip to take the hamstring to its end of ROM. If they hold the stretch at the same level of hip flexion for an extended period of time, the muscle will relax and the perceived intensity of the stretch will decrease (stress-relaxation). If they perform the same stretch, but this time move the leg into greater hip flexion once the stress-relaxation response has occurred, to maintain the feeling of discomfort, this is an example of creep. If the MTU is extended rapidly it will resist the stretch, rather than display properties of stress relaxation or creep (Alter, 2004). There are numerous papers evidencing viscoelastic responses in the MTU post-stretching (Kubo et al., 2001; Kubo et al., 2002: Guisard and Duchateau, 2004; Mahieu et al., 2007; Nakamura et al., 2012; Sobolewski et al., 2014; Blazevich et al., 2012), but there are also a significant number of researchers disputing these effects (Hoge et al., 2010; Konrad and Tilp, 2014a; Gajdosik et al., 2005; Magnusson et al., 1996, Folpp et al., 2006; Magnusson et al., 2000; Cornwell et al., 2002).

A theoretical passive tension-length, or stress-strain curve of an MTU being stretched

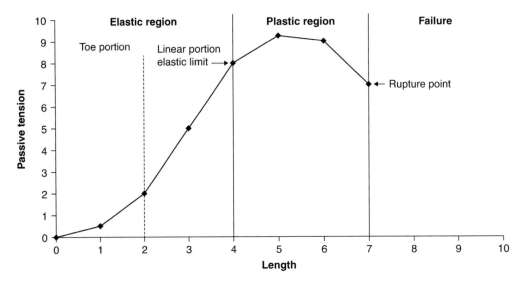

Fig. 5.2 Theoretical illustration of the passive length/tension curve for a musculotendinous unit (MTU). The elastic region begins at the initial length and ends at the elastic limit. In the plastic region, permanent deformation of the MTU will occur with application of tensile force beyond the elastic limit. Failure or rupture point is the last point on the curve. The length attained at the rupture point is the maximum length of the MTU. (Adapted from Weppler & Magnusson, 2010)

to failure is shown in Fig. 5.2. If the MTU is stretched within the elastic limit it will return to its normal resting length once the stretch is removed (Weppler and Magnusson, 2010; Stone *et al.*, 2006). However, if the MTU is stretched beyond the elastic limit, changes to the connective tissue elements of the MTU will be permanent (into the plastic region, see Fig. 5.2) (Weppler and Magnusson, 2010; Stone *et al.*, 2006). In practice, there is a dearth of evidence supporting the opinion that plastic deformation occurs as a result of normal stretching practices (Weppler and Magnusson, 2010).

According to the Hill muscle model (Hill, 1938; see 'Strength and Power' chapter), the contractile element is intricately woven together by a parallel elastic component (PEC) (Gadjosik, 2001). When the muscle is relaxed the PEC is responsible for the resting tension in the muscle, as well as the passive behaviour of the muscle when it is stretched (Purslow,

1989; Siff, 2004). The perimysium, the connective tissue that surrounds the fasciculus, is thought to be predominantly responsible for the force resisting the stretch when a muscle is stretched beyond its resting length (Purslow, 1989). When a muscle is active the PEC transmits the muscular force to the skeleton (Potach and Chu, 2016). In relation to the component parts of the MTU, passive stretch is thought to have more of a pronounced effect on the PEC (Latash and Zatsiorski, 1993), however, there is a growing body of evidence suggesting that increased tendon compliance is at least partially responsible for increases in MTU extensibility (Herbert *et al.*, 2002; Wilson *et al.*, 1992; Witvrouw, 2004; Ryan *et al.*, 2008; Magnusson *et al.*, 1996a). Differentiating between muscle and tendinous responses to changes in MTU extensibility is essential to our understanding of how increases in passive ROM can impact performance and injury.

Neuromuscular Relaxation

The range of motion available at a joint is not only determined by the mechanical properties of the MTU, but also the degree of muscle activation that acts to resist the imposed stretch (Siff, 2003; Moir, 2016). Voluntary activation of muscle promotes active stiffness, an essential quality for athletic performance. This will not be discussed in this chapter. However, involuntary muscle activation, through stimulation of muscle spindles and Golgi tendon organs (GTOs), is traditionally considered important to explain changes in passive MTU extensibility in response to a number of techniques to increase ROM.

Muscle spindles lie in parallel to the muscle fibres and are responsible for protecting the muscles from stretches that are extreme in terms of the degree of lengthening, the rate of lengthening, or both (Watkins, 1999, pp.237–240). Involuntary, neuromuscular 'stretch reflexes' have been shown to activate in the muscle during short, rapid stretches in the mid-range position, resulting in a contraction of short duration (Chalmers et al., 2004). Slow lengthening of the MTU via static and PNF stretches is not considered to elicit a stretch reflex response (Magnusson, 1996b; Chalmers, 2004) on the basis that minimal surface EMG responses (<1 per cent MVC) have been reported (Herda et al., 2011; Chalmers, 2004).

Golgi tendon organs (GTOs) are another major receptor found at the musculo-tendinous junction (Alter, 2004) that have been implicated in some strategies to increase ROM such as proprioceptive neuromuscular facilitation (PNF) stretching. Because of their location, GTOs are extremely sensitive to change in tension in the associated muscle fibres (Alter, 2004) and if activated can reduce the excitability of contracting muscle. This process, which causes an increase in the extensibility of the MTU, is termed autogenic inhibition (Sharman et al., 2006). Despite traditional beliefs, it has been proposed that GTO reflex activation is not operational in proprioceptive neuromuscular facilitation (PNF) techniques (Sharman et al., 2006).

Gender Differences in Viscoelastic Properties of the MTU (passive stiffness)

Stiffness refers to the extent of the resistance offered by the MTU in response to lengthening (Fouré et al., 2011). Changes in MTU stiffness reported after controlled stretching techniques (SS and PNF) are thought to occur directly via viscoelastic relaxation, but more ballistic techniques could, in theory, alter stiffness indirectly through reflexive responses in the MTU.

Passive MTU stiffness is calculated by a change in tension per unit change in length (Stone et al., 2006; Weppler and Magnusson, 2010; Ryan et al., 2008) with an increase in MTU stiffness being demonstrated by a leftward shift in the tension/length curve (see Fig. 5.2). Theoretically, a very stiff MTU will record a greater passive tension at the same absolute joint angle and will require more force to stretch it to a given length (Stone et al., 2008; Moir, 2016), potentially inhibiting MTU extensibility.

Passive MTU stiffness is influenced by muscle cross-sectional area (CSA) (Weppler and Magnusson, 2010; Magnusson et al., 1997; Ryan et al., 2009; Fouré et al., 2011) and the relative contribution of connective tissue to the MTU complex (Kjaer and Hanson, 2008; Douglas et al., 2015; Fouré et al., 2011). Since females typically demonstrate a lower physiological CSA compared to males (higher muscle volume, fascicle angles, fascicle length and CSA of Type II fibres) (Fouré et al., 2011; Ryan et al., 2009) and are purported to differ in connective tissue physiology (Kjaer and Hanson, 2008), it is entirely possible that female responses to interventions aimed at decreasing MTU passive stiffness and

115

improving MTU extensibility could be different (Gadjosik et al., 2006; Kubo et al., 2003). The mechanisms responsible for differences in connective tissue between genders is not well understood, although oestrogen and other hormonal fluctuations that occur throughout the menstrual cycle have been suggested (Fouré et al., 2011; Knapp, 2016).

STRETCH TOLERANCE

The sensory theory advocates that MTU extensibility can be explained more by a reduced sensation of stretch, discomfort or pain perception at a given ROM (Magnusson et al., 1996b and 1998a; Halbertsma et al., 1996; Weppler and Magnusson, 2010; Folpp et al., 2006; Stone et al., 2006; Konrad and Tilp, 2014a; Hoge et al., 2010), rather than because of any of the suggested mechanical theories. Muscle length increases in response to any of the mechanical mechanisms would produce a long-lasting rightward shift in the passive tension/length curve (see Fig. 5.2). However, several authors have demonstrated that tissue properties remained unchanged after a period of stretching, with only an increase in end-range joint angles and applied tension (Magnusson et al., 1996b and 1998a; Halbertsma et al., 1996; Folpp et al., 2006; Konrad and Tilp, 2014a; Hoge et al., 2010). All synovial joints have four types of receptor nerve endings (Alter 2004). Type III mechanoreceptors are situated within the intrinsic and extrinsic ligaments of the joints and are activated when high tensions are generated in the joint ligaments at the extremes of joint movement (Alter 2004). Type IV nerve endings are nociceptors that become active when articular tissue is placed under discernable mechanical deformation (Alter, 2004; Khals and Ge, 2004). Activation of Type III and IV afferents will increase the sensation of pain in the individual. In a study comparing high-level international athletes (four men, two women), who participated in

one to two intensive training sessions per day, to untrained controls, the nociceptor reflex at rest was higher (P<0.05) in athletes (Guieu et al., 1992). A study comparing gender differences in MTU stiffness and ROM after an acute bout of static stretching (SS) (9 × 135s of constant angle dorsiflexion, 10s rest between stretches) found that females experienced an increase in stretch tolerance, but males did not. This led to the conclusion that 'men may have to stretch for a longer duration or at a greater intensity to achieve similar increases in ROM as women.' (Hoge et al., 2010).

Not surprisingly, comparisons between flexible and non-flexible subjects have shown that not only is the joint angle that provokes a maximal stretch sensation lower for non-flexible subjects (Magnusson et al., 1997), but this is accompanied with lower peak torque and final stiffness measurements. The fact that EMG activity and viscoelastic stress relaxation responses were similar across groups provides evidence to support the sensory theory (Magnusson et al., 1997). In a recent publication (Sands and Neal, 2016a) stretch tolerance was described as 'an ability, therefore, a learned skill regulated by the CNS and PNS, to move a body part through a ROM against the resistance offered by antagonist muscles and associated connective tissues.'

WHY IS FLEXIBILITY IMPORTANT FOR INJURY PREVENTION IN THE FEMALE ATHLETE?

Research suggests that the relationship between flexibility and injury risk is best illustrated as an inverted bell-shaped curve, with individuals at both extremes of the flexibility scale (either very low or very high) coming with a higher injury risk than those with 'average' flexibility (Parrott and Zhu, 2013; Knapik et al., 2001; Hryosomallis, 2013;

Hrysomallis, 2009; Gleim and McHugh, 1997).

Hypomobility, defined as a decrease in the normal range of movement of a joint, can be an adaptive mechanism because of pain (Falsone *et al.*, 2014, p.62), persistent poor posture (perhaps through lifestyle habits) or chronic exposure to sport-specific movements that can lead to more permanent changes to the joint capsule and MTU. Conversely, hypermobility can be defined as an increase in the normal range of movement of a joint (Falsone *et al.*, 2014, p.62). In some sports, particularly aesthetic sports such as gymnastics, diving and dance, there are specific flexibility rules and extreme ROM requirements that go well beyond what is considered a 'normal' ROM (Moir, 2016; p.291). Gymnastics is an early specialization sport, with female gymnasts starting flexibility training at an early age and continuing this practice for potentially decades (Sands *et al.*, 2016b; Steinberg *et al.*, 2012; Gannon and Bird 1999). Some authors have stated (Sands *et al.*, 2016b) that 'flexibility is perhaps the single greatest discriminator of gymnastics from other sports.' The competitive advantage that hypermobility affords in these sports is not necessarily an injury risk provided there is sufficient stability to control the ROM (Sands 2016a; Falsone *et al.*, 2014). It is worth noting that because mobility is joint-specific, athletes often present with both hypo and hypermobility in different joints (Sands 2016b).

A decreased ROM/lack of mobility could lead to overextension injuries where the MTU is stretched beyond its normal active limit into dangerous loading positions (Stone *et al.*, 2006; Parrott and Zhu). Sport-specific demands of repetitive movements on slightly hypomobile joint(s) can cause micro damage to the MTU unit that could lead to overuse injuries such as tendonitis (Parrott and Zhu; Behm *et al.*, 2015). In cases of more extreme degrees of overextension exceeding the elastic limit of the MTU, see Fig. 5.1) this could cause

a partial tear or a complete rupture of the MTU (Stone *et al.*, 2006). Furthermore, in some types of sports, typically combat-based sports, a lack of flexibility can also make it difficult to escape from possible submission attempts (Costa *et al.*, 2011), which could then lead to MTU injuries or others of a more serious nature.

From a muscular standpoint, eccentric strength will provide a protective effect in the prevention of muscle strain injuries (Cleather and Brandon, 2007). Stronger muscles will provide greater energy absorbance before damage occurs (Opar *et al.*, 2012; Comfort *et al.*, 2009; Cleather and Brandon, 2007) and may prevent the limbs moving into dangerous extremes of ROM. A reduction in tendon stiffness can alter the force-length relationship, such that a more compliant tendon would shorten the muscle length for any given joint ROM. At long muscle lengths a more compliant tendon would favourably increase the force-generating capabilities of the muscle (increased capacity for cross bridge attachment), which will have a positive effect on muscle strain injury risk (Behm *et al.*, 2015). Lastly, a more compliant MTU and/or a larger ROM around a joint will also increase the distance and time through which forces can be absorbed so that deceleration forces are absorbed less abruptly and with greater control, further reducing injury potential (McNeal and Sands, 2006; Stojanovic and Ostojic, 2011).

However, most muscle strains typically occur during eccentric loading (muscle activated to resist stretch) within a normal ROM (Cleather and Brandon, 2007; Opar *et al.*, 2012; Comfort *et al.*, 2009). One mechanistic possibility responsible for the non-limit stretch injuries is increased muscle stiffness (Stone *et al.*, 2006; Witvrouw *et al.*, 2004). In a stiff MTU the rate at which the force (stress) resisting the stretch increases faster (see Fig. 5.2), which means that less force can be absorbed before injury of the MTU occurs and that the failure point of the tissue will be reached faster (Stone *et al.*, 2006). A more compliant passive tissue system may have a protective 'cushioning effect' (Witvrouw *et al.*, 2004; Gleim and McHugh, 1999). When a muscle is highly active (eccentric contraction), a more compliant tendon would allow greater absorbance of energy before forces are transmitted to the muscle fibres. This potentially reduces damage to the contractile elements, improving the ability of the MTU to resist strain injuries within the normal ROM (Ryan *et al.*, 2008; McNair *et al.*, 1996).

Although the effect of stretching and other techniques on whole MTU stiffness is not in agreement (Weppler and Magnusson 2010; Ryan *et al.*, 2008; Stojanovic and Ostojic, 2011), a greater understanding of the differential effect on tendon and muscle passive stiffness will further our understanding of ROM in relation to injury risk across a range of sports.

Whilst an increase in ROM is promoted to be injury-reducing, some authors speculate that strategies to increase ROM during warm-up (particularly SS and PNF) may actually increase the chances of injury (Shrier, 2007; Witvrouw *et al.*, 2004). The rationale for these statements is based predominantly around three findings. Firstly, if increases in ROM occur because of an increased stretch tolerance (Weppler and Magnusson, 2010), any stretch-induced increases in ROM may just be 'apparent', rather than 'real' changes. The analgesic effect of stretch tolerance may then encourage athletes to extend limbs more readily into ranges that can potentially damage musculo-tendinous structures. Secondly, voluntary activation of the muscles (central and/or afferent drive) is inhibited, lessening force output post-stretching (Behm *et al.*, 2015). And finally, there is the potential to delay force transmission to the skeleton via decreased tendon stiffness (Harrison-Gill, 2016). All of these effects would adversely affect coordination and co-activation of the muscles around the joints that protect the joint from injury.

FLEXIBILITY AND INJURY RISK – WHAT DOES THE RESEARCH SAY?

Training studies looking at the impact of stretching on sports injury prevention have increased by 15.7 per cent since 2000 (McBain *et al.*, 2011), a lag of approximately ten years since a published review by Shrier (1999) suggested that stretching prior to exercise is unlikely to reduce the risk of injury.

These findings were further confirmed in a recent systematic review (Behm *et al.*, 2015), that reported that static and PNF stretching had no overall effect on all-cause or overuse injuries (lower extremity only), although they did suggest that for activities requiring repetitive contractions (such as sprinting and running) there may be a benefit in reducing acute muscle injuries (Behm *et al.*, 2015). From the six studies that compared stretching and non-stretching groups, the authors calculated a 54 per cent risk-reduction (range of 25–94 per cent) in acute muscle injuries in favour of the stretch condition (Behm *et al.*, 2015). Whilst an increased range of movement resulting from stretching could be assumed to reduce certain types of muscle strain and sprain injuries, as previously discussed sports injuries are multirisk phenomena (Parkkari *et al.*, 2001). Numerous reviews (Schmitt *et al.*, 2012; Konstantinuous *et al.*, 2010; Prior *et al.*, 2009; Comfort *et al.*, 2009; McCall *et al.*, 2014; Nicholas and Tyler, 2002; Opar *et al.*, 2012; Heiderscheit, 2005; Gleim and McHugh, 1997; Baxter *et al.*, 2017; Witvrouw *et al.*, 2004; Magnusson and Renstrom, 2006; Konstantinuous *et al.*, 2010) and prospective studies (Owen *et al.*, 2013; Orchard *et al.*, 1997; Watsford *et al.*, 2010) often consider muscle strength, strength imbalances, and stiffness (energy storage/dissipation) qualities as strong predictors of muscle strain injury, with the relationship between ROM and injury being less clear. Moreover, if increases in ROM only occur because of an increased stretch tolerance (Weppler and Magnusson, 2010), any stretch-induced increases in ROM may not be expected to help reduce injury risk, depending on the mechanism of injury. For muscle strain injuries that are considered to be load dependent, rather than length dependent (Cleather and Brandon; Hrysomallis, 2013; Hrysomallis; 2009), it is logical that stretching per se may not prompt the breadth of adaptations required to significantly affect the relevant muscle-strain risk factors.

Muscle strain and sprain type injuries are common in female athletes (Knapp, 2016; Yang et al., 2012; Dick et al., 2007; Barber Foss et al., 2014; Steinberg et al., 2011; Clarsen et al., 2014; Marshall et al., 2007), just like they are in male athletic populations (Hrysomallis, 2013; Theriault and Lachance, 1998; King et al., 2014). A descriptive epidemiological study of 573 male and female NCAA Division I athletes, participating in 16 collegiate sports teams during the 2005–2008 season, concluded that more than 29.3 per cent of all injuries (1317) were overuse injuries, with female athletes having a higher rate of overuse injuries, compared to the male athletes (24.6 vs 13.3 per 10,000 athlete exposures) (Yang et al., 2012).

There is evidence to support the 'bell-shaped' curve of injury in relation to the extremes of joint ROM in female athletic populations. In a cross-sectional study involving thirty-four (eleven female athletes) competitive flatwater kayakers (Johansson et al., 2015), those that reported shoulder pain during the last season (45 per cent of subjects) had significantly lower internal rotation (p=0.009) than those who reported no pain. When an additional seventeen kayakers who were currently 'pain-free', but had experienced shoulder pain earlier than the previous season were included in the analysis,

significantly lower values of internal rotation remained in the pain group compared to those athletes who had never experienced pain (p=0.017). A study looking at the association between joint range of movement and patellofemoral pain in 1,359 female dancers (Steinberg et al., 2012), found that those who demonstrated hypomobility were at significantly less risk of developing patellofemoral pain than those with average ROM in ankle plantarflexion (p=0.001) and ankle/foot pointe (p=0.001), hip external rotation (p=0.014), abduction (p=0.001) and extension (p=0.000), lumbar back and hamstrings (p=0/000). Since joint ROM is typically higher in dancers than the normal population (Kadel et al., 2005) it could be implied that an average ROM for dancers infers a level of hypermobility in a normal population. In contrast, a study looking at injury prediction in female competitive gymnasts (Steel et al., 1986) showed no link between hypermobility and injury, although five independent variables (non-related to ROM measures) were suggested to be able to predict 'high risk' gymnasts with reasonable confidence (70 per cent). A prospective study looking at the relationship between pre-season ROM and muscle strain injury in thirty-six elite male soccer players found that those players who sustained a strain injury in the hip and knee flexors demonstrated lower pre-season ROM (p<0.05) than non-injured players in these muscle groups (Bradley and Portas, 2007).

Whilst these studies demonstrate some relationship between ROM and injury risk, we also know that there are multiple ways of developing ROM. Training interventions typically looking at ROM often refer to the effects of stretching on injury risk. What is not clear about this is whether those stretching are doing so because they are already injured, or because it is a normal part of their practice. Previous injury is a key confounding variable in these types of studies, which is not often considered (Shrier, 2007), plus stretching practice is not necessarily synonymous with ROM, meaning that some athletes display a large ROM, but spend little time stretching and vice versa. At the beginning of the chapter, we also recognized that flexibility and mobility are distinctly different qualities, suggesting that stretching alone may confer no benefit to injury prevention. Several researchers are now investigating multifactorial neuromuscular training strategies, which target injury prevention (Herman *et al.*, 2012; Andrews *et al.*, 2013), that typically involve a warm-up including sport-specific agility drills, landing techniques, balance exercises, strengthening and stretching. Young female football players who have adopted the FIFA 11+ prevention strategy have shown significant reductions in overall (RR 0.67, CI 0.32-0.72) and overuse (RR 0.45, CI 0.28-0.71) lower limb injuries as well as knee injuries (RR 0.48, CI 0.32 -0.72) (Soligard *et al.*, 2008).

WHY IS FLEXIBILITY IMPORTANT FOR SPORTS PERFORMANCE IN FEMALE ATHLETES?

Massiss (2009) suggested that establishing a greater ROM about a joint(s) in already powerful athletes may be the 'missing piece of the power jigsaw'. This statement is based on two biomechanical principles of work and power (Knudson, 2009; Haff and Nimphius, 2012). Work is the application of force to move an object from a start point to an end point (Work = Force × Distance travelled; Haff and Nimphius, 2012), whilst power is the ability to do a certain amount of work over a period of time (Power = Work/Time; Knudson, 2009). This means that a female athlete with a greater movement arc (ROM from full flexion to full extension) will be able to apply a force over a greater distance (therefore perform more work) than a female athlete with a lesser ROM.

If these athletes are comparable in strength terms, this means that the athlete with a greater ROM will be able to make better use of their current force-generating capacities (do more work) than the athlete with less ROM, provided the task does not constrain the window of time available to apply force (for example, stretch-shortening cycle activities). Similarly, if an athlete is able to do more work because of an increased ROM, by definition, they will be able to generate a greater power output. Populations of athletes that may benefit from the work and power advantages afforded by an increased ROM would be those involved in throwing (Borsa *et al.*, 2008) and kicking events (Akbulut and Agopyan, 2015).

Stretch-shortening cycle (SSCs) activities are an intrinsic component of most sporting performances and are generally considered to be an 'energy saving' mechanism (Witvrouw *et al.*, 2004; Turner *et al.*, 2010). Stretching of the SEC prior to shortening enhances performance (Wilson and Flanagan, 2008; Turner *et al.*, 2010; Wilson *et al.*, 2008) via a process of storage and release of mechanical work (elastic energy) and activation of the neural stretch reflex, induced by muscle spindle activation (Carter *et al.*, 2015; Wilson and Flanagan, 2008). MTU stiffness is strongly correlated to a decreased ground contact time in SSC-type activities leading to a larger release of elastic energy, which has been stored in the eccentric phase of the movement. MTU stiffness also improves force transmission because in order for muscular contraction to produce movement, the force generated by the muscle must first be transmitted to the SEC. The slack must be taken out of the SEC before the contractile force is transmitted to the skeletal system, a time lag known as the electromechanical delay (EMD) (Watsford *et al.*, 2010; Wilson *et al.*, 1994; Costa *et al.*, 2012). A more compliant MTU would increase the EMD (Hoge *et al.*, 2010; Van Hooren and Bosch, 2016), which could have a detrimental effect on performances that require a rapid rate of force development. Although there is a lack of clarity around whether stretching can either increase or decrease MTU compliance (Weppler and Magnusson, 2010) there is the additional consideration that females may already demonstrate a lower MTU stiffness as previously discussed (McMahon et al., 2012; Fouré et al., 2011, Hoge et al., 2010). This means that interventions that reduce MTU stiffness further may have greater adverse consequences for performance outcomes, especially those that involve fast SSCs.

FLEXIBILITY AND SPORTS PERFORMANCE – WHAT DOES THE RESEARCH SAY?

It is obvious that in sports such as diving and gymnastics, the individuals who participate in these require much greater ROM than those involved in other sports such as triathlon and football and it is often cited that females are 'more flexible' than males (Kibler and Chandler, 2003; Kibler et al., 1989). However, the optimal ROM required to improve performance and minimize injury potential in any sport is both joint (Siff, 2004; Moir, 2016; Maffulli et al., 1994; Yoon, 2001; Smith, 2010) and position or discipline specific (such as artisitic vs. rhythmic gymnastics) (Yoon, 2002; Smith, 2010; Johnstone and Ford, 2010). A recent cross-sectional study (Slater et al., 2016) on 343 male (n=60) and female (n=283) figure skaters (members of the US Figure Skating Association) provided evidence that flexibility assessments varied based on skating discipline. Pair skaters demonstrated a greater front-split distance than dance (p=0.024) and synchronized skaters (p=0.009). In the seated reach test, singles and pair skaters had a greater reach distance than dancers (p≤ 0.05), with singles also showing a greater reach than synchronized skaters (p=0.007). Interestingly, there were no differences in flexibility measures reported across the three different levels of skaters (novice, junior and senior)

(Slater et al., 2016). In agreement with this was a study exploring the physiological attributes of sixty-one female volleyball players from the best and the second-best volleyball leagues in Greece (Nikolaidis et al., 2012). No significant differences between age groups (under fourteen, fourteen to eighteen and over eighteen years) were found for the sit and reach test.

In contrast to this, there is evidence to demonstrate that flexibility can be a discriminating variable between different levels of athletes (Sell et al., 2007; McCullough et al., 2009). In swimmers who use the front crawl stroke, it has been estimated that the flutter-kicking action can contribute approximately 10 per cent to the total stroke speed, as well as contributing to keeping the body in a more streamlined position to reduce drag (Watkins et al., 1983). A study comparing ten female NCAA Division I swimmers and ten female recreational swimmers over 50m found significant moderate correlations between ankle plantarflexion and flutter-kicking speed (r=0.509), reinforcing the point that ankle flexibility plays a crucial role in flutter-kick capability (McCullough et al., 2009). Another cross-sectional study looking at the flexibility characteristics of male golfers (n=257) across three proficiency levels (Handicap <0, 1-9 and 10-20) found that the best golfers (<0) had significantly (p<0.05) greater shoulder, hip and torso flexibility than golfers in the low-proficiency group (HCP 10-20) (Sell et al., 2007). In a separate golf study (Wells et al., 2009), significant correlations were found between sit and reach measures in twenty-four Canadian Golf Team members (nine female, fifteen men) and driver carry distance (r=-0.36; P=0.04), five-iron ball speed (r=-0.41; P=0.02), five-iron carry distance (r=-0.44; P=0.01) and score or total shots per round (r=0.43; P=0.03). The weak to moderate correlations found in the latter study suggest that other factors aside from flexibility may be bigger determinants of golf performance. However,

121

there were no significant differences in flexibility measures between males and females.

The literature exploring the relationship between ROM and success in sport and between the sexes is mixed in its findings. Aside from the fact that there are huge methodological differences between studies, as well as the fact that there is limited longitudinal data to see how increases in ROM change performance outcomes, there are a few comments worth noting in relation to the concept of 'optimal' rather than 'maximal' ROM. Firstly, perhaps the reason why flexibility does not always differentiate between levels of performer could be due to the fact that once you have achieved the required ROM to perform the techniques required of the sport safely, additional ROM may only serve to produce an inherent joint laxity that could just increase injury risk. Secondly, although females are thought to be more flexible than males when comparing general populations (Tremblay et al., 2009; Rikli and Jones, 1999; Hands et al., 2008; Santos et al., 2014), athletes performing in the same sport will require the same ROM, provided the rules and the demands of the sport are the same. This may explain why in athletic populations a disparity in ROM between the sexes becomes less evident.

Although flexibility and mobility are clearly linked to athletic performance, with a warm-up and stretching being considered an integral part of an athlete's training, there is much debate around how, when and what types of stretching exercises should be integrated into the programme. There are essentially three periods when stretching is prescribed to athletes: as part of the warm-up, immediately post-workout and as a separate, discrete workout.

The aim of the pre-activity warm-up is to optimize performance by preparing the athlete mentally and physically for training or competition (Jeffreys, 2007; Woods Bishop, 2003a and 2003b), with RAMP (raise, activate,

mobilize and potentiate) being a well-accepted method of achieving both the temperature-related (such as increased nerve conduction velocity, increased MTU compliance, enhanced anaerobic energy provision, increased thermoregulatory strain and altered force–velocity relationship) and non-temperature related mechanisms (increased baseline oxygen comsumption, post-activation potentiation, plus effects of acidaemia) (Bishop, 2003a; Jeffreys, 2007) responsible for this. Whilst many types of stretching can induce the ROM changes required for the exercise session (Behm et al., 2015), there are a growing number of reviews suggesting that some types of stretching, in particular static and PNF stretching, may hinder performance (Baxter et al., 2017; Behm et al., 2015; Pratt, 2014; Harrison Gill, 2016; Kallerud and Gleeson, 2013; Behm and Chaouachi, 2011; Simic et al., 2013; Rubini et al., 2007; Kay and Blaxzevich, 2012). A summary of the findings of the most recent review is found in Table 5.1.

DOSE RESPONSE RELATIONSHIPS

The main conclusion of the most recent review (Behm et al., 2015; see Table 5.1) was that both SS (−3.7 per cent) and PNF (−4.4 per cent) induced small to moderate performance decrements when tested on average 3 to 5 minutes after the completion of the stretching intervention, whereas DS induced small to moderate performance enhancements (+1.3 per cent). Secondly, that performance deficits were greater with SS durations of >60 seconds per muscle group (−4.6 per cent) compared to those ≤ 60 seconds (−1.1 per cent) (Behm et al., 2015). This confirms the findings from several previous review papers that have highlighted a dose-response relationship between performance deficits and higher volumes of SS (Kallerud and Gleeson; Behm and Chaouachi, 2011; Rubini et al., 2007). Because of the heterogeneous nature of the studies involving the use of DS stretching, and the lack of numbers and breadth of literature exploring the effects of PNF methods, a dose-response relationship between the volumes of these types of stretching on performance has not yet been established (Behm *et al.*, 2015). However, there is a suggestion that performance decrements through the use of PNF (−6.4 per cent) may be more substantial than those using SS (−2.3 per cent).

DIFFERENT EFFECTS OF STRETCHING IN STRENGTH AND POWER-BASED PERFORMANCES

The detrimental effect of pre-activity stretching on performance has been shown to be dependent on the characteristic of the test measure (Kallerud and Gleeson, 2013; Behm and Chaouachi, 2011); Simic *et al.*, 2013; Rubini *et al.*, 2007; Kay and Blazevich, 2012). A meta-analytical review exploring pre-exercise SS and its effects on maximal muscular performance (Simic *et al.*, 2013) identified a total of 104 studies for inclusion (61 measures for strength, 12 measures for power and 57 measures for explosive, rate of force development performance) which revealed the pooled estimate for the acute effects of SS on strength (−5.4 per cent), power (−1.9 per cent) and explosive (−2.0 per cent) performance. The review presented in Table 5.1 also supports these findings. Longer durations of SS prior to strength-based activities (≥ 60s, −5.1 per cent) is shown to have a much more marked effect on performance than that of shorter duration stretches (<60s, −2.8 per cent), with large detrimental effects evident for all types of muscle contraction (concentric −4.4 per cent, eccentric, −4.2 per cent and isometric −6.3 per cent). Furthermore, regardless of stretch duration, the effects of SS on strength-based activities are far greater than for power-speed

tasks (<60s 0.15 per cent vs ≥60s 2.6 per cent). Pre-activity DS generally shows no adverse effects on strength performance or power-speed tasks, with negligible differential effects on either concentric (0.4 per cent) or eccentric (−1.2 per cent) muscle contraction. The number of studies looking at pre-activity PNF stretching is relatively small, when compared to those looking at SS or DS with studies showing large variability in effects. However, there is some similarity in these findings to those studies using the SS mode of stretching with larger detrimental effects on strength-based activities (−5.5 per cent), compared to power-speed movements (−1.6 per cent). The fact that SS is part of the PNF process may partly explain these findings.

A systematic review (Kallerud and Gleeson, 2013), on performances involving stretch-shortening cycles (SSCs), suggested that the negative acute effects of SS may be less pronounced in activities involving longer SSCs which have a lesser reliance on the storage and release of elastic energy (in other words those activities that require a stiffer MTU). Although this view was supported by other authors (Behm and Chaouachi *et al.*, 2011), only small-to-moderate effect sizes (d=0.15-0.5) were reported, suggesting that actual decrements in performance in practice are limited (Kallerud and Gleeson, 2013).

The relatively large decrements (up to ~8 per cent) in force output associated with SS and PNF is significant for more advanced athletes when the margins separating performers are small. Evidence looking at performance effects with more chronic long-term stretching programmes (typically three to eight weeks in duration) have shown that strength and power-based activities may actually be enhanced (Stone *et al.*, 2006; Rubini *et al.*, 2007; Kallerud and Gleeson, 2013; Kokkonen *et al.*, 2007), although generally evidence is lacking to support any definitive conclusions.

Chronic training effects are achieved by the

Type of Performance Task	Research summary	Observation	Practical Application
Effects of Static Stretching on Performance			
Power-speed tasks	26 studies, 38 power-speed based measures, <60 s of SS.	• 29 ↔, 4 ↓, 5 ↑in performance • Trivial change in performance (-0.15%).	Short duration SS (<60s) shows a greater number of significant improvements than reductions in jumping, sprint running and cycling performance.
	28 studies (44 measures) using ≥ 60s of SS.	• 27 ↔, 17 ↓, no study reported performance improvements. • Compared with short duration SS (<60s), mean reductions in performance marginally greater (-2.6%).	Longer duration SS (≥60s) show a greater likelihood and magnitude of effect on performance, changes likely small to moderate.
Strength	14 studies, 22 maximal strength-based measures, <60s of SS	• 16 ↔, 6 ↓, no study reported performance improvements. • Moderate reductions in performance (-2.8%)	Mean changes for strength greater than power-speed-based tasks regardless of SS duration
	72 studies, 166 measures, ≥60s of SS	• 73↔, 92↓, 1 ↑ • Compared with shorter duration SS (<60s), mean reductions in performance (-5.1%) were greater.	Substantially longer stretch durations used in strength-based studies. Possible evidence of a dose-response relationship.
Contraction types	Eccentric strength: 9 studies, 23 measures	• Moderate to large reductions measuring concentric (-4.4%), eccentric (-4.2%), isometric (-6.3%) strength performance. • <60s vs. ≥60s negative dose response effect: concentric (<60s -1.5%; ≥60s -4.8%); isometric (<60s -4.5%; ≥60s -6.8%) strength. • Eccentric strength: ≥ 60s -4.2% ;15 ↔, 8↓	No dose-response effects possible for eccentric strength, as no studies investigated SS durations <60s. Most muscle strain injuries occur during eccentric actions, influence of <60s SS durations remains to be studied (likely small negative effect).
Muscle length	5 studies examined muscle length adopted during testing on subsequent strength performance.	• 5 studies (4 examined knee flexors, 1 knee extensors). • 5↓at short muscle lengths (-10.2%) • 5↑at longest muscle lengths (+2.2%)	Reductions in maximal force may be notable in activities performed at shorter muscle lengths. Performance may be enhanced at longer muscle lengths; muscle strain injuries are more likely to occur with the muscle at a longer, rather than a shorter length.

out of 75 studies.	(-3.7%), knee flexors (-6.3%) and plantar flexors (-5.6%). • <60 SS vs. ≥60s SS, dose response in knee extensors (-2.6 vs. -3.8%), knee flexors (-4.8% vs. -6.4%), plantar flexors (-3.5% vs. -5.9%).	Dose dependent effect of stretch; similar moderate to large mean changes for all muscle groups. Large 95% CI in several findings indicating substantial variability among studies.

Effect of Dynamic stretching on performance

Strength and Power measures	Strength-based performances (18 measures), power-based tests (51 measures)	• ↑ 1.1% strength-based activities. • ↑ (2.1%) for jump performances (18 measures). • ↑ (1.4%) running, sprinting or agility (17 measures).	Lack of movement velocity between test measure and DS activity; part of the positive effect of DS comes from allowing practice at tasks similar to those in the tests.
Contraction type	11 studies: concentric (16 measures); eccentric (3 measures)	• ↑ (0.4%) concentric force or torque. • ↓ (-1.2%) eccentric force.	Extensive variability in eccentric measures, so values may not be truly reflective. Limited data show inconsequential contraction type-dependent effects of DS on force production.
Effect of movement frequency	Stretch frequency and perceived intensity or ROM studied.	• Dynamic leg swings at 100.min-1 ↑VJH and DJ heights (6.7-9.1%) more than at 50.min-1 (3.6%). • Combinations of fast and lower DS ↑VJH (4.9%), quadriceps eccentric and concentric torque (~7-15%), leg extension power (10.1%) and ↓ Wingate peak power and time to peak power. • Inconsistent results obtained from ballistic or bobbing methods; short durations ↔; long durations (20 mins) ↓ leg press 1-RM (2.2%) and (~5-7%) in knee flexion and extension 1-RMs.	↑ performance with faster and/or more ballistic stretches. Substantial variability in reported findings, no firm conclusions.

125

Effect of magnitude of DS movement	Described as DS through active ROM, exaggerated movements, bobbing, bouncing, ballistic bouncing movements, mild stretch.	• Movement through active or maximal ROM ↔ (or trivial) performance changes in 6 studies, ↓1 study, ↑3 studies. • Bobbing movements near end ROM, ↓2 studies. • Exaggerated movements ↓1 study, ↔ 1 study	No identifiable trend as to the effects associated with DS through a maximal or nearly maximal ROM.
Effects of Proprioceptive Neuromuscular Facilitation (PNF) Stretching on Performance			
Power-Speed Tasks	3 studies, 4 VJ measures (SJ and CMJ heights)	• 1 study, large-moderate significant ↓ (-5.1%), 5 ↑in performance. Effect not evident 15min post-stretch. • ↔ 2 studies • 1 study did not report mean change in jump measures or pre- and post-stretch results.	Analysis of available data revealed a small ↓ (-1.6%). Impact on jump data likely to be trivial or small.
Strength	8 studies, 19 findings	• 16↔, ↓3 • Large mean performance reduction (-5.5%)	Large 95% CI indicating highly variable impact on muscle strength
Contraction types	5 studies concentric (11 findings), 4 studies isometric, 8 findings.	• Concentric, ↓ (-2.1%) • Isometric ↓ (-8.3%) • No studies on eccentric strength	Eccentric strength is a factor influencing muscle strain injury, therefore, more research needed.

↔ no significant changes in performance; ↑ significant improvements in performance ↓significant decreases in performance; CI (Confidence Interval); SS (Static Stretching); DS (Dynamic Stretching); ROM (Range of Motion); RM (Repetition-Maximum); DJ (Drop Jump); SJ (Static Jump);

Table 5.1 The effects of pre-activity stretching on strength and power performance. (Adapted from Behm *et al*, 2015)

accumulation of adaptation to acute training bouts. There is no doubt that stretching and other modalities can increase ROM but, as discussed, some modalities can have detrimental effects on performance (SS, PNF) if they are performed in the pre-activity routine. It would, therefore, make sense for your female athletes to perform these activities during sessions that are separate to those targeting strength and power development, either at the end of the day or as part of a recovery session. Inclusion of additional ROM exercises immediately at the end of S&C sessions would delay nutritional recovery and may not be necessary if the majority of the session has already included a full range of motion exercises.

MEASURING RANGE OF MOTION

In a clinical setting, goniometric measurements (either manual or electric) are typically used to assess ROM at a specific joint, but a more integrated approach would be to assess ROM using some kind of movement assessment. The latter will give a more global measure of mobility, but typically ROM assessments for athletes involve both functional and static measures. This is particularly useful when athletes display defective movement patterns, because a judgement can be made as to whether it is a ROM deficit or a strength and motor control issue. For female athletes this may be particularly relevant because they are more likely to have the necessary range, but not the strength to control or realize the ROM during sports performance (Nassib et al., 2017; Wyon et al., 2013). It is also worth noting that improvements in ROM do not necessarily transfer to mobility in more functional movement patterns (Moreside and McGill, 2013), which reinforces the need for flexibility and mobility measures in female athletes.

It has been shown that joint laxity is more prevalent in the female athletic population. The Beighton and Horan Joint Mobility Index (Boyle et al., 2003) is a generalized joint laxity test that can be used to identify female athletes with this condition, but it will not be discussed further here.

What to Measure

Static measures of joint ROM can be either passive or active in nature. In a passive ROM test the S&C coach will take the joint to its end ROM, based on physiologic end-feel (NASM, 2014, p.149), without any assistance from the athlete. In an active ROM test the athlete voluntarily takes the joint to its end range and holds the position. It is worth remembering here that ROM is joint-specific and if one joint lacks ROM then adjacent joints will compensate (those above and below that being measured), suggesting that all joints in the kinetic chain must be considered from an injury standpoint (NASM, 2014). When deciding what to measure though, time often dictates how many ROM tests you can include in your battery of tests, so careful consideration of what are the essential measures from an injury and performance perspective is required.

There are a number of movement screen protocols that are commonly used by strength and conditioning coaches, including the Functional Movement Screen (FMS™) (Cook et al., 2006a, 2006b) and the Athletic Ability Assessment (AAA; McKeown et al., 2014). Although these tests may be suitable as a musculoskeletal screen, the evidence supporting their ability to improve injury risk is not well established, with some authors reporting no link to injury (Bond et al., 2017) and others making recommendations that they are a valuable tool that can predict injury risk throughout the season (Duke et al., 2017; Ransdell and Murray, 2016; Webb, 2016; Chorba et al., 2010). A recent systematic review (Dallinga et al., 2012) exploring whether screening tools can predict injuries in the lower extremities in team sports players, suggested that different screening tools could be useful in the prediction of injuries to the knee, ACL, hamstring, groin and ankle. However, this was surpassed by a more recent paper entitled, 'Why screening tests to predict injury do not work – and probably never will..' (Bahr, 2016). The conclusion of this paper was that 'although [there have been] a number of tests demonstrating a statistically significant association with injury risk, such tests are unlikely to be able to predict injury with sufficient accuracy' (Bahr, 2016).

Although movement screens do provide an objective measure of 'quality' of movement, a strength and conditioning coach is essentially a 'movement' coach, and as such will be performing movement screens routinely, every time they coach. They can also be time-consuming to administer and evaluate and they may not offer a sensitive enough measure of improvement (McCunn, 2015), in other words often an athlete's movement has clearly improved but the movement screen scoring system is not sufficient to differentiate the improvement between the two time points. A smarter and more time-efficient approach (better cost-benefit ratio) might be just to capture movement quality by videoing movements during training and track these over time; this way no 'sensitivity' is lost in the measure.

However, if you have just been introduced to a new athlete this might be a good place to start, with the athlete immediately getting some feedback about their movement competencies (McCunn, 2015), as well as providing you with a basis for appropriate exercise prescription.

TRAINING METHODS TO IMPROVE RANGE OF MOTION IN FEMALE ATHLETES

Stretching

Stretching has been defined as the 'act of applying tensile force to lengthen muscle and connective tissue' (Stone *et al.*, 2006). Every athlete will consistently incorporate some form of stretching into their training regimen. Although the methods are distinctly different (see Table 5.2), the goal is the same regardless, an increase in acute or chronic ROM. Of the three most common forms of stretching, ballistic and PNF techniques could be expected to have more of an effect on tendon stiffness than static stretching methods, although this is debated in the literature (Konrad and Tilp, 2014b).

Static stretching

Static stretching is an effective (Mojock *et al.*, 2011; Power *et al.*, 2004; Behm *et al.*, 2015; Alter, 2004; Allison *et al.*, 2008; Kokkonen *et al.*, 2007; Paradisis *et al.*, 2014) commonly used technique that takes and holds the joint to an extreme ROM position whilst the athlete remains relaxed. Athlete sensation is used to determine the end position and has been defined in many different ways including the 'point of mild discomfort' (Bradley *et al.*, 2007), 'threshold of discomfort' (Behm *et al.*, 2006), 'just before pain' (Bazett-Jones *et al.*, 2005) and 'maximal' (Cornwell *et al.*, 2002) to name a few. However, often times in the research the intensity of the stretch is inadequately defined or not specified at all (Mojock *et al.*, 2011; Serra *et al.*, 2013; Perrier *et al.*, 2011). Stretch tolerance (Behm *et al.*, 2015; Magnusson *et al.*, 1996a) and autogenic inhibition, via activation of the Golgi tendon organ (GTO) (Bandy and Saunders, 2001; Fowles *et al.*, 1999), have been mechanisms suggested for further improvements in ROM after SS. However, inhibition through GTO stimulation is thought to be transient, returning to control values within a few seconds of completion of the stretch (Guissard and Duchateau, 2006; Chalmers, 2004).

The stretched position is usually held at a point of discomfort for 15–30 seconds to facilitate connective tissue elongation and for less than 60 seconds to help minimize the negative effects of SS on sports performance (Behm et al., 2015). It has been suggested that constant tension (initiating 'creep') stretches are more effective at improving ROM than constant angle stretches (MTU held at constant length, leading to 'stress relaxation'), because they provide a constant pressure on

the MTU (Trajano et al., 2014; Yeh et al., 2005). Although there is some evidence to support this theory, the stretch durations used are typically too long to reflect usual athlete practice (30 minutes of stretch) (Yeh et al., 2005). However, in a more recent study (Herda et al., 2014), one 30-second bout of either constant angle or constant torque stretches produced similar increases in ROM, but only the constant torque condition showed significant reductions in MTU stiffness, suggesting that 'how' you perform SS can produce different outcomes that might relate to injury and performance outcomes. Continuous (1 × 5 min) versus intermittent (5 × 1 min) stretching has also been studied

Method	Classification	Description
Static Stretching	Active	Athlete actively (via muscle action) takes the joint to its end range and holds the position.
	Passive	Slowly taking the joint to end range (based on physiologic end-feel) with assistance from a trainer or tester. No muscle contraction.
Dynamic Stretching	Ballistic	Passive momentum (i.e. bouncing or bobbing movements at end range), used to exceed static ROM.
	Active	Stretching the muscles actively through functional ranges, with muscle action used to exceed static ROM.
	Proprioceptive Neuromuscular Facilitation	Involves cycles of contracting, relaxing and stretching a muscle. Two types: **Contract-Relax:** Target muscle (TM) taken to end range passively, followed by SS of TM, before being taken passively to an increased range. **Contrax-Relax-Agonist-Contract:** Similar to Contract-Relax method, except following the contraction of the TM, a shortening action of the antagonist muscle is used to place the TM into a new position of stretch.

Table 5.2 Description of commonly used stretching methods. (Adapted from Siff, 2003, pp. 173-192; NASM 2014, pp. 219-329, Sharman et al. 2006)

(Trajano *et al.*, 2014) and there is a suggestion that continuous stretch protocols are more effective at increasing ROM, possibly due to a greater viscoelastic relaxation response (Trajano *et al.*, 2014). These improvements in ROM were accompanied by less of a post-stretch induced force deficit (isometric plantar flexion, continuous −14.3 per cent versus −23.8 per cent for intermittent stretch), these deficits still being present 30 minutes post exercise in the intermittent group only (−5.6 per cent). Although these stretch durations may not be practical in strength and conditioning settings, other authors have shown that (Ryan *et al.*, 2010) the majority of viscoelastic effects occur within the 15–20 seconds of the stretch, which is meaningful for the S&C coach.

SS induced performance deficits have already been outlined. However, a recent systematic review (Behm *et al.*, 2015) highlighted the fact that when strength and performance measures were evaluated more than 10 minutes post-stretch, the performance decrements were trivial unless extreme stretching regimens were incorporated into the study design. For example, in a study investigating the effects of 15 minutes of SS on sprint and jump measures in male soccer players, explosive performances were negatively affected for at least 24 hours (Haddad *et al.*, 2013) post-stretch. Another relevant point to make here is that there is evidence to suggest that the detrimental effects of pre-activity SS can be offset by inclusion of more dynamic and specific components to the warm-up (Chaouachi *et al.*, 2010; Samson *et al.*, 2012). This suggests that a well-designed RAMP warm-up (Jeffreys, 2007) can both target SS, to gain the benefits of increased ROM, plus improve performance through the use of more dynamic movements that can produce potentiating effects (Taylor *et al.*, 2009).

Ballistic stretching

In a ballistic stretch the momentum of the moving body segment is used to create a rhythmical 'bouncing' or 'bobbing' movement at the end of ROM. In general, ballistic stretching is not considered to be the preferred method of stretching for athletes on the assumption that the movement may initiate the stretch reflex, via muscle spindles activation (Guissard *et al.*, 1988). Reflexive contraction of a muscle that is being intermittently stretched may cause damage and create injury to the muscle (Shrier, 2000), which is counterproductive to the whole concept that stretching is injury-reducing.

Dynamic stretching

Dynamic stretching is considered a more 'functional' type of stretching because it typically involves multi-muscle, multi-joint movements that more closely mimic the sports movements to be used in the main part of the training session. Specificity of DS movements, including velocity and range of movement, are suggested to transfer into the actual sports performance with greater success (Behm *et al.*, 2015; Covert, 2010; Man and Jones, 1999). In contrast to ballistic stretching, the ROM at end range is controlled (Fletcher *et al.*, 2010), so that overextension of the limb is avoided. Modern warm-up routines tend to use DS methods that progressively increase in intensity and range of movement to adequately prepare the body for training (Jeffreys, 2007). Because the evidence suggests that DS does not have adverse effects on strength and power performance (Behm *et al.*, 2015; Kallerud and Gleeson, 2011; McGowan *et al.*, 2015; Bishop 2003a and 2003b, Woods *et al.*, 2007) DS often replaces SS in a warm-up. However, because DS is believed to be less effective than SS or PNF at increasing ROM (Shrier, 2007), for sports that require extreme ROMs, DS is sometimes used to compliment SS in pre-activity routines.

PNF

When compared to SS and DS, PNF stretching is often considered to be a more superior method of improving ROM (Sharman *et al.*, 2006; Chalmers *et al.*, 2004, Rowlands *et al.*, 2003; O'Hora *et al.*, 2011; Miyahara *et al.*, 2013), although it is not usual practice in pre-activity routines since it is a relatively aggressive form of stretching that could induce microdamage to the muscle (Butterfield and Herzog, 2006) and also requires partner or band assistance. Autogenic inhibition (through isometric contraction of the target muscle) and reciprocal inhibition (through activation of the antagonist muscle) are the two mechanisms that are commonly cited to be responsible for the greater effectiveness of PNF stretching (Sharman *et al.*, 2006;), although the evidence to support these mechanisms is currently lacking (Sharman *et al.*, 2006; Moore and Hutton, 1980; Osternig *et al.*, 1987). The SS elements of PNF stretching means that viscoelastic changes in the MTU and an increase in stretch tolerance may largely explain the resultant increases in ROM.

From the discussion on injury and performance it is clear that both adequate ROM and stiffness are important trainable qualities for female athletes. A four-week study of PNF stretching (three times per week) in active women (Rees *et al.*, 2007) has shown that PNF methods can both increase ankle joint ROM (7.8 per cent) as well as improve maximal isometric strength (26 per cent) and MTU stiffness (8.4 per cent, $p<0.001$) due to adaptations in the maximal isometric components of the stretching method. This suggests that PNF may be both effective and provide a broader range of training adaptations than just an increase in ROM, which would be beneficial to female athletic populations.

Warm-Up

An increase in muscle temperature following warm-up can improve athletic performance (McGowan *et al.*, 2015; Bishop 2003a and 2003b; Woods *et al.*, 2007; Jeffreys, 2007). From a mobility perspective it can be helpful in reducing muscle stiffness by the breakage of stable bonds between the actin and myosin filaments (Bishop, 2003a), but it can also potentially offset the negative effects of any stretch-induced performance decrements. A 1°C increase in muscle temperature has been shown to improve the subsequent exercise performance in the range of 2–5 per cent, depending on the speed and type of the contraction (McGowan *et al.*, 2015).

Resistance Training

By definition, full range resistance training is a form of dynamic stretching that challenges flexibility. Athletic groups that consistently (weekly training over a number of years) undergo training that requires extreme ranges of movements under loaded conditions provide evidence of its effectiveness (for example weightlifters and gymnasts). At the other end of the spectrum, a group of untrained volunteers (male and female) following a five-week programme of resistance training (three sessions per week) or SS (nine stretches, thirty-second holds) showed similar improvements in hamstring, hip flexion and hip extension flexibility (Morton *et al.*, 2011). This was supported in a further study (Kim *et al.*, 2011) involving a four-week training programme that included traditional and superslow resistance training in college-aged women. Both methods of resistance training were shown to be equally effective for improving flexibility. Eccentric training in particular has been shown to produce superior gains in muscle strength compared to concentric only and traditional strength training methods and may promote an increase in longitudinal hypertrophy, by the addition of sarcomeres in series (Douglas *et al.*, 2015; Bridgemann *et al.*, 2015). The increase in fascicle length associated with this can have important implications for mitigating injury risk (Opar *et al.*, 2012; Comfort *et al.*, 2009).

The question this poses is, if your athletes regularly engage in a well-designed stretching programme and have been training for long enough to adapt to the stretch-strength stimulus, is there a requirement to do additional ROM training? Every strength session an athlete does is a flexibility-strength workout, and as such will lead to increases in not only ROM over time, but more importantly concurrent increases in strength over that full range. This includes developing strength at more extreme joint angles when the ability to generate force is less because of suboptimal length-tension relationships in the muscle (Watkins, 1999, pp.241), a phenomenon known as active insufficiency (Sands and McNeal, 2016a). Strength will provide the necessary stability and motor control required to safely realize any new ROM (improved mobility as well as flexibility) in a sport-specific movement pattern. In female athletes, who typically are less strong than their male counterparts (see 'Strength and Power' chapter) this can be an important injury reduction and performance outcome that is necessary.

A thorough needs analysis of the needs of the sport and the athlete could also identify particular types of flexibility/mobility that can be effectively improved through the use of resistance training. These include flexibility speed (ability to produce efficient full ROM at speed), static and dynamic flexibility strength (ability to produce efficient and powerful static or dynamic movements over full ROM) and static and dynamic flexibility endurance (ability to sustain or repeatedly produce efficient full range of movement) (Siff, 2003). In these instances it is very obvious that

'stretching' only will not adequately deliver the flexibility/mobility needs of most female athletes.

Myofascial Release

Fascia has been described as the 'glue' that holds all other bodily tissues together (Falsone, 2014, p.63). It is a form of connective tissue that surrounds muscles, blood vessels and nerves that can reduce ROM if it becomes restricted (Barnes, 2007). A natural consequence of the repetitive movements that athletes perform creates dysfunction within the fascial system, which leads to an inflammatory response in the body, initiating the cumulative injury cycle (Fig. 5.3, NASM, 2014). The associated muscle spasms result in 'knots' or 'trigger points' (microspams) that create inextensible, weak adhesions in the soft tissues that not only can produce pain, but can reduce ROM and negatively affect performance (for example by decreased endurance, coordination and strength) (Barnes, 2007, NASM, 2014).

Self-myofascial release (SMR) techniques are becoming increasingly commonplace in athletes' programmes as a method of addressing and alleviating the detrimental effects of fascial restrictions and overactive muscle microspams (Sullivan *et al.*, 2103), including pain and restricted ROM (MacDonald *et al.*, 2012). There are a number self-myofascial release devices of varying sizes and degrees of firmness (for example rollers, peanuts, balls, handheld rollers), with smaller and more rigid tools being capable of reaching deeper layers of fascia. A number of studies have shown significant acute (Sullivan *et al.*, 2013; Škarabot *et al.*, 2015; Behara *et al.*, 2017) and chronic (Junker and Stöggl, 2015) improvements in ROM as a result of SMR techniques being used. Furthermore, SMR (3 × 30s with 10s intra-set rest) has been shown to produce additive effects on ROM when paired with SS (6.2 per cent SS vs 9.1 per cent for SMR

+ SS), (Škarabot *et al.*, 2015), with effects comparable to those seen with a more traditional contract-relax PNF method of stretching (Junker and Stöggl, 2015). Moreover, studies also measuring strength and power performances have shown that the increases in ROM as a result of SMR have not produced concomitant reductions in performance (Cheatham *et al.*, 2015) in either maximal voluntary contraction force (Sullivan *et al.*, 2013, Behara *et al.*, 2017) or vertical jump measures (Behara *et al.*, 2017).

There are two main mechanisms hypothesized to explain the increased ROM with SMR techniques. Firstly, the mechanical stress induced by the pressure from rolling is proposed to reduce scar tissue and fascial adhesions (MacDonald *et al.*, 2013) by increasing the thixotropic nature of the fascia (in other words it becomes more gel-like and pliable due to rehydration of the fascia) (Barnes, 2007, Curran *et al.*, 2008). Secondly, that the Golgi tendon organs are stimulated during compression associated with rolling that causes a reduction in muscle spindle activity, thereby decreasing muscle tension (Junker and Stöggl, 2015; Fama and Bueti, 2011). In a recent systematic review

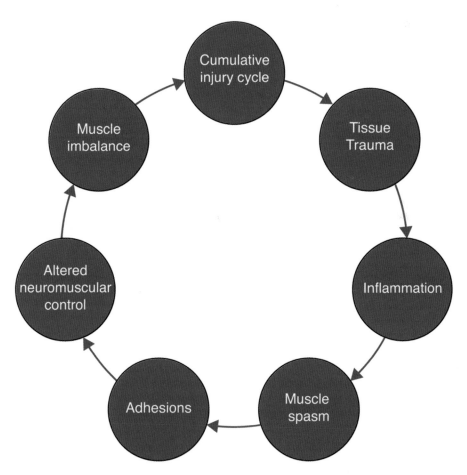

Fig. 5.3 Cumulative injury cycle. (Adapted from NASM, 2014, p 205)

Updog	Downdog	Long lunge with spinal rotation	Crescent moon lunge
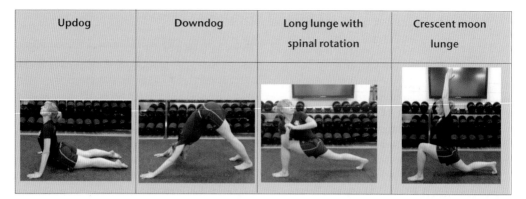			

Table 5.3 Yoga-based mobility exercises for thoracic extension and spinal rotation.

(Cheatham *et al.*, 2015), it was concluded that although SMR techniques were effective for enhancing joint ROM, there seemed to be no consensus opinion on the optimal prescription for inclusion. However, one further consideration is the notion of myofascial chains, meaning that there is only one fascial network throughout the body (Barnes *et al.*, 1997), so in theory, modifications to the fascia via SMR in one area of the body could have positive adaptations to adjacent tissues, transferring the effects along the myofascial chain. There is preliminary research to support this concept (Wilke *et al.*, 2016) using SS as the modality for increasing ROM, with lower limb stretching of the gastrocnemius and hamstring muscles producing increases in cervical flexion and extension ROM (Wilke *et al.*, 2016).

Yoga

Yoga-based activity is a functional, time and equipment efficient strategy that can improve flexibility and mobility (Noradechanunt *et al.* 2016; Tracy and Hart, 2013) in athletes. The focus on alignment, holding of static postures and dynamic flow between postures means that it is an effective way of improving not just ROM, but multiple fitness qualities that can improve dynamic flexibility. The practice involves multi-muscle, multi-joint movements that challenge all the soft tissues that can potentially limit flexibility/mobility in sport-specific postures. Yoga is particularly well received by female athletes and can easily be incorporated in warm-ups.

For example, kyphosis of the thoracic spine is a common sport-specific postural deficit for female golf athletes. They spend hours in the golf 'address' position, which in combination with carrying their golf bags, and lifestyle habits, typically leads to an anterior dominant posture (thoracic kyphosis). Technically, they also require an ability to separate the upper torso from the pelvis at the top of the backswing to create an X-factor stretch (Hellström, 2009), to maximize the force they can impart on the golf ball. The following four stretches (see Table 5.3) could be included into a golfer's dynamic warm-up routine to address these sport-specific postural imbalances and improve spinal rotation.

ADDITIONAL PROGRAMMING CONSIDERATIONS

Benchmarking

Although there are tables proposing norm values for general populations (Moir, 2016, p.291), there is insufficient normative data for specific athletic populations. Sport-specific data that provides an indication of minimum and maximum values of desired ROMs (active and passive), desired arcs of movement, or levels of accepted asymmetry to optimize performance and reduce injury potential is limited. This may only become evident after a consistent effort by the whole support team to collect, analyse and interpret flexibility/mobility measures alongside injury (prevalence and incidence) data in the environment in which they work.

Adherence

Adherence to flexibility/mobility programmes is often low, particularly if programmed to take place unsupervised. A review (forty-seven studies identified) looking at the benefit of targeted lower limb injury prevention programmes in Australian football showed adherence statistics ranging between 10–92 per cent (Andrews et al., 2013). Within this paper, the studies incorporating the exercise programme within usual training sessions, or as part of the warm-up or cool-down reported higher levels of adherence than those that did not (Andrew et al., 2013).

Therefore, higher levels of adherence to a flexibility/mobility programme are likely if the methods used to improve these qualities are consistently applied within a strength and conditioning training session, across all elements of the session (warm-up, main body and cool-down).

Education

Finally, despite the growing evidence challenging the practice of traditional methods of flexibility training to performance and injury outcomes, SS stretching is still a common practice in many sports-specific coaches' practice (Judge et al., 2012; Duehring et al., 2009; Gee et al., 2011; Ebben et al., 2004; Judge et al., 2013; Judge et al., 2009; Simenz et al., 2005; Popp et al., 2015). This suggests either a 'lag' between research and current coaching practices (Judge et al., 2014) or a sufficient lack of clarity in the flexibility/mobility literature to convince coaches to change their practice (Pratt, 2014). What this means is that strength and conditioning coaches need to educate athletes and sport-specific coaches on the mobility requirements of their female athletes and guide them on the most efficient methods of achieving the desired outcomes. With more attention to education, attendance and adherence to flexibility/mobility outcomes may be better achieved in your female athlete groups.

Table 5.4 aims to summarize the discussion of the chapter on how best to address flexibility/mobility issues in your female athletes. It is important to emphasize that 'one size does not fit all', but trial and error will help you identify which combination of strategies may best serve your athletes' requirements.

CONCLUSION

Whilst flexibility is a relatively simple concept, mobility is much more complex. There is a general lack of coherent findings and prescription recommendations on the best way(s) of achieving adequate ROM/mobility whilst preserving performance outcomes and reducing injury potential in female athletes. For example, data looking at the effects of

Flexibility/ Mobility Consideration	Key Take Home Messages & Exercise Prescription
Menstrual cycle	**Muscle stiffness may be influenced by hormonal fluctuations across the menstrual cycle.** • Less muscle stiffness and increased joint laxity potentially around ovulation (Park et al, 200; Schultz et al, 2005). • May be particularly problematic for female athletes who already demonstrate laxity tendencies. • Attention to detail in observation and coaching feedback will prevent negative effects of laxity translating into deficient movement kinetics that could increase injury potential. • Athletes with a history of using oral contraceptives less affected by laxity responses across the menstrual cycle than those that do not. • Practically, difficult to determine where female athletes are in their menstrual cycle.
Self-Myofascial Release	**Inhibit overactive muscle, so it can be lengthened.** • Perform 5 full range sweeps, friction 'trigger points' and repeat another 5 full range sweeps. • Perform before RAMP, no more than 5 minutes. • Choose the appropriate size and firmness of SMR tool. • Can be used post-exercise to promote recovery (MacDonald et al, 2014; Pearcey et al, 2015)
Active warm-up session	**Perform pre-activity to physiologically (movement preparation) and psychologically prepare for the exercise** • Follow RAMP protocol (Raise, Activate, Motivate and Potentiate), exercises should progress from general to specific, low- to high-intensity, 15-20mins duration. • Sport that require extreme range of motion may need a longer warm-up.
Passive warm-up	**Maintain the benefits of increased muscle temperature on flexibility/mobility and performance.** • Muscle temperature reduces significantly ~ 15-20mins post-exercise (McGowan et al, 2015). • Use devices such as heated garments and blizzard survival jackets. • Useful when there is a lengthy time period between the end of the warm –up and the main exercise session. For example, during competition.

Static stretching	Consider carefully whether static stretching is beneficial in pre-activity routines, as it can reduce strength and explosive strength performance.

Include if:

- Performance requires extreme ROMs such as gymnastics.
- Working with athletes that do not have sufficient ROM to be able to execute the exercise techniques safely. For non-elite populations, ROM will be more important than strength and power outcomes.
- Can be used to disinhibit overactive muscles restricting movement.
- If the SS has a psychological effect on the athlete and removal of the activity would have detrimental effects on performance.

To minimize adverse performance decrements:

- SS induced reduction in stiffness (Mizuno et al, 2013), recovers quicker (within 15mins post-stretch), than stretch effects on ROM. Complete maximal exercise >10mins post-SS.
- Include a high intensity skill based warm-up post static stretch (Taylor et al, 2009).
- Choose the exercise that most closely mimics the position you are trying to improve. E.g., if you want to improve the bottom of a squat position, performance stretches in that position.

SS Prescription:

- Stretch prescription < 60secs per muscle group (typically 15-30 secs per rep) 'to the point of discomfort', stretches targeted to needy areas only.
- Older athletes may need a longer time to achieve required ROM outcomes through stretching (Sobolewski et al, 2014).
- Within a squad, consider needs of starting vs bench players.

Dynamic stretching	**Preferred method of stretching in the warm-up can enhance performance.**

- Gradually increase ROM and intensity through RAMP protocol, making movements as specific as possible in relation to movement pattern and velocity.
- Female athletes engaging in power activities need to continue to perform DS in warm-up, but elicit maximal exercise response within 5 mins of complete for optimal effect
- 8-10 exercises per session, 1-3 sets, 10-15 reps per set.
- Within a squad, consider needs of starting vs bench players.

137

Resistance training	**Include full ROM resistance training to improve flexibility-strength:** • Specific training stimulus that correlates strongly with actual sports performance. • Set and rep range reflected in specific strength prescription fitting of session objectives. Warm up sets (5 reps) of resistance exercise can be included with increasing load in Potentiation part of the warm-up. • Increased fascicle length important for injury prevention and return to play.
Injury prevention	**Pre-activity stretching (SS & PNF) can have a positive effect on muscle strain injuries:** • Longer (total) stretch interventions (> 5 mins) have a greater potential to reduce injury risk. • If decreased MTU stiffness is required for the performance, stretching should be performed within 20mins prior to start of exercise or competition (Ryan et al, 2008)
Proprioceptive neuro-muscular facilitation	**Useful strategy to improve ROM, increase strength and MTU stiffness:** • Typically performed as a part of a discrete, stand-alone flexibility session due to detrimental effect on strength and power. • Contract-Relax: hold stretch for 10s, relax for 10s, isometric contraction 6-10s, further stretch for 10s (Moir, 2016). • Agonist-Contract technique: Use Contract-Relax as above, then contract agonist for 5s, hold stretch for 10s.
Periodization	**Include flexibility/mobility training in your periodized plan - this can vary considerably across the season:** • Prepare for times during the season where inadequate ROM may occur, possibly due to increased sport-specific training. • For travelling athletes, the training modality used to maintain adequate ROM will change according to access to coaching and facilities.

Table 5.4 Implementation considerations for a flexibility/mobility programme in female athletes.

acute SS on performance decrements show large between-study differences in post-stretch changes, ranging from +5 per cent to −20.5 per cent (Behm *et al.*, 2015), with individual responses rarely reported. For a coach, working out which protocols work for your female athletes (through monitoring and testing) within the training and competitive environments you work will help you customize this element of training prescription.

REFERENCES

Akbulut, T., and Agopyan, A. (2015) Effects of an eight week proprioceptive neuromuscular facioitation stretching programme on kicking speed and range of motion in young male soccer players. *Journal of Strength and Conditioning Research*, 29(12), pp.3412–3423.

Allison, S.J., Bailey, D.M., and Folland, J.P. (2008) Prolonged static stretching does not influence running economy despite changes in neuromuscular function. *Journal of Sports Science*, 26(14), pp.1489–1495.

Alter, M.J. (2004) *Science of Flexibility*, 3rd edition. Champaign: Human Kinetics.

Andrew, N., Gabbe, B.J., Cook, J., Lloyd, D.G., Donnelly, C.J., Nash, C. and Finch, C.F. (2013) Could targeted exercise programmes prevent lower limb injury in community Australian football? *Sports Medicine*, 43, pp.751–763.

Bahr, R. (2016) Why screening tests to predict injury do not work – and probably never will... a critical review. *British Journal of Sports Medicine*, 50(13), http://dx.doi.org/10.1136/bjsports-2016-096256 [accessed 12 Sept. 2017]

Bandy, W.D. and Sanders, B. (2001) *Therapeutic Exercise: Techniques for Intervention*. Philadelphia: Lippincott Williams and Wilkins.

Barber-Foss, K.D., Myer, G.,D. and Hewett, T.E. (2014) Epidemiology of basketball, soccer and volleyball injuries in middle-school female athletes. *The Physician and Sportsmedicine*, 42(2), pp.146–153.

Barnes, M.F. (1997) The basic science of myofascial release: Morphologic change in connective tissue. *Journal of Bodywork and Movement Therapy*, 1, pp.231–238.

Barnes, K.R. and Kilding, A.E. (2015) Strategies to improve running economy. *Sports Medicine*, 45, pp.37–56.

Baxter, C., Lars, R., McNaughton, M.C., Sparks, A., Norton, L. and Bentley, D. (2017) Impact of stretching on the performance and injury risk of long-distance runners. *Research in Sports Medicine*, 25(1), pp.78–90.

Bazett-Jones, D.M., Gibson, M.H., McBride, J.M. (2008) Sprint and vertical jump performance are not affected by six weeks of static hamstring stretching. *Journal of Strength and Conditioning Research*, 22(1), pp.25–31.

Behara, B. and Jacobsen, B.H. (2017) The acute effects of deep tissue foam rolling and dynamic stretching on muscular strength, power, and flexibility in Division I Linemen. *The Journal of Strength and Conditioning Research,* 31(4), pp.888–892.

Behm, D.G., Bradbury, E.E., Haynes, A.T., Hodder, J.N., Leonard, A.M. and Paddock, N.R. (2006) Flexibility is not related to stretch induced force deficits in force or power. *Journal of Sports Science and Medicine,* 5(1), pp.33–42.

Behm, D.G., Blazevich, A.J., Kay, A.D. and McHugh, M. (2015) Acute effects of muscle stretching on physical performance, range of motion, and injury incidence in healthy active individuals: A systematic review. *Applied Physiology, Nutrition and Metabolism,* 41, pp.1–11.

Behm, D.G., and Chaouachi, A. (2011) A review of the acute effects of static and dynamic stretching on performance. *European Journal of Applied Physiology,* 111, pp.2633–2651.

Bell, D.R., Blackburn, T., Norcorss, M.F., Ondrak, K.S., Hudson, J.D., Hackney, A.C. and Padua, D.A. (2012) Estrogen and muscle stiffness have a negative relationship in females. *Knee Surgery, Sports Traumatology, Arthroscopy,* 20, pp.361–367.

Bishop, D. (2003a) Warm Up II. Performance changes following active warm-up and how to structure the warm-up. *Sports Medicine,* 33(7), pp.483–498.

Bishop, D. (2003b) Warm Up I. Potential mechanisms and the effects of passive warm-up on exercise performance. *Sports Medicine,* 33(6), pp.439–454.

Bond, C.W., Dorman, J.C., Odney, T.O., Roggenbuck, S.J., Young, S.W. and Munce, T.A. (2017) Evaluation of the Functional Movement Screen and a novel basketball mobility test as an injury prediction tool for collegiate basketball players. *Journal of Strength and Conditioning Research,* doi: 10.1519/JSC.0000000000001944 (Published ahead of print).

Borsa, P.A., Laudner, K.G. and Sauers, E.L. (2008) Mobility and stability adaptations in the shoulder of the overhead athlete. *Sports Medicine,* 38(1), pp.17–36.

Boyle, K.L., Witt, P. and Riegger-Krugh, C. (2003) Intra-rater and inter-rater reliability of the Beighton and Horan Joint Mobility Index. *Journal of Athletic Training,* 38, pp.281–285.

Bradley, P.S., Olsen, P.D. and Portas, M.D. (2007) The effect of static, ballistic and proprioceptive neuromuscular facilitation stretching on vertical jump performance. *Journal of Strength and Conditioning Research,* 21, pp.223–226.

Bridgemann, L.A., McGuigan, M.R. and Gill, N.D. (2015) Eccentric exercise as a training modality: A brief review. *Journal of Australian Strength and Conditioning,* 23(5), pp.52–64.

Brooks, T. and Cressey, E. (2013) Mobility training for the young athlete. *Strength and Conditioning Journal,* 35(3), pp.27–33.

Butterfield, T.A. and Herzog, W. (2006) Effect of altering starting length and activation timing of muscle on fibre strain and muscle damage. *Journal of Applied Physiology,* 100, pp.1489–1498.

Carter, J. and Greenwood, M. (2015) Does flexibility exercise affect running economy? A brief review, *Strength and Conditioning Journal,* 37(3), pp.12–21.

Challoumas, D., Artemiou, A.A. and Dimitrkakis, G. (2017) Dominant vs. non-dominant shoulder morphology in volleyball players and associations with shoulder pain and spike speed. *Journal of Sports Sciences,* 35(1), pp.65–73

Chalmers, G. (2004) Re-examination of the possible role of Golgi tendon organ and muscle spindle reflexes in proprioceptive neuromuscular facilitation muscle stretching, *Sports Biomechanics,* 3, pp.159–183

Chaouachi, A., Castagna, C., Chtara, M., Brughelli, M., Turki, O., Galy, O., Chamari,

K. and Behm, D.G. (2010) Effect of warm-ups involving static or dynamic stretching on agility, sprinting, and jumping performance in trained individuals. *Journal of Strength and Conditioning Research*, 24(8), pp.2001–2011.

Cheatham, S.W., Kolber, M.J., Cain, M. and Lee, M. (2015) The effects of self-myofascial release using a foam roller or roller massager on joint range of notion, muscle recovery, and performance: A systematic review. *The International Journal of Sports Physical Therapy*, 10(6), pp.827–837.

Chorba, R.S., Chirba, D.J., Bouillon, L.E., Overmyer, C.A. and Landis, J.A. (2010) Use of a functional movement screening tool to determine injury risk in female collegiate athletes. *North American Journal of Sports Physical Therapy*, 5(2), 47–54.

Clarsen, B., Bahr, R., Heymans, M.W., Engedahl, M., Midtsundstad, G., Rosenlund, L., Thorsen, G. and Mykleburst, G. (2014) The prevalence and impact of overuse injuries in five Norwegian sports: Application of a new surveillance method, *Scandinavian Journal of Medicine and Science in Sports*, DOI: 10.1111/sms.12223.

Cleather, D. and Brandon, R. (2007) Training the hamstrings for high speed running: Part 1- Theoretical considerations. *Professional Strength and Conditioning*, 6, pp.10–14.

Collins English Dictionary (2017) Available at: https://www.collinsdictionary.com/dictionary/english [accessed 21 Jan. 2017]

Comfort, P., Green, C. M. and Matthews, M. (2009) Training considerations after hamstring injury in athletes. *Strength and Conditioning Journal*, 31(1), pp.68–74.

Cooke, G., Burton, L. and Hoogenboom, B. (2006a) Pre-participation screening: the use of fundamental movements as an assessment of function – part 1. *North American Journal of Sports Therapy*, 1, pp.62–72.

Cooke, G., Burton, L. and Hoogenboom, B. (2006b) Pre-participation screening: the use of fundamental movements as an assessment of function – part 2. *North American Journal of Sports Therapy*, 1, pp.132–139.

Cornwell, A., Nelson, A. G. and Sidaway, B. (2002) Acute effects of stretching on the neuromechanical properties of the triceps surae muscle complex. *European Journal of Applied Physiology*, 86(5), pp.428–434.

Costa, P.B., Medeiros, H.B.O. and Fukuda, D.H. (2011) Warm-up, stretching, and cool-down strategies for combat sports. *Strength and Conditioning Journal*, 33(6), pp.71–79.

Costa, P.B., Ryan, E.D., Herda, T.J., Walter, A.A., Hoge, K.M. and Cramer, J.T. (2012) Acute effects of passive stretching on the electromechanical delay and evoked twitch properties: A gender comparison. *Journal of Applied Biomechanics*, 28, pp.645–654.

Covert, C.A., Alexander, M.P., Petronis, J.J. and Davis, D.S. (2010) Comparison of ballistic and static stretching on hamstring muscle length using an equal stretching dose. *Journal of Strength and Conditioning Research*, 24, pp.3008–3014.

Crockett, H.C., Gross, L.B., Wilk, K.E., Schwartz, M.L., Reed, J., O'Mara, J., Reilly, M.T., Meister, K., Lyman, S. and Andrews, J.R. (2002) Osseous adaptation and range of morion at the glenohumeral joint in professional baseball pitchers. *American Journal of Sports Medicine*, 30, pp.20-26.

Curran, P.F., Fiore, R.D. and Crisco, J.J. (2008) A comparison of the pressure exerted on soft tissue by 2 myofascial rollers. *Journal of Sports Rehabilitation*, 17(4), pp.432–442.

Dallinga, J.M., Benjaminse, A. and Lemmink, K.A.P.M. (2012) Which screening tools can predict injury to the lower extremities in team sports? A systematic review. *Sports Medicine*, 42(9), pp.791–815.

Dick, R., Hertel, J., Agel, J., Grossman, J. and Marshall, S.W. (2007a) Descriptive epidemiology of collegiate Men's Basketball Injuries: National Collegiate Athletic Association Injury Surveillance System, 1988–1989 through 2003–2004. *Journal of Athletic Training*, 42(2), pp.194–201.

Dick, R., Lincoln, A.E., Agel, J., Carter, E.A.,

Marshall, S.W. and Hinton, R.Y. (2007b) Descriptive epidemiology of collegiate women's lacrosse injuries: National collegiate athletic association injury surveillance system 1988–1989 through 2003–2004. *Journal of Athletic Training*, 47(2), pp.262–269.

Douglas, J., Pearson, S., Ross, A. and McGuigan, M. (2015) Chronic adaptations to eccentric training: A systematic review. *Sports Medicine*, 47(5), pp.917–941.

Duehring, M.D., Feldmann, C.R. and Ebben, W.P. (2009) Strength and conditioning practices of United States high school strength and conditioning coaches. *Journal of Strength and Conditioning Coaches*, 23(8), pp.2188–2203.

Duke, S.R., Martin, S.E. and Gaul, C.A. (2017) Pre-season Functional Movement ScreenTM predicts risk of time loss injury in experienced male rugby union athletes. DOI: 10.1519/JSC.0000000000001838 (Published ahead of print).

Ebben, W.P., Carroll, R.M. and Simenz, C.J. (2004) Strength and conditioning practices of national hockey league strength and conditioning coaches. *Journal of Strength and Conditioning Research*, 18(4), pp.889–897.

Eiling, E., Bryant, A.L., Petersen, W., Murphy, A. and Hohmann, E. (2007) Effects of menstrual cycle hormone fluctuations on musculotendinous stiffness and knee joint laxity. *Knee Surgery, Sports Traumatology, Arthroscopy*, 15, pp.126–132.

Falsone, S. (2014) Optimising flexibility, in Joyce, D. and Lewindon, D. (ed.) *High performance training for sports*. United States: Human Kinetics, pp.61–70.

Fama, B.J. and Bueti, D.R. (2011) *The acute effect of self-myofafascial release on lower extremity plyometric performance:* Theses and Dissertations, Paper 2. Fairfield, CT: Sacred Heart University.

Fatouros, I.G., Kambas, A., Katrabasas, I., Leontsini, D., Chatzinikolaou, A., Jamurtas, A.Z., Douroudos, I., Aggelousis, N. and Taxildaris, K. (2006) Resistance training and detraining effects on flexibility performance in the elderly are intensity-dependent. *Journal of Strength and Conditioning Research*, 20(3), pp.634–642.

Feldbauer, C.M., Smith, B.A. and Van Lunen, B. (2015) The effects of self-myofascial release on flexibility of the lower extremity: A critically appraised topic. *International Journal of Athletic Therapy and Training*, 20(2), pp.14–19.

Fletcher, J.R., Esau, S.P. and MacIntosh, B.R. (2010) Changes in tendon stiffness and running economy in highly trained distance runners. *European Journal of Applied Physiology*, 110, pp.1037–1046.

Folpp, H., Deall, S., Harvey, L.A. and Gwinn, T. (2006) Can apparent increases in muscle extensibility with regular stretch be explained by changes in tolerance to stretch? *Australian Journal of Physiotherapy*, 52, pp.45–50.

Fouré, A., Cornu, C., McNair, P.J. and Nordez, A. (2011) Gender differences in both active and passive parts of the plantar flexor series elastic component stiffness and geometrical parameters of the muscle-tendon complex. *Journal of Orthopaedic Research*, DOI: 10.1002/jor.21584.

Fowles, J.R., Sale, D.G. and MacDougall, J.D. (1999) Reduced strength after passive stretch of the human plantar flexors. *Journal of Applied Physiology*, 89, pp.1179–1188.

Gajdosik, R.L. (2001) Passive extensibility of skeletal muscle: review of the literature with clinical implications. *Clinical Biomechanics*, 16(2), pp.87–101.

Gajdosik, R.L., Lentz, D.J., Mcfarley, D.C., Meyer, K.M. and Riggin, T.J. (2006) Dynamic elastic and static viscoelastic stress-relaxation properties of the calf muscle-tendon unit of men and women. *Isokinetic Exercise Science*, 14, pp.33–44.

Gannon, L.M. and Bird, H.A. (1999) The quantification of joint laxity in dancers and gymnasts. *Journal of Sports Sciences*, 17, pp.743–750.

Gee, T.I., Olsen, P.D., Berger, N.J., Golby, J. and Thompson, K.G. (2011) Strength and conditioning practices in rowing. *Journal of Strength and Conditioning Research*, 25(3), pp.668–682.

Gleim, G. and McHugh, M.P. (1997) Flexibility and its effect on sports injury and performance. *Sports Medicine,* 24, pp.289–297.

Guieu, R., Blin, O., Pouget, J. and Serratrice, G. (1992) Nociceptive threshold and physical activity. *Canadian Journal of Neurological Sciences,* 19, pp.69–71.

Guissard, N., Duchateau, J. and Hainaut, K. (1988) Muscle stretching and motorneuronal excitability. *European Journal of Applied Occupational Physiology,* 58, pp.47–52.

Guissard, N. and Duchateau, J. (2006) Neural aspects of muscle stretching. *Exercise and Sports Science Reviews,* 34, pp.154–158.

Haddad, M., Dridi, A., Chtara, M., Chaouachi, A., Wong, D.P., Behm, D. and Chamari, K. (2014) Static stretching can impair explosive performance for at least 24 hours. *Journal of Strength and Conditioning Research,* 28(1), pp.140–146.

Haff, G.G. and Nimphius, S. (2012) Training principles for power. *Strength and Conditioning Journal,* 34(6), pp.2–12.

Halbertsma, J., van Bolhuis, A. and Goeken, L. (1996) Sport stretching: Effects on passive muscle stiffness of short hamstrings. *Archives of Physical Medicine and Rehabilitation,* 77, pp.688–692.

Hands, B.P., Larkin, D., Parker, H., Straker, L. and Perry, M. (2008) The relationship between physical activity, motor competence and health-related fitness in 14-year-old adolescents. *Scandinavian Journal of Medicine and Science in Sports,* 19(5), 655–663.

Harrison Gill, A. (2016) Stretching the truth of literature on the effects of static and dynamic stretching protocols on strength and power performance. *Journal of Australian Strength and Conditioning,* 24(7), pp.61–67.

Heiderscheit, B.B., Hoerth, D.M., Chumanov, E.S., Swanson, S.C., Thelen, B.J. and Thelen, D.G. (2005) Identifying the time of occurrence of a hamstring strain injury during treadmill running: A case study. *Clinical Biomechanics,* 20, pp.1072–1078.

Hellström, J. (2009) Competitive elite golf. *Sports Medicine,* 39(9), pp.723–741.

Herbert, R.D., Moseley, A.M., Butler, J.E. and Gandevia, S.C. (2002) Change in length of relaxed muscle fascicles and tendons with knee and ankle movements in humans. *Journal of Physiology,* 539, pp.637–645.

Herda, T.J., Costa, P.B., Walter, A.A., Ryan, E.D. and Cramer, J.T. (2014) The time course of the effects of constant angle and constant torque stretching on the muscle tendon unit. *Scandinavian Journal of Medicine in Sports,* 24(1), pp.62–67.

Herman, K.B., Barton, C., Malliaras, P. and Morrissey, D. (2012) The effectiveness of neuromuscular warm-up strategies, that require no additional equipment, for preventing lower limb injuries during sports participation: a systematic review. *BMC Medicine,* 10(75), pp.1–12.

Hewett, T.E., Zazulak, B.T. and Myer, G.D. (2007) Effects of the menstrual cycle on anterior cruciate ligament injury risk. *The American Journal of Sports Medicine,* 35(4), pp.659–668.

Heyward, V.H. (1984) *Designs for fitness: A guide to physical fitness appraisal and exercise prescription.* Minneapolis, MN: Burgess.

Hibberd, E.E. and Myers, J.B. (2013) Practice habits and attitudes and behaviours concerning shoulder pain in high school competitive club swimmers. *Clinical Journal of Sports Medicine,* 23(6), pp.450–455.

Hill, A.V. (1938) The heat of shortening and the dynamic constants of muscle. *Proceedings of the Royal Society B,* 126, pp.136–195.

Hoge, K.M., Ryan, E.D., Costa, P.B., Herda, T.J., Walter, A.A., Stout, J.R. and Cramer, J.T. (2010) Gender differences in musculotendinous stiffness and range of motion after an acute bout of stretching. *Journal of Strength and Conditioning Research,* 24(10), pp.2618–2626.

Hrysomallis, C. (2009) Hip adductors' strength and flexibility and injury risk. *Journal of Strength and Conditioning Research,* 23(5), pp.1514–1517.

Hrysomallis, C. (2013) Injury incidence and prevention in Australian Rules Football.

Sports Medicine, 43, pp.339–354.

Jeffreys, I. (2007) Warm-up Revisited – The 'Ramp' Method of Optimising Performance Preparation. *Professional Strength and Conditioning,* 6, pp.15–19.

Jeffreys, I. (2016) Warm-up and flexibility training, in Haff, G.G. and Triplett, N.T. (eds.) *Essentials of Strength and Conditioning* (4th ed.). Champaign. IL: Human Kinetics, pp.317–350.

Jeffreys, I. (2017) RAMP warm-ups: more than simply short-term preparation. *Professional Strength and Conditioning,* 44, pp.17–24.

Johansson, A., Svantesson, U., Tannerstedt, J. and Alricsson, M. (2016) Prevalence of shoulder pain in Swedish flatwater kayakers and its relevance to range of motion and scapula stability of the shoulder joint. *Journal of Sports Sciences,* 34(10), pp.951–958.

Johnstone, J.A. and Ford, P.A. (2010) Physiologic profile of professional cricketers, *Journal of Strength and Conditioning Research.* 24(11), pp.2900–2907.

Judge, L.W., Craig, B., Baudendistal, S. and Bodey, K.J. (2009) An examination of the stretching practices of Division I and Division III college football programmes in the midwestern United States. *Journal of Strength and Conditioning Research,* 23(4), pp.1091–1096.

Judge, L.W., Bellar, D., Craig, B., Petersen, J., Camerota, J., Wanless, E. and Bodey K. (2012) An examination of preactivity and postactivity flexibility practices of national collegiate athletic association Division I tennis coaches. *Journal of Strength and Conditioning Research,* 26(1), 184–191.

Judge, L.W., Petersen, J.C., Bellar, D.M., Craig, B.W., Wanless, E.A., Benner, M. and Simon, L.S. (2013a) An examination of preactivity and postactivity stretching practices of cross country and track and field distance coaches. *Journal of Strength and Conditioning,* 27(9), 2456–2464.

Judge, L.W. and Craig, B. (2014) The disconnect between research and current coaching practices. *Strength and*

Conditioning Journal, 36(1), pp.46–51.

Junker, D.H. and Stöggl, T.L. (2015) The foam roll as a tool to improve hamstring flexibility. *The Journal of Strength and Conditioning Research,* 29(12), pp.3480–3485.

Kadelm N.J., Donaldson-Fletcher, E.A., Gerberg, L.F. and Micheli, L.J. (2005) Anthropometric measurements of young ballet dancers, examining body composition, puberty, flexibility, and joint range of motion with non-dancer controls. *Journal of Dance Medicine and Science,* 9(3–4), pp.84–89.

Kallerud, H. and Gleeson, N. (2013) Effects of stretching on performances involving stretch-shortening cycles. *Sports Medicine,* 43, pp.733–750.

Kay, A.D. and Blazevich, A.J. (2012) Effect of acute static stretch on maximal muscle performance: A systematic review. *Medicine and Science in Sports and Exercise,* 44(1), pp.154–164.

Kay, A.D., Richmond, D., Talbot, C., Mina, M., Barross A.W. and Blazevich, A.J. (2016) Stretching of active muscle elicits chronic changes in multiple strain risk factors. *Medicine and Science in Sports and Exercise,* 48(7), pp.1388–1396.

Khals, P.S. and Ge, W. (2004) Encoding of tensile stress and strain during stretch by muscle mechano-nociceptors. *Muscle and Nerve Review,* 30, 216–224.

Kibler, W.B., Chandler, T.J., Uhl, T.L. and Maddux, R.E. (1989) A musculoskeletal approach to the preparticipation physical examination: Preventing injury and improving performance. *The American Journal of Sports Medicine,* 17(4), pp.525–531.

Kibler, W.B. and Chandler, T.J. (2003) Range of motion in junior tennis players participating in an injury risk modification programme. *Journal of Science and Medicine in Sport,* 6(1), pp.51–62.

Kim, E., Dear, A., Ferguson, S.L., Seo, D. and Bemben, M.G. (2011) Effects of 4 weeks of traditional resistance training vs. superslow training on early phase adaptations in strength, flexibility, and aerobic capacity in college-aged women. *Journal of Strength and Conditioning Research*, 25(11), pp.3006–3013.

King, D., Gissane, C., Clark, T. and Marshall, S.W. (2014) The incidence of match and training injuries in rugby league: A pooled data analysis of published studies. *International Journal of Sports Science and Coaching*, 9(2), pp.417–431.

Kjaer, M. and Hansen, M. (2008) The mystery of female connective tissue. *Journal of Applied Physiology*, 105, pp.1026–1027.

Knapp, K.A. (2016) Self-care modalities: Improved performance and decreased injury for female athletes. *Strength and Conditioning Journal*, 38(2), pp.70–78.

Knudson, D.V. (2009) Correcting the use of the term 'power' in the strength and conditioning literature. *Journal of Strength and Conditioning Research*, 23, pp.1902–1908.

Kokkonen, J., Nelson, A.G., Eldredge, C. and Winchester, J.B. (2007) Chronic static stretching improves exercise performance. *Medicine and Science in Sports and Exercise*, 39(10), pp.1825–1831.

Konrad, A. and Tilp, M. (2014a) Increased range of motion after static stretching is not due to changes in muscle and tendon structures. *Clinical Biomechanics*, 29, pp.636–642.

Konrad, A. and Tilp, M. (2014b) Effects of ballistic stretching training on the properties of human muscle and tendon structures. *Journal of Applied Physiology*, 117(1), pp.29–35.

Koutedakis, Y. and Jamurtas, A. (2004) The dancer as a performing athlete: Physiological considerations. *Sports Medicine*, 34(10), pp.651–661.

Kubo, K., Kanehisa, H. and Fukunaga, T. (2002) Gender differences in the viscoelastic properties of tendon structures. *European Journal of Applied Physiology*, 88, pp.520–526.

Kubo, K., Kanehisa, H. and Fukunaga, T. (2003) Gender differences in the viscoelastic properties of tendon structures. *European Journal of Applied Physiology*, 88, pp.520–526.

Latash, M.L. and Zatsiorski, V.M. (1993) Joint stiffness: myth or reality? *Human Movement Science*, 12, pp.653–692.

Leite, T., de Souza Teixeira, A., Saavedra, F., Leite, R.D., Rhea, M.R. and Simão, R. (2015) Influence of strength and flexibility training, combined or isolated, on strength and flexibility gains. *Journal of Strength and Conditioning Research*, 29(4), pp.1083–1088.

MacDonald, G.Z., Penney, M.D., Mullaley, M.E., Cuconato, A.L., Drake, C.D., Behm, D.G. and Button, D.C. (2013) An acute bout of self-myofascial release increases range of motion without a subsequent decrease in muscle activation or force. *Journal of Strength and Conditioning Research*, 27, pp.812–821.

MacDonald, G.Z., Button, D.C., Drinkwater, E.J. and Behm, D.G. (2014) Foam rolling as a recovery tool after an intense bout of physical activity. *Medicine and Science in Sports and Exercise*, 46(1), pp.131–142.

Maffuli, N., King, J.B. and Helms, P. (1994) Training in elite young athletes (the training of young athletes [TOYA] study): Injuries, flexibility and isometric strength. *British Journal of Sports Medicine*, 28, pp.123–135.

Magnusson, P., Simonsen, E., Aagaard, P. and Kjaer, M. (1996a) Biomechanical response to repeated stretches in human hamstring muscle in vivo. *American Journal of Sports Medicine*, 24, pp.622–628.

Magnusson, P., Simonsen, E., Aagaard, P., Sorensen, H. and Kjaer, M. (1996b) A mechanism for altered flexibility in human skeletal muscle. *Journal of Physiology*, 497, pp.291–298.

Magnusson, P., Simonsen, E., Aagaard, P., Boesen, J., Johannsen, F. and Kjaer, M. (1997) Determinants of musculoskeletal flexibility: viscoelastic properties, cross-sectional area, EMG and stretch tolerance. *Scandinavian Journal of Medicine and Science in Sports*, 7(4), pp.195–202.

Magnusson, P, Aagaard, P. Simonsen, E. and Bojsenmoller, F. (1998a) A biomechanical evaluation of cyclic and static stretch in human skeletal muscle. *International*

Journal of Sports Medicine, 19, pp.310–316.

Magnusson, P. (1998b) Passive properties of human skeletal muscle during stretch manoeuvres. A review. *Scandinavian Journal of Medicine and Science in Sports,* 8, pp.65–77.

Magnusson, P. and Renstrom, P. (2006) ECSS position statement: The role of stretching exercises in sports. *European Journal of Sports Sciences,* 6, pp.87–91.

Mann, D.P. and Jones, M.T. (1999) Guidelines to the implementation of a dynamic stretching programme. *Strength and Conditioning Journal,* 21(6), pp.53–55.

Marek, S.M., Cramer, J.T. Fincher, A.L., Massey L.L., Dangelmaier, S.M., Purkayastha, S., Fitz, K.A. and Culbertson, J.Y. (2005) Acute effects of static and proprioceptive neuromuscular facilitation stretching on muscle strength and power output. *Journal of Athletic Training,* 40(2), pp.94–103.

Marshall, S.W., Covassin, T., Dick, R. Nassar, L.G. and Agel, J. (2007) Descriptive epidemiology of collegiate women's gymnastics injuries: National collegiate athletic association injury surveillance system, 1988–1989 through 2003–2004. *Journal of Athletic Training,* 42(2), pp.234–240.

Massis, M. (2009) Flexibility – the missing link in the power jigsaw? *Professional Strength and Conditioning,* 14, pp.16–19.

McCullough, A.S., Kraemer, W.J., Volek, J.S., Solomon-Hill Jr., G.F., Hatfield, D.L., Vingren, J.L., Ho, J., Fragala, M.S., Thomas, G.A., Häkkinen, K. and Maresh, C.M. (2009) Factors affecting flutter kicking speed in women who are competitive and recreational swimmers. *Journal of Strength and Conditioning Research,* 23(7), pp.2130–2136.

McBain, K., Shrier, I., Schultz, R., Meeuwisse, W.H., Klügl, Garza, D. and O'Matheson, G.O. (2011) Prevention of sports injury I: a systematic review of applied biomechanics and physiology outcomes research. *British Journal of Sports Medicine,* DOI: 10.1136/bjsm.2010.080929.

McCall, A., Carling, C., Davison, M., Nedelec, M., Le Gall, F., Berthoin, S. and Dupont, G. (2015) Injury risk factors, screening tests and preventative strategies: a systematic review of the evidence that underpins the perceptions and practices of 44 football (soccer) teams from various premier leagues. *British Journal of Sports Medicine,* 49, pp.583–589.

McCunn, R. (2015) The case for movement screening – the usefulness depends on the application. *The Sport and Exercise Scientist,* 45, pp.21.

McGowan, C.J., Payne, D.B. and Thompson, K.G. (2015) Warm-up strategies for sport and exercise: Mechanisms and applications. *Sports Medicine,* 45, pp.1523–1546.

McHugh, M.P., Connolly, D.A., Eston, R.G., Kremenic, I.J., Nicholas, S.J.and Gleim, G.W. (1999) The role of passive muscle stiffness in symptoms of exercise-induced muscle damage, *American Journal of Sports Medicine.* 27(5), pp.594–599.

McHugh, M.P. and Cosgrave, C.H. (2010) To stretch or not to stretch: the role of stretching in injury prevention and performance. *Scandinavian Journal of Medicine and Science in Sports,* 20, pp.169–181.

McKeown, I., Taylor-McKeown, Woods, C. and Ball, N. (2014) Athletic ability assessment: A movement assessment protocol for athletes. *The International Journal of Sports Physical Therapy,* 9(7), pp.862–873.

McMahon, J.J., Comfort, P. and Pearson, S. (2012) Lower limb stiffness: Considerations for female athletes. *Strength and Conditioning Journal,* 34(5), pp.70–73.

McNair, P., Dombroski, E., Hewson, D. and Stanley, S. (2000) Stretching at the ankle joint: viscoelastic responses to holds and continuous passive motion. *Medicine and Science in Sports and Exercise,* 33, pp.354–358.

McNeal, J.R. and Sand, W.A. (2006) Stretching for performance enhancement. *Current Sports Medicine Reports,* 5, pp.141–146.

Miyahara, Y., Naito, H., Ogura, Y., Katamoto, S.

and Aoki, J. (2013) Effects of proprioceptive neuromuscular facilitation stretching and static stretching on maximal voluntary contraction. *Journal of Strength and Conditioning Research*, 27(1), pp.195–201.

Mizuno, T., Matsumoto, M. and Umemura Y. (2013) Viscoelasticity of the muscle–tendon unit is returned more rapidly than range of motion after stretching. *Scandinavian Journal of Medicine and Science in Sports*, 23(1), pp.23–30.

Moir, G.L. (2016) *Strength and Conditioning: A Biomechanical Approach*. Burlington, MA (US): Jones and Bartlett Learning, pp.287–322.

Mojock, C.D., Kim, J.S., Eccles, D.W. and Panton, L.B. (2011) The effects of static stretching on running economy and endurance performance in female distance runners during treadmill running. *Journal of Strength and Conditioning Research*, 25(8), pp.2170–2176.

Moore, M.A. and Hutton, R.S. (1980) Electromyographic investigation of muscle stretching techniques. *Medicine and Science in Sports and Exercise*, 12, pp.322–329.

Moreside, J.M. and McGill, S.M. (2013) Improvements in hip flexibility do not transfer mobility in functional movement patterns. *Journal of Strength and Conditioning Research*, 27(10), pp.2635–2643.

Morton, S.K., Whitehead, J.R., Brinkert, R.H. and Caine, D.J. (2011) Resistance training vs. static stretching: Effects on flexibility and strength. *Journal of Strength and Conditioning Research*, 25(12), pp.3391–3398.

Myer, G.D., Ford, K.R., Paterno, M.V., Nick, T.G. and Hewett, T.E. (2008) The effects of generalised joint laxity on risk of anterior cruciate ligament injury in young female gymnasts. *American Journal of Sports Medicine*, 36(6), pp.1073–1080.

Nakamura, M., Ikezoe, T., Takeno, Y. and Ichihashi, N. (2012) Effects of a 4 week static stretching programme on passive stiffness of human gastrocnemius muscle-tendon unit in vivo. *European Journal of Applied Physiology*, 112, pp.2749–2755.

NASM (2014) NASM *Essentials of Corrective Exercise Training*. Baltimore, Philadelphia: Lippincott Williams and Wilkins, pp.205–239.

Nassib, S.H., Mkaouer, B., Riahi, S.H., Wali, S.M. and Nassib, S. (2017) Prediction of gymnastics profile through an international program evaluation in womens' artistic gymnastics. doi: 10.1519/JSC.0000000000001902, Published ahead of print.

Nawata, K., Teshima, R., Morio, Y., Hagino, H., Enokida, M. and Yamamoto, K. (1999) Anterior-posterior knee laxity increased by exercise: Quantitative evaluation of physiological changes. *Acta Orthopaedica Scandinavica*, 70, pp.261–264.

Nelson, R.T. and Bandy, W.D. (2005) An update on flexibility. *Strength and Conditioning Journal*, 27(1), pp.10–16.

Nicholas, S.J. and Tyler, T.F. (2002) Adductor muscle strains in sport. *Sports Medicine*, 32(5), pp.339–344.

Nikolaidis, P.T., Ziv, G., Arnon, M. and Lidor, R. (2012) Physical characteristics and physiological attributes of female volleyball players – the need for individual data. *Journal of Strength and Conditioning Research*, 26(9), pp.2547–2557.

Noradechanut, C., Worsley, A. and Groeller, H. (2016) Thai Yoga improves physical function and wellbeing on older adults: A randomised controlled trial. *Journal of Science and Medicine in Sport*, DOI: 10.1016/j.jsams.2016.10.007.

O'Hora, J., Cartwright, A., Wade, C.D., Hough, A.D. and Shum, G.I. (2011) Efficacy of static stretching and proprioceptive neuromuscular facilitation stretch on hamstrings length after a single session. *Journal of Strength and Conditioning Research*, 25, pp.1586–1591.

Opar, D.A., Williams, M.D. and Shield, A.J. (2012) Hamstring strain injuries: Factors that lead to injury and re-injury. *Sports Medicine*, 42(3), pp.209–226.

Orchard, J., Marsden, J., Lord, S. and Garlick,

D. (1997) Preseason hamstring muscle weakness associated with hamstring muscle injury in Australian footballers. *American Journal of Sports Medicine*, 23, pp.81–85.

Osternig, L.R., Robertson, R., Troxel, R.K. and Hansen, P. (1987) Muscle activation during proprioceptive neuromuscular facilitation (PNF) stretching techniques. *American Journal of Physical Medicine*, 66, pp.298–307.

Owen, A.L., Wong, D.P., Dellal, A., Paul, D.J., Orhant, E. and Collie, S. (2013) Effect of an injury prevention programme on muscle injuries in elite professional soccer. *Journal of Strength and Conditioning Research*, 27(12), pp.3275–3285.

Palmer, T.B., Thompson, B. J., Hawkey, M.J., Conchola, E., Adams, B.M., Akehi, K., Thiele, R.M. and Smith, D.B. (2014) The influence of athletic status on the passive properties of the muscle-tendon unit and traditional performance measures in Division I female soccer players and non-athlete controls. *Journal of Strength and Conditioning Research*, 28(7), pp.2026–2034.

Paradisis, G.P., Pappas, P.T., Theodorou, A.S., Zacharogiannis, E.G., Skordilis, E.K. and Smirniotou, A.S. (2004) Effects of static and dynamic stretching on sprint and jump performance in boys and girls. *Journal of Strength and Conditioning Research*, 28, pp.154–160.

Park, S.K., Stefanyshyn, D.J., Ramage, B., Hart, D.A. and Ronsky, J.L. (2008) Relationship between knee joint laxity and knee joint mechanics during the menstrual cycle. *British Journal of Sports Medicine*, 43, pp.174–179.

Parkkari, J., Kujala, U.M. and Kannus, P. (2001) Is it possible to prevent sports injuries? Review of controlled clinical trials and recommendations for future work. *Sports Medicine*, 31(14), pp.985–995.

Parrott, J. and Zhu, X. (2013) A critical view of static stretching and its relevance in physical education. *The Physical Educator*, 70, pp.395–412.

Pearcey, G.E.P., Bradbury-Squires, D.J.,

Kawamoto, J.E., Drinkwater, E.J., Behm, D.G. and Button, D.C. (2015) Foam rolling for delayed onset muscle soreness and recovery of dynamic performance measures. *Journal of Athletic Training*, 50(1), pp.5–13.

Perrier, E.T., Pavol, M.J. and Hoffman, M.A. (2011) The acute effects of a warm-up including static or dynamic stretching on countermovement jump height, reaction time and flexibility. *Journal of Strength and Conditioning Research*, 25(7), pp.1925–1931.

Pope, R.P., Herbert, R.D., Kirwan, J.D. and Graham, B.J. (2000) A randomised trial of-pre-exercise stretching for prevention of lower-limb injury, *Medicine in Science and Sports and Exercise*, 32, pp.271–277.

Popp, J.K., Bellar, D., Hoover, D.L., Craig, B.W., Leitzelar, B.N., Wanless, E.A. and Judge, L.W. (2015) Pre- and post-activity stretching practices of collegiate athletic trainers in the United States, *Journal of Strength and Conditioning Research*, DOI: 10.1519/JSC.0000000000000890.

Potach, D.H. and Chu, D.A. (2016) Program Design and Technique for Plyometric Training, in Haff, G.G. and Triplett, N.T. (Eds) *Essentials of Strength and Conditioning* (4th ed.). Champaign. IL: Human Kinetics, pp.317–350.

Power, K., Behm, D., Cahill, F., Carroll, M. and Young, W. (2004) An acute bout of static stretching. Effects on force and jumping performance. *Medicine and Science in Sports and Exercise*, 36, pp.1389–1396.

Pratt, D. (2014) A critical review on the acute effects of various stretching methods on performance. *Professional Strength and Conditioning*, 35, pp.13–21.

Prior, M., Guerin, M. and Grimmer, K. (2009) An evidence-based approach to hamstring strain injury: A systematic review of the literature. *Sports: A multidisciplinary approach*, 1 (2), DOI: 10.1177/1941738108324962.

Purslow, P.P. (1989) Strain-induced reorientation of an intramuscular connective tissue network: implications for passive muscle elasticity. *Journal of*

Biomechanics, 22 (1), pp.21–31.

Ransdell, L.B. and Murray, T. (2016) Functional Movement Screen: An important tool for female athletes. *Strength and Conditioning Journal,* 38(2), pp.40–46.

Rees, S.S., Murphy, A.J., Watsford, M.L., McLachlan, K.A. and Coutts, A.J. (2007) Effects of proprioceptive neuromuscular facilitation stretching on stiffness and force-producing characteristics of the ankle in active women. *Journal of Strength and Conditioning Research,* 21(2), pp.572–577.

Rikli, R.E. and Jones, C.J. (1999) Functional fitness normative scores for community-residing older adults, ages 60–94. *Journal of Aging and Physical Activity,* 7, pp.162–181.

Rowlands, A.V., Marginson, V.F. and Lee, J. (2003) Chronic flexibility gains; Effect of isometric contraction during proprioceptive neuromuscular facilitation stretching techniques. *Research Quarterly for Exercise and Sport,* 74, pp.47–51.

Rubini, E.C., Costa, A.L., Gomes, P.S. (2007) The effects of stretching on strength performance. *Sports Medicine,* 37, pp.213–224.

Ryan, E.C., Beck, T.W., Herda, T.J., Hull, H.R., Hartman, M.J., Costa, P.B., Defreitas, J.M., Stout, J.R. and Cramer, J.T. (2008) The time course of musculotendinous stiffness responses following different durations of passive stretching. *Journal of Orthopaedic and Sports Physical Therapy,* 38(10), pp.632–639.

Ryan, E.D., Herda, T.J., Costa, P.B., Defreitas, J.M., Beck, T.W., Stout, J.R. and Cramer, J.T. (2009) Passive properties of the muscle tendon unit; The influence of muscle cross-sectional area. *Muscle Nerve,* 39, pp.227–229.

Ryan, E.D., Rossi, M.D. and Lopez, R. (2010) The effects of the contract-relax-antagonist-contract form of proprioceptive neuromuscular facilitation stretching on postural stability. *Journal of Strength and Conditioning Research,* 24(7), pp.1888–1894.

Ryan, E.D., Herda, T.J., Costa, O.B., Walter, A.A., Hoge, K.M., Stout. J.R. and Cramer, J.T. (2010) Viscoelastic creep in the human skeletal muscle-tendon unit. *European Journal of Applied Physiology,* 108, pp.207–211.

Ryan, E.D., Herda, T.J., Cosat, P.B., Walter, A.A. and Cramer, J.T. (2012) Dynamics of viscoelastic creep during repeated stretches. *Scandinavian Journal of Medicine and Science in Sports,* 22, pp.179–184.

Samson, M., Button, D.C., Chaouachi, A. and Behm, D.G. (2012) Effects of dynamic and static stretching within general and activity specific warm-up protocols. *Journal of Sports Science and Medicine,* 11, pp.279–285.

Sands, W.A. and McNeal, J.R. (2014) Mobility development and flexibility in youths, in Lloyd, R.S. and Oliver, R.S. (eds.) *Strength and Conditioning for Young Athletes, Science and Application.* New York: Routledge, pp.132–146.

Sands, W.A. and McNeal, J.R. (2016) Flexibility: Developing effective movement, in Jeffreys, I. and Moody, J. (eds.) *Strength and Conditioning for Sports Performance.* London and New York: Routledge, pp.387–403.

Sands, W.A., McNeal, J.R., Penitente, G., Murray, S.R., Nassar, L., Jemni, M., Mizuguchi, S. and Stone, M.H. (2016) Stretching the spine of gymnasts: A review. *Sports Medicine,* 46, pp.315–327.

Santos, R., Mota, J., Santos, D.A., Silva, A.M., Baptista, F. and Sardinha, L.B. Physical fitness percentiles for Portugese children and adolescents aged 10–18 years. *Journal of Sports Sciences,* 32(16), pp.1510–1518.

Saunders, P.U., Pyne, D.B., Telford, R.D. and Hawley, J.A. (2004) Factors affecting running economy in trained distance runners. *Sports Medicine,* 34, pp.465–485.

Schmidtt, B., Tyler, T. and McHugh, M. (2012) Hamstring injury rehabilitation and prevention of reinjury using lengthened state eccentric training: A new concept. *The International Journal of Sports Physical Therapy,* 7(3), pp.333–341.

Sell, T.C., Tsai, Y., Smoliga, J.M., Myers, J.B. and Lephart, S.M. (2007) Strength, flexibility, and balance characteristics of highly proficient golfers. *Journal of Strength and Conditioning Research,* 21(4), pp.1166–1171.

Serra, A.J., Silva Jr, J.A., Marcolongo, A.A., Manchini. M.T., Oliviera, J.V.A., Santos, L.F.N., Rica, R.L. and Bocalini, D.S. (2013) Experience in resistance training does not prevent reduction in muscle strength evoked by passive static stretching. *Journal of Strength and Conditioning Research,* 27(8), pp.2304–2308.

Sharman, M.J., Cresswell, A.G. and Riek, S. (2006) Proprioceptive neuromuscular facilitation: Mechanisms and Clinical Implications, *Sports Medicine,* 26(11), pp.929–939.

Shrier, I. (1999) Stretching before exercise does not reduce the risk of local muscle injury. A critical review of the clinical and basic science literature. *Sports Medicine,* 9, pp.221–227.

Shrier, I. Stretching before exercise: an evidence based approach. *British Journal of Sports Medicine,* 34(5), pp.324–325.

Shrier, I. (2007) Does stretching help prevent injuries? in MacAuley, D. and Thomas, B. (Eds) *Evidence Based Sports Medicine,* (2nd ed.). Oxford, UK: Blackwell Publishing, pp.36–58.

Shultz, S.J., Sander, T.C., Kirk, S.E. and Perrin, D.H. (2005) Sex differences in knee joint laxity change across the female menstrual cycle. *Journal of Sports Medicine and Physical Fitness,* 45(4), pp.594–603.

Siff, M. (2003) *Supertraining.* Denver USA: Supertraining Institute.

Simenz, C.J., Dugan, C.A. and Ebben, W.P. (2005) Strength and conditioning practices of national basketball association strength and conditioning coaches. *Journal of Strength and Conditioning Research,* 19(3), pp.495–504.

Simic, L., Sarabon, N. and Markovic, G. (2013) Does pre-exercise static stretching inhibit maximal muscular performance? A meta-analytical review. *Scandinavian Journal of Medicine and Science in Sports,* 23, pp.131–148.

Škarabot, J., Beardsley, C. and Štirn, I. (2015) Comparing the effects of self-myofascial release with static stretching on ankle range of motion in adolescent athletes. *The International Journal of Sports Physical Therapy,* 10(2), pp.203–212.

Slater, L.V., Vriner, M., Zapalo, P., Arbour, K. and Hart, J.M. (2016) Difference in agility, strength and flexibility in competitive figure skaters based on level of expertise and skating. *Journal of Strength and Conditioning Research,* 30(12), pp.3321–3328.

Smith, M.F. (2010) The role of physiology in the development of golf performance. *Sports Medicine,* 40(8), pp.635–655.

Sobolewski, E.J., Ryan, E.D., Thompson, B.J., McHugh, M.P. and Conchola, E.C. (2014) The influence of age on the viscoelastic stretch response. *Journal of Strength and Conditioning Research,* 28(4), 1106–1112.

Soligard, T.M., Mykleburst, G., Steffen, K., Holme, I., Silvers, H., Bizzini, M., Junge, A., Dvorak, J., Bahr, R. and Andersen, T.E. (2008) Comprehensive warm-up programme to prevent injuries in young female footballers: cluster randomised controlled trial. *British Medical Journal,* 337, doi:10.1136/bmj.a2469.

Steele, V. and White, J.A. (1986) Injury prediction in female gymnasts. *British Journal of Sports Medicine,* 20, pp.31–33.

Steinberg, N., Siev-Ner, I., Peleg, S., Dar, G., Masharawi, Y., Zeev, A. and Hershkovitz, I. (2012) Joint range of motion and patellofemoral pain in dancers. *International Journal of Sports Medicine,* 33, pp.561–566.

Stojanovic, M.D. and Ostojic, S.M. (2011) Stretching and injury prevention in football: Current perspectives. *Research in Sports Medicine,* 19, pp.73–91.

Stone, M., Ramsey, M.W., Kinser, A.M., O'Bryant. H.S., Ayers, C. and Sands, W.A. (2006) Stretching acute or chronic? The potential consequences. *Strength and Conditioning Journal,* 28(6), pp.66–74.

Sullivan, K.M., Silvey, D.B.J., Button, D.C. and Behm, D.G. (2013) Roller massager application to the hamstrings increases sit-and-reach range of motion within five to ten seconds without performance impairments. *The International Journal of Sports Physical Therapy*, 8(3), pp.228–236.

Taylor, D.C., Dalton, J.D., Jr., Seaber, A.V. and Jr. Garrett, W.E. (1990) Viscoelastic properties of muscle-tendon units. The biomechanical effects of stretching. *American Journal of Sports Medicine*, 18, pp.300–309.

Taylor, K.L., Sheppard, J.M., Lee, H. and Plummer, N. (2009) Negative effect of static stretching restored when combined with a sport specific warm-up component. *Journal of Science and Medicine in Sport*, 12, pp.657–661.

Thacker, S.B., Gilchrist, J., Stroup, D.F. and Kimsey, C.D. (2004) The impact of stretching on sports injury risk: A systematic review of the literature. *Medicine and Science in Sports and Exercise*, 36(3), pp.371–378.

Thériault, G. and Lachance, P. (1998) Golf Injuries: An overview. *Sports Medicine*, 26(1), pp.43–57.

Tracy, B.L. and Hart, C.E.F. (2013) Bikram yoga training and physical fitness in healthy young adults. *Journal of Strength and Conditioning Research*, 27(3), pp.822–830.

Trajano, G.S., Nosaka, K., Seit, L.B. and Blazevich, A.J. (2014) Intermittent stretch reduces force and central drive more than continuous stretch. *Medicine and Science in Sports and Exercise*, 46(5), pp.902–910.

Tremblay, M.S., Shields, M., Laviolett, M., Craig, C.L., Janssen, I. and Gorber, S.C. (2009) Fitness of Canadian children and youth: Results from the 2007–2009 Canadian Health Measures Survey. *Health Reports*, 21(1), 1–14.

Turner, A.N. and Jeffreys, I. (2010) The stretch-shortening cycle: Proposed mechanisms and methods for enhancement. *Strength and Conditioning Journal*, 32(4), 87–99.

Van Hooren, B., and Bosch, F. (2016) Influence of muscle slack on high-intensity sport performance: A review. *Strength and Conditioning Journal*, 38(5), pp.75–87.

Vescovi, J.D. (2011) The menstrual cycle and anterior cruciate ligament injury risk.

Sports Medicine, 41(2), pp.91–101.

Watkins, J. and Gordon, T.W. (1983) The effect of leg action on performance in sprint front crawl stroke, in Hollander, P.A., Huijing, P.A. and de Groot, G. (eds.) *Biomechanics and Medicine in Swimming*. Champaign, IL: Human Kinetics, pp.310–314.

Watkins. J. (1999) *Structure and function of the musculoskeletal system*. United States: Human Kinetics.

Watsford, M., Ditroilo, M., Fernandez-Pena, E., D'Amen, G. and Lucertini, F. (2010) Muscle stiffness and rate of torque development during sprint cycling. *Medicine and Science in Sports and Exercise*, 42, pp.1324–1332.

Webb, A. (2016) Review of the literature: Functional movement development for athletic performance. *Journal of Australian Strength and Conditioning*, 24(3), pp.23–40.

Wells, G.D., Elmi, M. and Thomas, S. (2009) Physiological correlates of golf performance. *Journal of Strength and Conditioning Research*, 23(3), pp.741–750.

Weppler, C.H. and Magnusson, S.P. (2010) Increasing muscle extensibility: A matter of increasing length of modifying sensation? *Physical Therapy*, 90(3), 438–449.

Wilke, J., Niedere, D., Vogt, L. and Banzer, W. (2016) Remote effects of lower limb stretching: preliminary evidence of myofascial connectivity? *Journal of Sports Sciences*, 34(22), pp.2145–2148.

Wilson, J.M. and Flanagan, E.P. (2008) The role of elastic energy in activities with high force and power requirements: A brief review. *Journal of Strength and Conditioning Research*, 22(5), pp.1705–1715.

Wilson, G., Murphy, A. and Pryor, J. (1994) Musculotendinous stiffness: Its relationship to eccentric, isometric and concentric performance. *Journal of Applied Physiology*, 76, pp.2714–2719.

Witvrouw, E., Danneels, L., Asselman, P., D'Have. T. and Cambier, D. (2003) Muscle flexibility as a risk factor for developing muscle injuries in male professional soccer players. *The American Journal of Sports Medicine,* 31(1), pp.41–46.

Witvrouw, E., Mahieu, N., Danneels, L. and McNair, P. (2004) Stretching and injury prevention: an obscure relationship. *Sports Medicine,* 34(7), pp.2058–2064.

Woods, K., Bishop, P. and Jones, E. (2007) Warm-up and stretching in the prevention of muscular injury. *Sports Medicine,* 37(12), pp.1089–1099.

Wyon, M., Felton, L. and Galloway, S. (2009) A comparison of 2 stretching modalities on lower-limb range of motion measurements in recreational dancers. *Journal of Strength and Conditioning Research,* 23(7), pp.2144–2148.

Yang, J., Tibbetts, A.S., Covassin, T., Cheng, G., Nayar, S. and Heiden, E. (2012) Epidemiology of overuse and acute injuries among competitive collegiate athletes. *Journal of Athletic Training,* 47(2), pp.198–204.

Yasuda, N. Glover, E.I., Phillips, S.M., Tarnopolsky, M.A. and MacDonald, M.J. (2005) Sex-based differences in skeletal muscle function and morphology with short-term limb immobilisation. *Journal of Applied Physiology,* 99, pp.1085–1092.

Yeh, C.Y., Tsai, K.H. and Chen, J.J. (2005) Effects of prolonged muscle stretching with constant torque or constant angle on hypertonic calf muscles. *Archives of Physical Medicine and Rehabilitation,* 86, pp.235–241.

Yoon, J. (2001) Physiological profiles of elite senior wrestlers. *Sports Medicine,* 32(4), pp.225–233.

CHAPTER 6
RECOVERY PRACTICES TO OPTIMIZE TRAINING ADAPTATION AND PERFORMANCE FOR FEMALE ATHLETES

Keith Barker MSc, ASCC

As athletes strive to optimize training adaptations and sports performance, efficient recovery following exercise is a key component to success. Athletic 'recovery' in this context may be considered as the return to homeostasis of the body's physiology and the replenishment of energy stores. The optimal training programme should find the balance between physiological stress, recovery and resulting adaptation for each individual athlete. There are many programme variables that may be manipulated in order to achieve this balance. Efficient post-exercise recovery becomes particularly important when training or competition programmes are extremely demanding. Deliberate recovery activities may be used in order to either reduce exercise-induced fatigue and muscle damage, accelerate post-exercise recovery to enable increased training load, or optimize in-competition performance when the time between competitions is compressed. Female athletes tend to respond slightly differently to exercise stress when compared to their male counterparts. Metabolic responses, thermoregulation, inflammation and repair processes all subtly differ between males and females, prompting the need for customized recovery practices to optimize training adaptation and performance for female athletes.

Recent years have seen the popularization of recovery interventions at all levels of sport, with practices such as ice baths, the use of compression garments, low-intensity exercise protocol, nutritional supplements and cryotherapy being utilized relatively widely. If an athlete is well conditioned to the demands of training and competition, they will recover more rapidly and be able to more effectively repeat performances. Before considering acute recovery interventions, athletes should first ensure they have appropriately planned training and rest time along with a good routine of nutrition, hydration and sleep. Without these key training and lifestyle components, any acute recovery intervention is likely to be relatively meaningless.

As training and competition requires athletes to undertake activities that leave them in a fatigued 'catabolic' state, it is important that the athlete and coach are aware of the athlete's physical states in order that appropriate training can be executed. Best practice planning of training and competition includes the strategic prescription of recovery 'training' integral to the training and competing processes. The strategic organization of recovery activities should be based upon the objective of each training or competition phase. Effective recovery from training and competition is complex, involving a range of physiological and psychological stressors. The specific nature of exercise stress plus external environmental stressors placed upon the athlete should be considered when making decisions regarding optimal post-exercise recovery interventions.

This chapter will outline the basis for recovery interventions and their place in the training and competition schedule for female athletes aiming to maximize their performance in a range of sports contexts. The range of recovery activities that may be utilized will be outlined and their possible applications identified. Practical recommendations for implementation are then provided.

PHYSIOLOGICAL OVERVIEW

Before considering recovery interventions the athlete should first ensure they are well conditioned for the training and competitions that they undertake. Lifestyle habits, sleep patterns and ongoing nutrition should all be positive and support the athlete's performance. In many aspects, best-practice recovery advice for female athletes does not differ significantly from that associated with their male equivalents. Female athletes do respond differently to exercise stress in several quite subtle ways that should be factored into decisions regarding optimal recovery practices. Post-exercise thermoregulation, blood pressure and flow, energy store depletion/repletion and inflammatory response can all be different for female athletes when compared to males.

Before embarking on the use of any acute recovery practices, it should first be established whether an intervention is necessary; is insufficient recovery limiting subsequent competition or training performance? Given time, in most cases, athletes will recover from exercise-induced stress without any need for additional intervention. For example, an amateur team sports athlete training Tuesday and Thursday and competing on a weekend will have 48 hours between sessions to recover naturally, which should be sufficient for muscle glycogen to be restored through normal healthy eating and muscle damage to be repaired, assuming training is appropriate and lifestyle habits are not negative.

The demand of high-load training or competition exercise commonly causes symptoms such as decreased neuromuscular function, muscle soreness and stiffness or swelling. Athletes training or competing whilst experiencing these symptoms are likely to be subject to reduced performance along with the possibility of elevated injury risk (Hargreaves, 2016; Cheung, Hume and Maxwell, 2003). If it is established that incomplete recovery is limiting an athlete's training or competition performance then the specific mechanism for performance reduction should be identified in order to address it effectively.

Appropriate recovery methods undertaken post-training or competition can enable an athlete to return to their normal physiological and psychological state as rapidly as possible. This is of particular value when a competition schedule allows limited time between events, or when a training phase prioritizes repeated exercise capacity. Traditional recovery practices include massage and stretching protocol. More recently, methods such as cryotherapy, neuromuscular electrical stimulation and compression garments have also become widely utilized by athletes from a range of sports.

Post-exercise fatigue may be central (nervous system fatigue or energy system depletion), peripheral mechanical, hormonal or psychological. Effective recovery methods must target the highest priority stresses in each specific scenario. The identification of the main performance-limiting stressors is key to the optimal recovery intervention, for example competing in a high-profile event may be physically easier than a typical training session, but the emotional and psychological stress of the event may limit subsequent performance, whereas a netball match involving a high volume of decelerations may mean that addressing muscle damage is the main problem. The fatiguing nature of environmental factors such as temperature, humidity, altitude, travel arrangements and associated sleep disruption should also be considered, particularly around competition performances. Table 6.1 summarizes a range of possible factors contributing to exercise-induced fatigue.

In pure sprint or pure endurance activities it may be straightforward to identify the key physiological stress, whereas in many more technical, tactical, intermittent or collision sports it may be far more complex. The athlete's physical state prior to the exercise along with its duration, intensity, modality and the environment in which exercise is performed are all to be considered when decisions are made regarding the most appropriate recovery intervention. When the reasons for impaired performance and the time available before the next training session or competition are identified, the best course of action to enable recovery can be implemented.

Immediately post-exercise, female athletes generally have a lower capacity to dissipate heat and return their body temperature to normal than males. This means that recovery practices that involve cooling the body such as cold-water immersion or cryotherapy may be particularly effective for females. A greater decrease in blood pressure following exercise also occurs in female athletes than in comparable males. Active recovery modalities that maintain blood flow could be of particular benefit to female athletes as they attempt to restore homeostasis and facilitate the efficient removal of metabolic waste products (Hausswirth and Le Meur, 2011).

The depletion of energy stores may occur during one prolonged exercise bout or competitive event, but may also steadily progress over days if habitual calorie intake doesn't match the total energy expenditure from training or performance. Some understanding of the energy demands of exercise undertaken is required if an athlete is to effectively match expenditure with intake. Given the tendency of some female athletes to restrict calorie intake in order to meet body mass or body composition goals, ensuring the

Energy Store Depletion	Metabolic By-Products	Neuromuscular Processes	Elevated Body Temperature
Adenosine triphosphate (ATP)	Hydrogen ions (H+)	Decreased CNS firing (both rate and intensity)	Very high core temperatures
Phosphocreatine (PC)	Inorganic phosphate (Pi)	Impaired sodium and potassium gradients	Increased rates of dehydration
Muscle glycogen	Adenosine diphosphate (ADP)		Redistribution of blood away from muscles to assist cooling
Blood glucose	Calcium ions (Ca2+)		
	Lactate		
	Magnesium ions (Mg2+)		

Table 6.1 Possible factors contributing to fatigue. (Modified from Hargreaves, 2015)

daily demands of energy expenditure are adequately met by intake is a priority to enable recovery and repeated performance.

Following brief bouts of intense exercise, female athletes have a greater capacity for recycling their supply of ATP than males, enabling more efficient recovery and readiness for subsequent intense bouts. Female athletes are also able to utilize fats as fuel more effectively than males during prolonged exercise, sparing glycogen and providing greater ability to maintain constant energy substrate stores both during and post-exercise (Tarnopolsky, 2008; Boisseau, 2004). Optimal post-exercise nutrition for female athletes may well therefore be slightly different to that which is optimal for their male counterparts.

For female athletes, their menstrual cycle may create a physiological or psychological state that dictates the need for a specific post-exercise recovery method or protocol; during the follicular phase of the menstrual cycle, female athletes will recover more easily from intense exercise, whereas during the luteal phase recovery is less efficient and restoring

hydration status post-exercise becomes a greater priority. Further detail of how the menstrual cycle may affect an athlete's performance is presented within Chapter 8 of this book. As presented by Kanaley et al. (1992), although the menstrual cycle causes significant changes in the hormonal environment, the influence of menstrual phases on exercise metabolism and the resulting depletion of energy stores is likely to be far less relevant to post-exercise recovery than other factors such as nutritional status, exercise intensity and the total energy demand of the exercise.

Female athletes tend to demonstrate an earlier post-exercise muscular inflammatory response to intense exercise than males (Clarkson and Hubal, 2001). Following intense exercise, recovery practices making use of cold exposure and/or compression to help reduce post-exercise inflammation would therefore appear to be particularly relevant to address this inflammatory response in female athletes. In tournament-type competition that requires an athlete to perform multiple high-intensity competitive efforts in one day, or repeated

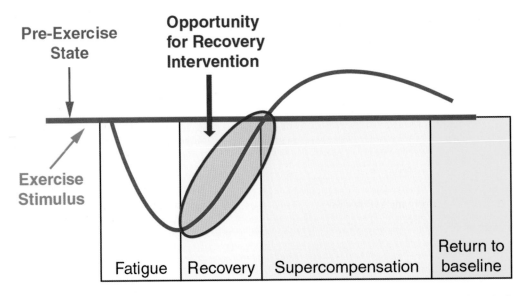

Fig. 6.1 The supercompensation cycle and opportunity for recovery intervention. (Adapted from Selye, 1960)

competition efforts over multiple days, female athletes would be well advised to consider the use of recovery modalities that involve cooling and compressing major muscle groups.

Based upon the fundamental training principle of 'supercompensation' (Selye, 1960), the training process requires athletes to be put into a state of physiological stress by an exercise stimulus, followed by adequate recovery, in order to elicit positive adaptation to the demands placed upon them. Without subsequent exposure to a similar exercise stimulus, the body will soon return to its pre-training state. However, if further training takes place during the positive supercompensation phase, then greater volume or higher intensities of exercise can be tolerated. Repeating this process over a sustained period can lead to sustained physical development.

Fig. 6.1 illustrates a theoretical model of the supercompensation cycle and the opportunity for positively affecting post-exercise recovery. Taking a strategic view of an athlete's training and intended adaptation, the chronic use of recovery interventions could limit the level of exercise-induced stress caused by training sessions or competition, so may in turn reduce the magnitude of any subsequent adaptation(s) or training effect. Existing scientific evidence around the chronic use of recovery strategies lacks clarity and is far from definitive. An example of the lack of clarity in the research evidence in this area relates to cold-water immersion with Roberts *et al.* (2015) reporting a blunting of adaptations to both resistance and endurance training such as reduced anabolic signalling, satellite cell proliferation and strength performance. Ihsan *et al.* (2014) contradict those findings in relation to endurance performance with cold application improving mitochondrial biogenesis and slightly improved subsequent performance in their subjects. Given the likelihood that there may be some dampening of training adaptation(s) when recovery methods are consistently applied over an extended period, it would be logical to avoid the use of recovery interventions during certain training phases when adaptation to training rather than short-term performance is the objective. There may also be circumstances in general preparation (accumulation) phases of training when inadequate recovery between training sessions is planned. In this case the objective may be to condition the athlete to function under fatigue, or to overload the exercise capacity of the athlete. This approach should generally be utilized on a short-term basis of no more than a few days, before some period of recovery is allowed.

The effectiveness of any recovery practice may vary significantly between individuals, both with regard to objective performance measures and the athlete's perception of its value. One athlete may really enjoy a specific recovery activity, feel better afterwards and associate it with a subsequent successful performance, whereas another athlete may have a very different experience of the same recovery protocol. Pragmatic considerations such as cost, potential for harm and whether the athlete enjoys doing it should be factored into the selection of optimal recovery methods on any individual basis.

Often athletes, teams and support staff use recovery interventions during both training and competition phases without substantive scientific support for their effectiveness, rather they follow fashionable approaches or they want to feel like they're doing everything they can. When determining optimal recovery protocol, an athlete should trial scientifically validated means in a dose-response approach during accumulation phases and competition rehearsals to establish the individual's response to specific methods and develop optimal protocol.

MONITORING OF ATHLETE RECOVERY AND READINESS TO PERFORM

Direct measures of performance or exercise capacity related to the demands of the athlete's sport may be used to indicate how well an athlete has recovered post-exercise. The problem with this in many scenarios is that the test itself places stress upon the athlete, adding to the level of fatigue. The 30cm drop jump reactive strength index is one measure that may be sensitive to certain types of fatigue and can be undertaken daily by the athlete without creating additional fatigue (Rechichi and Dawson, 2009). Examination of an athlete's exercise intensity in training on an ongoing basis is an excellent way of assessing fatigue-induced performance decrement. Analysis of time-motion data from GPS tracking in field sports, timed distance efforts in linear sports, loads lifted or bar velocity at heavy loads in the gym can indicate any significant drop-off in an athlete's peak output.

Heart rate variability (HRV) as an indicator of an athlete's physical state is popular in a range of sports contexts. HRV indicates the function of the parasympathetic nervous system and can be a relatively simple method of measuring how well an athlete is recovering post-exercise. HRV can be utilized to characterize the function of the autonomic nervous system. Greater HRV is indicative of greater parasympathetic system activity that slows systems down, returning the body to its normal state. Recent developments in HR monitoring and smartphone applications mean that it is now possible to measure HRV without expensive equipment. A smartphone application and compatible HR monitor can be effectively used by an athlete in a consistent daily monitoring routine.

Creatine kinase (CK) is an enzyme within the body that acts as a catalyst for the synthesis of adenosine triphosphate (ATP). Elevated levels of CK are commonly used by sports scientists as an indication of muscle damage from exercise. The rate at which post-exercise elevated CK returns to normal levels can be used as a measure of recovery. CK measurement requires specialist equipment and expertise that prohibits its application in most sports contexts.

The ratio between the concentration of testosterone and cortisol (T:C) is frequently used as an indicator of exercise-induced stress. Decreased testosterone and increased cortisol show disturbance in the anabolic-catabolic balance and are linked to performance decrement in most situations. The return of T:C ratio to pre-exercise level can be used to monitor an athlete's recovery. As the monitoring of T:C ratio requires laboratory analysis of saliva samples, this method is not a realistic approach for many athletes within their normal training regime and may only be utilized on a short-term basis by those athletes with the access to this level of sports science support.

'Omegawave' technology uses a chest strap, sensor and electrode cables for the forehead and hand and a smartphone application to assess the acute physical state of an athlete. In a 3–4 minute at-rest measurement, the athlete's heart rate, direct current potential of the brain (Omega), neuromuscular function, and reaction rate are assessed with the aim of identifying appropriate types and intensities of training or recovery activities for an individual athlete on a given day. Athletes may have success when their training is based around their daily Omegawave assessment but this requires significant flexibility and the athlete must be comfortable with frequently modifying their planned training, which isn't suitable in all circumstances.

The prohibitive cost of sophisticated technology and expert support staff mean that in most circumstances, it is often necessary to utilize a quick, easy and inexpensive means of monitoring an athlete's physical state. Daily wellness monitoring where an athlete responds on a Likert scale to quantify perceived levels of fatigue, soreness, sleep quality, and so on coupled with session durations and ratings of perceived exertion from training and competition can be used to monitor the state of the athlete and whether sufficient recovery is taking place between training sessions.

However an athlete chooses to monitor their physical state, a clear understanding of how competition and training activities impact upon subsequent fatigue and exercise performance can support the identification of when recovery activities are required and which intervention(s) would be most appropriate.

POPULAR RECOVERY PRACTICES

A range of acute recovery methods is currently popular with both professional and amateur athletes alike aiming to enhance post-exercise recovery. An understanding of recovery methods, the level of scientific support an athlete has, along with the resources and time available dictate the best course of action to promote athletic recovery. The most effective recovery intervention for any given situation will depend upon the athlete's physical state prior to exercise, the type and duration of exercise performed (and nature of the resulting stress), the time until the next training session or competitive event and the resources available. Popular recovery interventions utilized by athletes include active recovery modalities, hydrotherapy, compression garments, cryotherapy, neuromuscular electrical stimulation (NMES), massage, targeted nutrition and the use of nonsteroidal anti-inflammatory drugs (NSAIDs).

Active Recovery

Post-exercise 'active recovery' is routinely carried out by the majority of athletes either immediately post-exercise or during rest days in either training or competition phases. Maintaining blood flow through low to moderate intensity exercise post-training or competition can aid the removal of several metabolites (acidity, hydrogen, potassium and lactate) from in and around the muscles that have been stressed during strenuous training or competition and support the return to homeostasis (Lum, Landers and Peeling, 2010; Monedero and Donne, 2000; Takahashi and Miyamoto, 1998). Immediately following exercise, female athletes exhibit a more significant decrease in arterial blood pressure than their male counterparts (Carter et al., 2001), so it may well be the case that female athletes gain greater advantage from active recovery protocol than males.

The mode and duration of any active recovery undertaken should reflect the athlete's physical state and training status, for example a low-intensity 45-minute run may well have a positive effect upon the physical state of a marathon runner, but would likely have a negative impact upon the physical state of a weightlifter. Generally speaking, active recovery should involve low to moderate intensity non-impact exercise. Active recovery can be effective when performed either immediately post-exercise (cool-down) (approximately 15–20 minutes of activity), or as a separate recovery session within 24 hours (approximately 40–60 minute session). Researchers including Menzies et al. (2010) indicate that moderate intensities (70 per cent to 85 per cent HRmax) of recovery exercise are optimal for the clearance of metabolic by-products that may limit subsequent performance. The mode of recovery exercise should reflect the athlete's physical state and conditioning but should avoid rapid eccentric muscular actions, high-intensity impacts or jarring of the joints. Static cycling is a relevant mode of recovery exercise for many athletes, not least because access is often available and it avoids impact forces and the jarring of joints. Swimming or pool-based recovery sessions may provide both the benefits of active recovery (removal of waste products) and hydrostatic pressure from the water (thought to increase venous return and blood flow). Successful pool-based recovery studies are common, with examples such as that presented by Lum, Landers and Peeling (2010) who report benefits in the subsequent running performance of well-trained triathletes using a swim recovery session when compared to passive recovery.

Active recovery sessions can be most beneficial when performed between two intense exercise sessions that are closely scheduled (<1 hour) and there is insufficient time to return to homeostasis through passive rest. Active recovery is a low-risk and low-cost intervention that may reduce delayed onset muscle soreness (DOMS), help restore metabolic balance and improve mood state following intense exercise. Shown to be effective as a stand-alone method, active recovery may also be combined with other methods such as cold-water immersion or compression garments to maximize the recovery processes.

Post-Exercise Stretching

Historically, static and passive stretching have been a key component of post-exercise cooldown protocol for many athletes with the intention of reducing subsequent muscular stiffness and soreness. There is though very little scientific support for stretching as a recovery activity, in fact some stretching regimen may contradict the principles that underpin other effective recovery modalities (Herbert and Gabriel, 2002). In a comprehensive review of recovery methods, Barnett (2006) concludes that there is no benefit for stretching as a recovery modality. The premise of several recovery interventions is to maintain blood flow to replenish inter-muscular nutrients and remove waste metabolites. Rather than increasing blood flow, stretching may restrict it (Sands et al., 2013). If a high-intensity exercise bout has created muscle damage, the muscular tension applied by stretching protocol may exacerbate the muscle damage rather than limit damage and accelerate recovery.

If stretching is undertaken following high-intensity exercise, it should involve mild submaximal stretches rather than using the time immediately post-exercise to attempt to increase the range around joints or gain any increases in muscle length. Flexibility training should be planned into an athlete's training schedule, normally as a stand-alone session rather than trying to simultaneously achieve both increased ranges of movement and accelerated post-exercise recovery.

Water Immersion

A range of water immersion practices is commonly utilized as post-exercise recovery sessions by both individual and team sports athletes. However, the optimal water immersion protocols to assist short-term recovery of performance still remain unclear. Researchers such as Stanley, Buchheit and Peake (2012), Vaille et al. (2008) and Wilcock et al. (2006) report positive responses to water immersion post-exercise including changes in heart rate and blood flow along with effects on skin, core and muscle temperature. This impact upon changes in blood flow and temperature may have a positive impact upon post-exercise inflammation, immune function, muscle soreness and the athlete's perception of fatigue, all of which could be extremely relevant to the post-exercise recovery of female athletes.

As the compression applied by hydrostatic pressure during water immersion is thought to be a significant influence upon recovery, it may well be that the deeper the athlete is immersed, the greater the impact of the intervention. As one desired effect of immersion is to move internal fluids from the extremities and lower limbs towards the trunk, ideally an athlete should remain upright during immersion, which requires relatively deep water.

Post-exercise water immersion protocol are commonly classified according to water temperature:

- Cold-water immersion (CWI)
- Hot-water immersion (HWI)
- Contrast water therapy (CWT), alternating between hot and hot water immersion
- Thermoneutral water immersion (TWI).

Cold-water immersion (CWI)

The use of cold-water immersion (CWI) or 'ice baths' has been an extremely popular post-exercise recovery practice for many years. CWI can cause beneficial adjustments to blow flow that support effective recovery for subsequent exercise performance (McCarthy, Mulligan and Egaña, 2016; Hohenauer et al., 2015; Ihsan et al., 2014). Immediately post-exercise, female athletes generally have a lower capacity to dissipate heat and return their body temperature to normal than males (Kenny and Jay, 2007). The hormonal variations created by the menstrual cycle also modify the thermoregulatory response to exercise in female athletes. The rise in progesterone levels during the luteal phase (post-ovulation) elicits a rise in body and skin temperature that delays perspiration. This combination of factors means that recovery interventions that involve cooling the body such as cold-water immersion can be particularly effective for female athletes.

Immersion into very cold water stimulates the sympathetic nervous system and can invigorate an athlete but the use of CWT does not suit all athletes and in some cases may add further stress to that caused by the exercise itself. Gradual cooling may be more suitable for some individuals. The optimal duration of CMI may depend upon the water temperature and the time between the CWI and the subsequent competitive event or training session. Broadly speaking, athletes undertaking CWI as a recovery intervention should use cold-water immersion at 12°C or lower for at least 5 minutes. Athletes exerting the whole body during their training session or competitive event, for example playing hockey or rugby, should be fully immersed with only the head

showing while with athletes primarily exerting the lower body such as a cyclist or soccer player, immersion to above the waist may be equally effective.

Hot-water immersion

Hot-water immersion (HWI) as a post-exercise recovery method is not well evidenced and would appear to go against the principle of post-exercise cooling to limit inflammation, promote recovery and accelerate the restoration of homeostasis for females. The small number of studies that have investigated the efficacy of HWI as a recovery intervention report conflicting findings, leaving any benefits to athletic recovery unclear. With female athletes generally having a lesser ability to dissipate heat post-exercise than males, HWI does not appear to fit with the effective return to homeostasis.

Contrast water therapy (CWT)

Contrast water therapy (CWT) has been shown to positively impact upon post-exercise state in a range of scenarios when compared to passive recovery, although may not be as effective as CWI in some contexts (Versey et al., 2013; Hamlin, 2007). Those studies that have utilized full-body immersion in both hot and cold temperatures have tended to report most positive outcomes rather than those that have employed either partial immersion or hot showers instead of hot pools (Juliff et al., 2014). As a guide, post-exercise CWT protocol should involve the athlete spending equal time in hot and cold water. The hot water used should be approximately 38–40°C, with cold water at 15°C or lower. Each individual full-body immersion should be short duration (1–3 minutes) and the total immersion duration should be approximately 6–15 minutes.

Thermoneutral water immersion (TWI)

As the hydrostatic pressure created by water immersion and its impact upon inflammation and blood flow is an underpinning premise behind its use to support post-exercise recovery, thermoneutral water immersion may elicit some of the benefits demonstrated through CWI and CWT (Al Haddad et al., 2010). Thermoneutral immersion may be an effective post-exercise recovery intervention for some athletes but is currently not as well evidenced as either CWI or CWT protocol.

Water immersion summary

Various forms of water immersion have been demonstrated to improve post-exercise markers of recovery within sports science research with no clear optimal protocol being identified. Positive effects of water immersion are commonly reported at temperatures of 10–15°C for cold water, and when cold immersion is contrasted with hot (38–40°C) water. There is growing support for the benefits of water immersion at thermoneutral temperatures. Cold-water immersion or contrast water therapy for a duration of 10–15 minutes has frequently been shown to improve post-exercise recovery in a range of studies. In summary, vertical full-body immersion in cold (≤15°C) water for 10–15 minutes would appear to be an appropriate protocol to support the post-exercise recovery of female athletes. Combining CWI with other methods such as compression garments and targeted nutrition may result in an optimal recovery intervention for female athletes in specific scenarios.

Compression Garments

Compression has traditionally been a course of action to treat injuries and lymphatic and circulatory conditions. Compression garments are designed to improve venous return (blood flow) through the application of graduated compression to the limbs from proximal to distal, potentially accelerating the removal of muscle metabolites associated with reduced performance (hydrogen ions, lactate and potassium ions). The compression applied may also reduce the intramuscular space and support muscle structure, limiting inflammatory response and reducing subsequent muscle soreness (Jakeman, Byrne and Eston, 2010; Duffield et al., 2008; Ali, Caine and Snow, 2007). Compression tights or calf socks can also be valuable when worn during long-haul travel, as a means of limiting lower leg swelling and discomfort.

With some positive scientific evidence and a great deal of anecdotal support, compression garments can provide an athlete with a simple intervention that appears to have no negative effects on either subsequent performance or adaptation (Hill et al., 2013). For similar reasons to those that support water immersion, the impact upon post-exercise blood flow and inflammation, muscle soreness and an athlete's perception of fatigue, compression garments may improve the post-exercise recovery of female athletes in a range of contexts.

A wide range of commercially marketed compression garments is currently available but their efficacy as a recovery aid is heavily dependent upon how well they are fitted to the athlete (which may well change after repeated laundry). Lower-limb compression with tights or calf socks is appropriate for many travel and recovery scenarios. Upper-body compression could be of benefit to those athletes involved in contact sports, or where upper-body muscle damage is incurred. Bespoke fitted garments rather than off-the-shelf brands are less accessible to most athletes but are likely to provide a more effective recovery aid (MacRae et al., 2011). Guidance regarding the optimal protocol for the use of compression garments varies widely but they are normally best used in combination with targeted nutrition and other methods such as active recovery, cryotherapy or cold-water immersion.

Whole-Body Cryotherapy

Whole-body cryotherapy (WBC) involves brief exposures to air temperatures below −100°C in an environmentally controlled room or chamber. WBC protocol typically exposes an athlete to between −100˚C and −140˚C for a duration of 2–8 minutes. WBC should be undertaken within the early stages (within 24 hours) after intense exercise and may be repeated several times in the same day or multiple times over a number of weeks. Originally developed to treat chronic medical conditions, WBC is increasingly popular with professional athletes from a range of sports, although the associated cost and logistics make it inaccessible to most. Given the post-exercise thermoregulation challenge faced by female athletes, cryotherapy may be a particularly effective method enabling the return to homeostasis more rapidly than without any cooling being applied.

There is growing scientific evidence to support WBC as a recovery intervention. Those studies that exist suggest that WBC could have a positive influence on the reduction of inflammation and soreness, improved antioxidant capacity and autonomic function and the perception of enhanced recovery (Bleakley et al., 2014; Banfi et al., 2010). The majority of athletes who do not have access to WBC should consider the less expensive modes of cooling, such as local ice-pack application, ice vests or CWI, as they may offer similar physiological effects to WBC.

Massage

Massage is a popular post-exercise practice with athletes from a wide range of sports with both massage therapy and self-myofascial release (foam rolling) being commonly utilized for the purpose of recovery. Massage alone however is not well evidenced as an effective recovery method (Robertson, Watt and Galloway, 2004). Apart from the perceived benefits of massage and self-myofascial release on muscle soreness, few researchers have demonstrated positive effects on repeated exercise performance. As demonstrated in cycling studies by both Ogai et al. (2008) and Lane and Wenger (2004),

massage may be better than passive recovery between performances, but is likely to be less effective than other recovery options available to female athletes such as CWI or active recovery (Monedero and Donne, 2000).

Rather than being utilized as an acute post-exercise recovery method, instead it would be more relevant for most athletes to integrate massage and/or self-myofascial release into their training programme on a regular basis in order to optimize tissue condition rather than to accelerate rapid post- exercise recovery.

Neuromuscular Electrial Stimulation

Neuromuscular electrical stimulation (NMES) may be used in the post-exercise recovery process to either increase blood flow and the removal of metabolic by-products via visible muscle contractions, or to create an analgesic effect on muscle soreness. Specific levels of stimulation and positioning of electrodes can elicit one of these desired outcomes with 'motor threshold' protocol utilized to increase blood flow and 'sub-motor threshold' levels most commonly used to reduce the perception of muscle pain (Malone et al., 2014).

NMES may not be as effective as some other recovery methods and may require some investment in equipment, but it may provide an alternative that suits some athletes or that is suitable for specific contexts. There is not a universal recommendation on the optimal intensity of NMES that should be used during recovery from fatiguing exercise. However, it is likely that intensity needs to be comfortable but high enough to induce sufficient muscle contractions (to act as a muscle pump) for metabolite clearance, while not being too high, which will induce further muscular fatigue.

Non-Steroidal Anti-Inflammatory Drugs

The popular use of non-steroidal anti-inflammatory drugs (NSAIDs) to reduce muscular damage and inflammation is not proven to aid recovery, nor is the long-term impact upon adaptation to training known (Urso *et al*. 2013). The chronic use of NSAIDs is associated with several negative health side effects. The lack of evidence supporting their effectiveness as a recovery aid coupled with the potential health issues they may cause mean that NSAIDs should not be recommended as a means of enhancing post-exercise recovery.

Post-Exercise Nutrition

Timely targeted nutrition consisting of a mixture of carbohydrates, fats, proteins, electrolytes and fluid can contribute to post-exercise recovery rate in most circumstances. Post-exercise, there appears to be no difference between male and female athletes in their ability to replenish glycogen stores. Optimal timing of carbohydrate intake does not differ between genders, with all athletes advised to consume carbohydrates as soon as possible post-exercise to maximize glycogen store repletion. The intake of fats should be limited immediately post-exercise in favour of carbohydrate and protein intake (Hausswirth and Le Meur, 2011).

The function of post-exercise nutrition may be to enable some or all of the four processes below:

- Refuel – replenish the muscle and liver glycogen stores
- Rehydrate – replace the fluid and electrolytes lost through sweating
- Repair – synthesis of new muscle protein, red blood cells and other cellular components
- Immune support – allowing the immune system to handle the damage and challenges caused by the exercise stress.

The emphasis an athlete should place on each of these processes will vary according to the demands of the exercise undertaken.

Inadequate replacement of glycogen stores depleted during exercise will compromise subsequent performance. Post-exercise carbohydrate consumption is key immediately post-intense or prolonged exercise with common guidelines recommending an intake of 1–1.2g per kg of body weight within one hour of the exercise bout, as this is when the rate of glycogen synthesis is most rapid. Prolonged or high-intensity exercise also causes a substantial breakdown of muscle protein. The intake of essential amino acids from good quality protein foods within one hour post-exercise promotes the increase in protein rebuilding. Protein ingested after the first hour post-exercise can still support regeneration but its utilization is less effective in the recovery process.

Many athletes frequently complete intense training or competition in some degree of fluid deficit, which can negatively impact upon subsequent performance. Athletes should therefore incorporate strategies to restore fluid balance into their competition and training schedule, especially in situations where there is a limited amount of time before their next training session or competition performance. Athletes should aim to replace the fluids and electrolytes lost during exercise as soon as possible by consuming 125–150 per cent of their estimated fluid losses in the 4–6 hours after exercise. In brief periods of recovery between training sessions or competition performances, cool water (12–15°C) containing small amounts of carbohydrates, sodium and protein is optimal (Maughan and Shirreffs, 1997). When the time between performances is greater, fluid and electrolytes may be effectively recovered through a combination of water and solid food intake.

In most circumstances, the immune system is suppressed by the stress of intense exercise, which may place athletes at elevated risk of succumbing to an infectious illness post-exercise. Vitamins C and E, glutamine, zinc and

Recovery Method		Possible Benefits	Example Protocol
Active Recovery		• ↑ Blood flow accelerates the removal of metabolic by-products. Particularly relevant for females. • ↓ DOMS.	• 20 minutes static cycle or swim at 70% - 85% HRmax immediately post-exercise. • Particularly valuable between two intense exercise sessions that are closely scheduled (<1 hour).
Stretching		• Possible dilation of blood vessels but appears to offer little in the way of post-exercise recovery.	• If stretching is undertaken post-exercise, it should involve mild sub-maximal stretches.
Hydro-therapy	CWI	• ↓ Blood flow and tissue temperature. • ↓ Inflammation. ↓ DOMS. • Stimulates the sympathetic nervous system. • Assists thermoregulation which is particularly relevant for females.	• Vertical full-body immersion in cold (≤15°C) water for 12 – 15 minutes. • CWI should be undertaken within the early stages after intense exercise.
	HWI	• Not well evidenced.	• Not advised for female athletes as opposes the required post-exercise cooling.
	CWT	• ↓ Inflammation. ↓ DOMS. • Stimulates the sympathetic nervous system.	• Alternate between cold and hot, 2 mins / 2 mins X3 (12 minutes total). • Full-body immersions. Hot 38°C–40°C, cold ≤15°C.
	TWI	• May result in similar benefits to those provided by CWI.	• Vertical full-body immersion for 12 – 15 minutes.
Compression Garments		• ↓ DOMS. Fit of garment is key to benefit. Ideally custom fitted.	• Wear compression tights one hour after CWI (not during or any earlier). • Worn for up to 48 hours following exercise, including throughout the night, provided sleep isn't disrupted.
Whole Body Cryotherapy		• ↓ Inflammation. ↑ Perception of recovery. • Possible improvements in antioxidant capacity and autonomic function.	• Exposure to between -100°C and -140°C for a duration of 4 – 8 minutes. • WBC should be undertaken within the early stages after intense exercise. • Costs and resources required are prohibitive.
Massage		• Possibly ↓DOMS. • Poorly timed massage can negatively impact upon recovery.	• Not advised as a recovery intervention. Should be integrated in the training schedule as part of tissue maintenance regime. *...continued over*

Recovery Method	Possible Benefits	Example Protocol
Neuromuscular Electrical Stimulation	• ↑ Blood flow accelerates the removal of metabolic by-products. • ↓ DOMS.	• Comfortable intensity but high enough to induce muscle contractions for metabolite clearance. • Total duration of 10 – 15 minutes.
Targeted Nutrition & Hydration	• Replenish muscle and liver glycogen stores. • Rehydrate. • Synthesis of new muscle protein, red blood cells and other cellular components. • Immune support.	• Post-exercise carbohydrate consumption of 1-1.2g per kg of body weight **within** one hour of the exercise. • Consume 125%–150% of estimated fluid losses in the 4–6 hours post-exercise. Cool water (12-15°C) containing small amounts of carbohydrates, sodium and protein. • Consume good quality protein foods within one hour post-exercise. • Ensure diet routinely contains sufficient amounts of nutrients, vitamins and minerals. Supplementary glutamine and probiotics may be valuable for some athletes.
Non-steroidal anti-Inflammatory drugs	• No evidence to support use. • Chronic use associated with negative side effects	• Not advised.

Table 6.2 Summary of popular recovery methods and example protocol. (Modified from Howatson, Leeder & Van Someren, 2016)

probiotics may all support immune function, although their value when supplemented into an athlete's diet is largely unproven. An athlete should ensure their diet routinely contains sufficient amounts of nutrients, vitamins and minerals. Supplementary glutamine and probiotics may be valuable for athletes who engage in high volumes of training and competition.

SUMMARY

As several significant differences in the physiological responses to exercise and subsequent recovery processes exist between female and male athletes, it is appropriate to customize recovery practices specifically for female athletes in order to optimize post-exercise recovery. If regular and sufficient sleep, nutrition and hydration are not habitual then acute recovery practices will have limited impact. Understanding the specific demands of training and competition exertion and the athlete's performance levels will indicate whether a recovery intervention is required and if so, which method will be most relevant. Table 6.2 provides a concise summary of popular recovery methods with example protocol.

Taking a strategic view of the training process, short-term recovery and its potential impact upon longer-term adaptation should be balanced within periodization and prescription. The periodization of recovery interventions may mean that in key training phases, recovery interventions are not used. In a general preparation or accumulation phase of training, when chronic adaptation to training is the objective, then it may well be appropriate to limit or avoid the use of acute recovery practices. During tournament-type competitions or following specific training sessions when performance in the next competitive event or training session is of highest priority, then recovery interventions should be used.

Individual athlete responses to specific recovery protocol must be assessed and factored into decision-making. A successful recovery method should consider an athlete's personal preferences, for example pool recovery sessions might not be appropriate for an athlete who hates going in the pool or has a skin condition that is irritated by the pool water. Athlete engagement and belief in the value of any recovery intervention are integral to its successful implementation. It is important that athletes experiment with a variety of strategies and methods to identify the recovery options that work best for that individual. Novel or untried recovery methods should not be trialled around important competition performances; their value to the individual should be established during training phases prior to their use in competition.

REFERENCES

Al Haddad, H. *et al*. (2010) Effect of cold or thermoneutral water immersion on post-exercise heart rate recovery and heart rate variability indices. *Autonomic Neuro-science: Basic and Clinical* 156: 111–116.

Ali, A., Cain, M.P. and Snow, B.G. (2007) Graduated compression stockings: Physiological and perceptual responses during and after exercise. *Journal of Sports Science,* 25(4), 413–419.

Banfi, G. *et al*. (2010) Whole-Body Cryotherapy in Athletes. *Sports Medicine*, 40(6), 509–517.

Barnett, A. (2006) Using recovery modalities between training sessions in elite athletes. Does it help? *Sports Medicine,* 36(9), 781–796.

Bird, S.P. (2013) Sleep, Recovery, and Athletic Performance: A brief review and recommendations. *Strength and Conditioning Journal,* 35(5), 43–47.

Bleakley, C.M. *et al*. (2014) Whole-Body cryotherapy: empirical evidence and theoretical perspectives. *Open Access Journal of Sports Medicine.*

Boisseau, N. (2004) Gender differences in metabolism during exercise and recovery. *Science and Sports,* 19, 220–227.

Brown, J. and Glaister, M. (2014) The interactive effects of recovery mode and duration on subsequent repeated sprint performance. *Journal of Strength and Conditioning Research,* 28(3), 651–660.

Carter, S. *et al*. (2001) Short-term 17beta-estradiol decreases glucose r(a) but not whole body metabolism during endurance exercise. *Journal of Applied Physiology,* 90(1), 139–146.

Chatzinikolaou, A. *et al*. (2014) A microcycle of inflammation following a team handball game. *Journal of Strength and Conditioning Research,* 28(7), 1981–1994.

Cheung, K., Hume, P. and Maxwell, L. (2003) Delayed onset muscle soreness: treatment strategies and performance factors. *Sports Medicine,* 33, 145–164.

Clarkson, P.M. and Hubal, M.J. (2001) Are women less susceptible to exercise-induced muscle damage? *Current Opinion in Clinical Nutrition and Metabolic Care,* 4(6), 527–531.

Duffield, R. *et al.* (2008) The effects of Compression Garments on Intermittent Exercise Performance and Recovery on Consecutive Days. *International Journal of Sports Physiology and Performance,* 3, 454–468.

Greener, T. *et al.* (2013) Recovery. *Strength and Conditioning Journal,* 35(6), 86–88.

Halson, S.L. (2014) Sleep in elite athletes and nutritional interventions to enhance sleep. *Sports Medicine,* 44(Suppl. 1), S13–S23.

Hamlin, M.J. (2007) The effect of contrast water therapy on repeated sprint performance. *Journal of Science and Medicine in Sport,* 10(6), 396–402.

Hargreaves, M. (2016) Metabolic Factors in Fatigue. *Sports Science Exchange* 28(155), 1–5.

Hausswirth, C. and Le Meur, Y. (2011) Physiological and nutritional aspects of post-exercise recovery: Specific recommendations for female athletes. *Sports Medicine,* 41(10), 861–882.

Herbert, R.D. and Gabriel, M. (2002) Effects of stretching before and after exercising on muscle soreness and risk of injury: Systematic review. *British Medical Journal,* 325, 468–473.

Hill, J. *et al.* (2013) Compression garments and recovery from exercise-induced muscle damage: a meta-analysis. *British Journal of Sports Medicine,* 0,1–7. doi:10.1136/bjsports-2013-092456

Hohenauer, E. *et al.* (2015) The Effect of Post-Exercise Cryotherapy on Recovery Characteristics: A Systematic Review and Meta-Analysis. *PLoS ONE* 10(9), e0139028. doi:10.1371/journal.pone.0139028.

Howatson, G., Leeder, J. and Van Someren, K.A. (2016) The BASES Expert Statement on Athletic Recovery Strategies. *The Sport and Exercise Scientist,* 48, 6–7.

Howatson, G. and Van Someren, K.A. (2008) The prevention and treatment of exercise-induced muscle damage. *Sports Medicine,* 38, 483–503.

Ihsan, M. *et al.* (2014) Post-exercise muscle cooling enhances gene expression of PGC-1a. *Medicine and Science in Sports and Exercise,* 46, 1900–1907.

Jakeman, J.R., Byrne, C. and Eston, R.G. (2010) Lower limb compression garment improves recovery from exercise-induced muscle damage in young, active females. *European Journal of Applied Physiology,* 109(6), 1137–1144.

Johansson, P.H. *et al.* (1999) The effects of pre-exercise stretching on muscular soreness, tenderness, and force loss following heavy eccentric exercise. *Scandinavian Journal of Medicine and Science in Sports,* 9, 219–225.

Juliff, L.E. *et al.* (2014) Influence of contrast shower and water immersion of recovery in elite netballers. *Journal of Strength and Conditioning Research,* 28(8), 2353–2358.

Kanaley, J.A. *et al.* (1992) Substrate oxidation and gh responses to exercise are independent of menstrual phase and status. *Medicine and Science in Sports and Exercise.* 24(8), 873–880.

Kenny, G.P. and Jay, O. (2007) Sex differences in post-exercise oesophageal and muscle tissue temperature response. *American Journal of Physiology, Regulative, Integrated and Comparative Physiology,* 292(4), R1632–1640.

Lane, K.N. and Wenger, H.A. (2004) Effect of selected recovery conditions on performance of repeated bouts of intermittent cycling separated by 24 hours. *Journal of Strength and Conditioning Research,* 18(4), 855–860.

Lum, D., Landers, G. and Peeling, P. (2010) Effects of a Recovery Swim on Subsequent Running Performance. *International Journal of Sports Medicine,* 31, 26–30

MacRae, B.A. *et al.* (2011) Compression garments and exercise: Garment considerations, physiology and performance. *Sports Medicine,* 41(10), 815–843.

Malone, J.K. *et al.* (2014) Neuromscular electrical stimulation during recovery from exercise: A systematic review. *Journal of Strength and Conditioning Research,*

28(9), 2478–2506.

Maughan, R.J. and Shirreffs, S.M. (1997) Recovery from prolonged exercise: restoration of water and electrolyte balance. *Journal of Sports Science*, 15(3), 297–303.

McCarthy, A., Mulligan, J. and Egaña, M. (2016) Post-exercise cold water immersion improves high-intensity exercise performance in normothermia. *Applied Physiology, Nutrition and Metabolism*, 41(11), 1163–1170.

Menzies, P. *et al.* (2010) Blood lactate clearance during active recovery after an intense running bout depends on the intensity of the active recovery. *Journal of Sports Science*, 28(9), 975–982.

Mika, A. *et al.* (2007) Comparison of recovery strategies on muscle performance after fatiguing exercise. *American Journal of Physical Medicine and Rehabilitation*, 86, 474–481.

Monedero, J. and Donne, B. (2000) Effect of recovery interventions on lactate removal and subsequent performance. *International Journal of Sports Medicine*, 21(8), 593–597.

Nedelec, M. *et al.* (2012) Recovery in soccer Part II. *Sports Medicine*, 43, 9–22.

Nunes, J.A. *et al.* (2014) Monitoring training load, recovery-stress state, immune-endocrine responses, and physical performance in elite female basketball players during a periodized training program. *Journal of Strength and Conditioning Research*, 28(10), 2973–2980.

Ogai, R. *et al.* (2008) Effects of petrissage massage on fatigue and exercise performance following intensive cycle pedalling. *British Journal of Sports Medicine*, 42, 834–838.

Pasiakos, S.M. *et al.* (2014) Effect of protein supplements on muscle damage, muscle soreness and recovery of muscle function and physical performance: a systematic review. *Sports Medicine*, 44, 655–670.

Paulsen, G. *et al.* (2014) Vitamin C and E supplementation hampers cellular adaptation to endurance training in humans: a double-blind, randomised, controlled trial. *Journal of Physiology*, 592, 1887–1901.

Scanlan, A.T. *et al.* (2014) The relationship between internal and external training load models during basketball training. *Journal of Strength and Conditioning Research*, 28(9), 2397–2405.

Rechichi, C. and Dawson, D. (2009) Effect of oral contraceptive cycle phase on performance in team sport players. *Journal of Science and Medicine in Sport*, 12(1), 190–195.

Roberts, L.A. *et al.* (2015) Post-exercise cold water immersion attenuates acute anabolic signalling and long-term adaptations in muscle to strength training. *Journal of Physiology*, 593, 4285–4301.

Robertson, A., Watt, J.M. and Galloway, S.D. (2004) Effects of leg massage on recovery from high intensity cycling exercise. *British Journal of Sports Medicine*, 38(2), 173–176.

Sands, W.A. *et al.* (2013) Stretching and its effects on recovery: A review. *Strength and Conditioning Journal*, 35(5), 30–36.

Selye, H. The Story of the Adaptation Syndrome. Montreal, PQ: *ACTA Medical*, 1952 (Russian edition by Medgiz, Moscow, 1960).

Stanley, J., Buchheit, M. and Peake, J.M. (2012) The effect of post-exercise hydrotherapy on subsequent exercise performance and heart rate variability. *European Journal of Applied Physiology*, 112, 951–961.

Takahashi, T. and Miyamoto, Y. (1998) Influence of light physical activity on cardiac responses during recovery from exercise in humans. *European Journal of Applied Physiology*, 77, 1137–1144.

Tarnopolsky, M.A. (2000) Gender differences in metabolism; nutrition and supplements. *Journal of Science and Medicine in Sport*, 3(3), 287–298.

Tarnopolsky, M.A. (2008) Sex differences in exercise metabolism and the role of 17-beta estradiol. *Medicine and Science in Sports and Exercise*, 40(4), 648–654.

Urso, M.L. (2013) Anti-inflammatory

169

interventions and skeletal muscle injury: benefit or detriment? *Journal of Applied Physiology,* 115, 920–928.

Vaile, J., Halson, S., Gill, N. and Dawson, B. (2008) Effect of hydrotherapy on the signs and symptoms of delayed onset muscle soreness. *European Journal of Applied Physiology.* 102, 447–455.

Versey, N.G., Halson, S.L. and Dawson, B.T. (2013) Water immersion recovery for athletes: effect on exercise performance and practical recommendations. *Sports Medicine,* 43(11), 1101–1130.

CHAPTER 7
TRAINING YOUNG FEMALE ATHLETES

Rhodri S. Lloyd, PhD, ASCC, CSCS*D[1,2,3]; Lucy Kember, MSc[1]; John M. Radnor, MSc, ASCC[1]; Jon L. Oliver, PhD[1,2]

[1]Cardiff School of Sport, Cardiff Metropolitan University, UK; [2]Sport Performance Research Institute New Zealand, Auckland University of Technology, New Zealand; [3]Centre for Sport Science and Human Performance, Waikato Institute of Technology, New Zealand

Over the last decade there has been a greater attention on increasing female participation rates in sports and identifying potential female sporting talent from a young age. Campaigns such as 'Girls4Gold' by UK Sport and the English Institute of Sport, and the more recent 'This Girl Can' are examples of recent initiatives. Current data show an increase in participation in female sport over the last decade (95). In light of the increase in participation, and in order to maximize the talent pool at the elite levels of sport, it is generally accepted that sporting pathways should be designed to develop well-rounded athletes from a young age (63). In conjunction with sports coaches and sports medicine professionals, the strength and conditioning coach has a vital role to play in ensuring that young female athletes are suitably prepared for the physical rigors of sports. Similarly, in the event that female athletes choose to exit sporting systems due to injury, loss of interest, or to pursue an alternative career, the strength and conditioning coach should have provided them with the 'tools' to facilitate life-long engagement in recreational physical activity.

Recently, the International Olympic Committee (14) and the National Strength and Conditioning Association (59) have published consensus and position statements respectively advocating the use of a long-term approach to the athletic development of youth. This is of particular importance considering the two emerging corollaries within the paediatric literature. Firstly, there is an alarmingly high number of youth who fail to meet global physical activity recommendations and consequently present with negative health profiles, including overweight/obesity, physical illiteracy, and low fitness levels (22–24, 42, 73, 83, 92). In juxtaposition are those young athletes that are at risk of overuse injury due to high volumes of competition and an absence of preparatory conditioning (51, 52, 84). Whether the child accumulates insufficient or excessive amounts of exercise, or falls somewhere between these opposing ends of the spectrum, it is generally accepted that the young bodies of modern-day youth are often ill-prepared to tolerate the demands of sports or physical activity.

Owing to the unique physical and psychosocial characteristics associated with youth, practitioners should design and deliver training programmes that are developmentally appropriate for the individual. As opposed to chasing short-term gains in a particular performance test (for example increases in the one-repetition maximum squat test), practitioners should initially seek to develop a depth and breadth of movement skills in combination with rudimentary levels of muscle

SLOW COOK, DON'T FLASH FRY!

A long-term philosophy to the development of athleticism in young females requires the strength and conditioning coach to adopt a patient and understanding approach to training. An analogy to reflect this process can be seen in the difference between flash frying a piece of meat that leaves the middle raw and under-cooked (poor, weak mover), versus a slow cooking process that renders the meat tender and cooked all the way though (good, strong mover).

strength in young female athletes, to ensure they possess robust and resilient athletic qualities that enable them to move in a variety of ways, and in a range of different environments.

DEVELOPMENTAL PHYSIOLOGY OF YOUNG FEMALE ATHLETES

It has often been stated that youth are not 'miniature adults', and consequently practitioners should not simply superimpose adult-based training programmes on a child or adolescent. The current evidence base shows that children differ to adults in terms of their acute cardiorespiratory response to exercise (5), metabolic and hormonal responses during exercise (17), ability to voluntarily activate muscle (30), and the manner in which they recover from high-intensity exercise (34). Despite these clear child-adult differences, of greater interest to practitioners working with young athletes is the way in which developmental processes dynamically affect individuals as they transition in a non-linear fashion throughout childhood and adolescence.

Childhood

Childhood reflects the developmental period of life from the end of infancy to the beginning of adolescence, with the term 'children' referring to girls and boys (generally up to the age of eleven and thirteen years, respectively) who have not developed secondary sex characteristics (60). During childhood, both girls and boys will experience rapid development in their central nervous systems (CNS), with most children reaching 95 per cent of their adult sized system by the age of seven (65). It is this natural development of the CNS that explains how children demonstrate observable improvements in gross motor control programmes for tasks such as walking, running and jumping. While these motor control programmes are adapted, and refined through late childhood and adolescence, it is imperative that children are afforded the opportunities to learn a broad range of fundamental movement techniques, under the guise of a qualified practitioner, while they possess a heightened degree of neural plasticity (38, 74). This is especially the case given the negative trajectories of low motor skill competency in childhood leading to lower levels of physical activity later in life (85, 99, 100). In addition to the development of the CNS, muscular (104), skeletal (55), and cardiovascular and respiratory systems (65) develop at similar rates in both girls and boys

HOW YOUNG SHOULD GIRLS START IN A STRENGTH AND CONDITIONING PROGRAMME?

The answer is simple; if a child is ready to participate in sport, then they are ready to engage in some form of strength and conditioning. Very young girls should learn to control their own bodyweight, using fun-based, gymnastics-based activities targeted at improving coordination and muscle strength. However, with improvements in technical competency and increased psychosocial maturity, girls should be encouraged to participate in more recognized forms of neuromuscular training involving a range of resistance training equipment situated within appropriate strength and conditioning facilities.

throughout childhood. The similarities in development of the various systems of the body result in both boys and girls showing comparable rates of development in measures of physical fitness. For example, muscle strength develops in a similar fashion for both sexes during childhood (19) with the same pattern emerging for measures of sprint speed (18) and endurance (15).

Adolescence

Adolescence refers to a period of life between childhood and adulthood. Although adolescence is a more difficult period to define in terms of chronological age due to differential maturation rates (65), girls twelve to eighteen years and boys fourteen to eighteen years are generally considered adolescents. Literature has clearly demonstrated that individuals of the same chronological age (single time point away from the date of birth) can differ markedly with respect to biological maturity (11, 54). Significant inter-individual variance exists for the level (magnitude of change), timing (onset of change), and tempo (rate of change) of biological maturation. Dependent on these variables, children will be viewed as either biologically ahead of their chronological age (early-maturing individual), 'on-time' with their chronological age (average maturer), or behind their chronological age (late-maturing individual) (65). Because girls mature approximately two years earlier than boys, they consequently spend less time in preadolescent growth and experience smaller growth rates, resulting in females attaining shorter adult height (94).

It is during adolescence that sex differences in athletic performance materialize, with boys demonstrating accelerated gains in physical fitness, especially in terms of muscular strength and power (15, 20, 60, 89). These performance changes are best explained by the increase in muscle size and strength

witnessed in males relative to females during the adolescent years (53, 86, 91), most likely owing to the greater rise in anabolic hormones (for example testosterone, growth hormone, IGF-1) in males (91). In addition, girls are likely to experience smaller growth in internal organs, blood volume and a greater relative increase in fat mass. These sex differences in physiology and anatomy should be considered by practitioners as they may dictate training responsiveness and importantly, the relative injury risk in young female athletes. For example, research has shown that abnormal joint mechanics may be amplified when musculoskeletal growth occurs in the absence of corresponding neuromuscular adaptation (36, 45). Adolescent girls do not experience a naturally occurring neuromuscular spurt in the same way as their male counterparts; therefore relevant training (for example motor skill training, strength and power training) plays a key role in 'triggering' a training-induced spurt (46, 77).

TRAINABILITY OF YOUNG FEMALE ATHLETES

When examining the trainability of youth, it becomes clear that girls experience gains in fitness following different training interventions, including aerobic (4, 7), sprint (67) and resistance (13) training. Closer inspection of the data shows that absolute changes in performance are likely to be greater in males, but when normalized, some of these adaptations may become less divergent between sexes.

Resistance training

Meta-analytical data has shown that girls are consistently able to improve muscular strength in response to resistance training interventions, and that the efficacy of resistance training does not differ between sexes (13). This was corroborated by Lesinski *et al.* (57) who showed that both boys and girls made similar gains in muscular strength and vertical jump performance in response to strength and power training. The authors did however report that girls had significantly larger improvements in sport-specific performance (for example throwing, hitting and/or kicking velocities) compared with boys in response to resistance training programmes (57). Thus, despite the misplaced controversies around girls participating in resistance training (97), it would appear that their trainability in response to this training modality is at least equal, if not higher than boys. Mechanistically, neural adaptations will be primarily responsible for the training-induced changes seen in both boys and girls during childhood; however, as adolescence manifests, males are likely to experience a greater contribution from increases in muscle cross-sectional area (26) and potentially preferential muscle fibre-type distribution (37) owing to their elevated levels of anabolic hormones (39, 60). The manner in which sex and maturity interact with resistance training is an area that requires further exploration to better understand the training responsiveness of females. However, given the many benefits associated with resistance training, it should form a central training component of any strength and conditioning programme for female athletes irrespective of maturity status.

Aerobic training

The majority of published literature examining the responsiveness of youth to aerobic training has utilized boys as participants; however data has shown that girls can also make worthwhile improvements in VO_2peak that are comparable to those reported previously in samples of boys (71). Where data has directly examined sex differences in responsiveness to aerobic training, it is apparent that girls demonstrate a similar adaptive response to boys (6, 7, 82). For example, Obert *et al.* (82)

reported 15 per cent and 8 per cent improvements in VO_2peak in boys and girls respectively in response to a 13-week training programme involving 3 × 1-hour sessions per week and > 80 per cent HRmax. Similarly, prepubertal girls and boys made comparable gains in VO_2peak (7.2 per cent and 9.5 per cent respectively) following a 7-week training programme, inclusive of 2 × 30 minute sessions per week working at 100–130 per cent maximal aerobic speed (6). Mechanistically, it is unclear what drives aerobic training-induced adaptations in VO_2peak in boys versus girls. The available evidence is largely based on boys, and suggests that increased stroke volume, and thus cardiac output, are typically due to increased heart volume and contractility (64). However, the increased anabolic profile and related physiological benefits (for example increased VO_2, muscle size and strength, and maximal arterio-venous oxygen [A-VO$_2$] difference) associated with the pubertal spurt may help explain further adaptations during adolescence (68). Much like resistance training, the manner in which training, sex and maturation interact to augment the aerobic training responsiveness remains unclear.

INJURY RISKS IN YOUNG FEMALE ATHLETES

The physical, physiological and psychological demands associated with training intensity and competition are rapidly increasing within modern-day young athletes (52). The rapid growth in youth elite sport places increasing pressures on adolescents to become fitter, faster and stronger, often at the detriment of progressive and structured training programmes. Furthermore, coaches may disregard the importance of holistic physical development and maturation in adolescents, which may lead to a lack of physical preparation and the inability to tolerate the rigors of sports or physical activity. Exposure to the risk of injury and long-term impairments to health are therefore increased, and although adolescents may be considered as a single entity, it should be noted that young female athletes can still fall prey to the same injuries that affect the female adult.

Early Specialization

Early specialization refers to the concept of a child participating in year-round intensive training within a single sport or physical activity at the exclusion of others (59). Research has identified that early specialization in one sport can increase risk of injury and serious overuse injury in young athletes, regardless of training volume and age (40, 52). Spending a greater amount of time participating in competitive sports compared to unstructured free play (> 2:1 ratio), training in excess of eight months per year in a single sport, and accumulating a weekly training volume greater than a child's chronological age have been identified as thresholds above which the potential for overuse injury is increased (52). Athletes that specialize in one sport are more likely to expose their neuromuscular system and musculoskeletal tissues to only one set of motor patterns (59, 78), which inevitably may lead to the development of muscular imbalances. Such an important finding highlights the significant responsibility of coaches and parents on the monitoring of young females, and keeping average weekly training volume lower than age in years for adolescent athletes. This is especially important around the time of the pubertal growth spurt where rapid periods of growth may heighten the risk of injury.

Injuries

Injuries are an unfortunate consequence of any sports participation and activity; however, there are common musculoskeletal conditions that are more frequent in female athletes compared to their male counterparts, regardless of age. Injuries can be categorized into two main groups: acute trauma or overuse injuries (49). Overuse injuries are defined as the breakdown and damage of tissues that are a result of repetitive sub-maximal loading on the musculoskeletal system with inadequate recovery time for adaptation (29). Overuse injuries that are particularly prevalent in female athletes include: 1) stress fractures, 2) patellofemoral pain syndrome (PFPS) and 3) anterior cruciate ligament (ACL) ruptures (43, 49).

1) Stress Fractures

Besides menstrual disturbances (2, 8, 103), other common mechanisms that induce stress fractures in young female athletes include alterations to bone formation (independent of low bone mineral density), low calcium intake, greater or sudden increases in training load, low body fat or BMI, and a change in footwear or training surface (2). An athlete suspected of a stress fracture may present with gradual onset of pain (aggravated by exercise), local tenderness on palpation, and possible bruising. The recognition of such symptoms is crucial for early intervention, load modification and rehabilitation, consequently minimizing the need for possible surgery. Although conservative treatment will require relative rest, the majority of stress fractures affect the lower extremities, thus allowing

---

'VITAMIN D IS KEY'

In addition to engaging in physical acitivity, it is imperative that young females adopt a good lifestyle and consume a healthy diet. Vitamin D plays a vital role in bone mass accrual and calcium regulation for all adolescents. Athletes who have inadequate exposure to sunlight, low vitamin D levels, or are recovering from a stress fracture may be encouraged to increase their vitamin D intake. Alternatively, safe exposure to a little ray of sunshine goes a long way.

conditioning of other areas of the body to be maintained through alternative training.

2) Patellofemoral pain syndrome (PFPS)

Despite its high incidence, the source of pain and treatment guidelines of PFPS remain unclear. It is believed that an increased Q-angle (angle between the anterior superior iliac spine and midpoint of the patella), vastus medialis (VMO) and hip weakness, training overload, altered gluteus activity, and patellofemoral malalignment (9, 88, 102) are the primary precursors for PFPS. Furthermore, the resultant biomechanical abnormalities may increase susceptibility of female athletes to the development of other overuse injuries, such as medial tibial stress syndrome (2). Conservative treatment is the most effective strategy for young athletes with PFPS, with current literature emphasizing the importance of hip strengthening, and flexibility of the iliotibial band and iliopsoas (9). Prevention strategies should include regular monitoring of adequate training loads, regular soft tissue release of tight structures (for example sports massage) and neuromuscular training with an emphasis on correct jumping and landing mechanics. Additionally, specific warm-up strategies should include activation exercises targeting the gluteus medius and VMO, such as mini-band walks, lateral planks, single leg glute-bridges, and partial range single leg squats.

3) Anterior cruciate ligament (ACL) ruptures

Adolescent girls are two to ten times more likely to suffer injuries to the ACL compared to their male counterparts (75). Non-contact mechanisms account for 60–80 per cent of ACL injuries, especially in movements involving cutting, jumping, and single leg landings (1, 16, 56, 90). Females are predisposed to a greater risk of ACL injury due to anatomical structures, fluctuating hormone levels, muscle imbalances, and poor neuromuscular function (1, 76, 90, 105). Anatomically, females have a smaller ACL (within a smaller notch), wider pelvis, greater Q-angle and greater ligament laxity than males (1). Research has suggested possible links between hormonal cycling, joint laxity and neuromuscular imbalances in female athletes (76). While a true mechanism is unknown, it is believed that sex hormone receptors (for example oestrogen, testosterone and relaxin) may influence the structure, metabolism and mechanical properties of the ACL (90). Although such differences might play a role in injury susceptibility, these risk factors are deemed non-modifiable, and therefore focus should be placed on more modifiable mechanisms (1).

Muscular strength and neuromuscular control are crucial components of functional knee stability during the execution of sports movements. The ability to control rotation of the lower limb in pivoting and landing movements requires large amounts of knee stability and co-contraction of the hamstring and quadriceps groups. Longer hamstring electromechanical delay (EMD) may negatively influence the muscle's ability to rapidly stabilize the knee, therefore increasing the chances of ACL injury (70). Younger girls present longer EMD than older girls (27), and the effects of fatigue are significantly greater in the younger population. Additionally, females have been shown to activate their quadriceps more than males during landing and pivoting movements, demonstrating less hip and knee flexion and therefore a lower hamstring to quadriceps ratio (31, 44). Given the detrimental effects of poor muscular strength and neuromuscular control, injury prevention strategies should be based around such mechanisms in order to reduce the prevalence of ACL injuries in young female athletes.

A current meta-analysis of fourteen ACL injury prevention studies has shown significantly greater reduction of knee injuries

'KNOWLEDGE IS POWER'

The biggest issue with poor movement competency is education. Athletes often don't think about how they move, or how they 'look' when performing simple tasks such as landing or pivoting. Simple cueing and education of correct techniques will often see dramatic improvements in movement patterns. The power of knowledge may reduce the risk of injury!

in female athletes who are exposed to neuromuscular training compared to controls (80). Results also showed that greater reductions in injury risk were evident in mid-teens (fourteen to eighteen years) compared to late teens (eighteen to twenty years) and early adults (>twenty years) (80), further highlighting the importance of implementing injury prevention strategies as early as possible in a young athlete's life. Prevention strategies should emphasize a focus on lower body and hip strengthening, proprioceptive balance training, dynamic stabilization during jumping and landing, movement education during deceleration and cutting manoeuvres and preseason conditioning.

THE FEMALE ATHLETE TRIAD

The female athlete triad is often seen in physically active girls and women and involves an individual presenting with one or more of the following inter-related symptoms: 1) menstrual dysfunction, 2) low bone mineral density, and 3) low energy availability (25). Prolonged negative energy balance supresses oestrogen and this leads to increased bone reabsorption, and this can be exacerbated where the diet is also low in calcium (girls trying to restrict their calorie intake are likely to avoid calcium). Adolescent athletes are at particular risk of developing one or more of the triad components due to the critical period of bone mass accumulation and maturation (25, 81, 103). In addition, the prolonged

presence of one component increases the likelihood of developing other triad conditions, with potentially irreversible consequences if left untreated (25). It is thought that athletes participating in any sport may be at risk of the triad; however, those that participate in endurance sports or those events that are based on aesthetics, weight-class categories, or an emphasis or reward for leanness, are at a much greater risk (8).

Triad components

Menstrual dysfunction (for example anovulation, luteal phase defects, amenorrhea [primary or secondary] and oligomenorrhea) is seen in roughly 54 per cent of female adolescent athletes who regularly participate in sport (48, 103). The presence of menstrual irregularities is commonly associated with inadequate energy availability, increases in training volume, and overtraining. As a result of these, a cascading effect can stimulate compensatory mechanisms such as weight loss, metabolic hormone alterations, or energy conservation. A regular assumption is often made that such disruptions to menstrual functions are normal amongst athletic adolescents partaking in intense training. However, symptoms must not be ignored and may result in negative consequences to cardiovascular health and premature osteoporosis (72, 81).

Bone growth and development is critical during childhood and adolescence, with peak gains occurring approximately one year after the age of peak linear growth (65). Athletic amenorrhea can lead to lower bone mineral density, with approximately 4 per cent per year of bone loss apparent in the first two or three years' menstrual dysfunction (2). Subsequent loss in bone mineral density can predispose athletes to the risk of stress fractures and development of osteoporosis. It is also thought that early specialization in specific non-weight bearing sports can lead to altered adaptations in bone mass accrual. Literature has identified that swimmers exhibit lower levels of BMD compared with gymnasts, despite greater levels of body disfaction and menstrual dysfunction (93, 103).

The term 'energy availability' is defined as dietary energy intake minus exercise energy expenditure, corrected for fat-free mass (FFM) (81). Optimal energy availability for a female adult is 45 kcal/kg FFM per day, with adolescents often requiring increased levels due to the period of growth and development (72, 81). Energy availability <30 kcal/kg FFM per day can adversely affect bone remodelling and may disrupt menstrual function and bone mineral density (103). Previous literature has suggested that athletes who fit this element of the triad will commonly present with abnormal eating behaviours or clinical eating disorders such as anorexia nervosa and bulimia nervosa (101). Developing an eating disorder may manifest from prolonged periods of dieting, weight fluctuations, coach changes, injury, and casual weight comments from coaches, parents, friends and peers (98).

The significant relationship between each component of the triad emphasizes the importance of a holistic approach to monitoring female adolescent athletes. Elevated training levels ≥ 12h/wk, reduced BMD, late age at menarche, and low energy availability independently or combined, pose the greatest risk to developing bone stress injuries (8, 81, 103). The interrelationship between high training volumes and insufficient energy intake are largely consequences of inadequate knowledge and understanding of specific elevated calorie need. Education and interventions need to be implemented based on the individual athlete and must include one or a combination of strategies to be effective. Such strategies must address specific nutritional and weight requirements (including specifications for weight gain), menstrual restoration, psychological support, training volumes, and

'STOP, LOOK AND LISTEN'
To identify adolescent athletes susceptible to the triad, coaches must have the skills to recognize the risk factors; STOP, LOOK and LISTEN. STOP: Ensure that prevention and intervention strategies have been considered and incorporated into training plans. LOOK: Educate staff, parents and athletes on the signs and symptoms, including weight loss and amenorrhea. Be mindful of patterns and behaviours associated with training volume and calorie restrictions. This could be monitored with general wellness questionnaires. LISTEN: Adolescents at risk may give indirect indications through passing comments with teammates, coaches or medical staff. Be aware of information regarding eating habits, menstrual cycles and volume of sports participation.

activity limitations (8). Early diagnosis is the critical step in the prevention of immediate and long-term health consequences [12], highlighting the importance of a multidisciplinary collaboration. If weight loss or clinical eating disorders are suspected, it is essential that athletes are referred to the appropriate medical or nutritional professionals rather than coaching staff. Prehabilitation, biomechanical analysis and bespoke strength and conditioning programmes should be implemented to reduce the risk of injury and reverse the development of the negative consequences associated with the female athlete triad.

PUTTING IT ALL TOGETHER: TRAINING PRESCRIPTION FOR THE YOUNG FEMALE ATHLETE

Developing a Culture

Research has shown that females may naturally be less confident in their abilities to perform resistance training compared with males (87), thus as a practitioner it is important to develop a culture in which they feel comfortable. Data indicates that confidence and motivation will be reduced in young females if they perceive resistance training to be a masculine activity (58). Therefore, it is important to educate the athlete early within the strength and conditioning programme, explaining the process of resistance training including the physiological changes, potential muscle soreness, and the benefits of strength training for improved performance and injury prevention. By educating young females about the benefit of strength training, coaches can increase motivation, address fears and dispel misconceptions. In order to increase confidence, it is important to set achievable expectations, striking a balance between the challenge of the task and the athlete's skill level (32). Training goals should be based predominantly on the process of the resistance-training programme, as females focus more on the performance of tasks rather than the outcome (41). When providing feedback and setting individualized goals (especially early in the programme), technique and task-related improvements should be the priority focus rather than personal records.

'ALL FOR ONE, AND ONE FOR ALL'

The female behavioural response can sometimes be characterized by patterns of immersing within social groups to seek shared encouragement from peers when confronted by challenging scenarios. This is different to the behavioural response typically witnessed in males ('fight or flight'), which results in a more aggressive and forthright reaction. It is important for practitioners to develop a culture that enables the former response to drive a sense of collegiality and teamwork, and to promote encouragement and enthusiasm amongst young female athletes. Positive encouragement and verbal persuasion by coaches and other athletes can improve confidence in young female athletes, especially if it is interpreted by the athlete as being realistic.

Programming

The prescription of resistance training should always be individualized, based on factors such as technical competency, biological age, and specific injury risk factors. It is imperative that the prescribed training is part of a holistic training programme, that is appropriate for the developmental stage of the athlete (33). The Youth Physical Development (YPD) model offers an overview of holistic physical development, identifying the relevant training priorities associated with each stage of development (61). Importantly, the YPD model recognizes that all fitness qualities are trainable throughout childhood and adolescence; however, the importance of strength and movement competency as training priorities are emphasized during all stages of development.

To take advantage of the heightened degree of neural plasticity and neuromuscular maturation (79), childhood appears to be the optimal time to develop motor skill competency. The ability of the young athlete to manage their own bodyweight in a variety of positions is important for general athleticism. The use of the body as a form of resistance also provides a suitable training stimulus for the simultaneous development of fundamental motor skills and muscle strength. Basic bodyweight movements based around the athletic motor skills competencies (AMSC; Fig. 7.1) should be incorporated; allowing young girls to learn the correct movement patterns for squatting, lunging, pushing, pulling, jumping, landing, and bracing (62). Gymnastics-based movements can offer young girls an enjoyable training method in which to learn movement skills and build relative strength (10). For example, simple gymnastic shapes such as the arch, dish, straddle, pike, and tuck can be included as part of the warm-up, prior to more structured training based around the AMSC. Additionally, the use of animal shapes and crawls can be

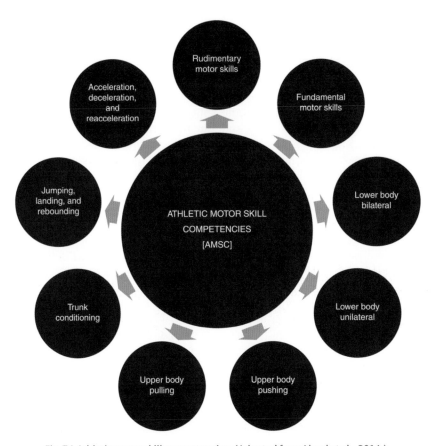

Fig.7.1 Athletic motor skill competencies. (Adapted from Lloyd et al., 2014.)

utilized to promote trunk stability in various planes of movement.

A number of programming principles can remain similar for both boys and girls. Regardless of sex, compound exercises such as squats, deadlifts, lunges, and step-ups should be staple exercises for most strength and conditioning programmes. However, the strength and conditioning coach should be aware of the physiological differences between males and females when programming and coaching exercises. Considering that females display a larger Q-angle than males (35), particular attention should be paid to technical competency in both unilateral and bilateral lower-body exercises, ensuring that knee

valgus is minimized at all times. Considering that females display greater knee valgus when landing and cutting (35, 66), it is paramount to teach good mechanics in a controlled environment, and where necessary regress tasks or use relevant cues to correct technique and enable optimal movement competency.

As females tend to place a larger emphasis on the process rather than the outcome of tasks (41), the use of unilateral exercises that are more technically demanding and require an increased level of stability (12) may be of greater benefit to girls, at least in the early stages of the programme. Additionally, research has demonstrated that greater activation of the gluteus medius can be achieved through the use of unilateral exercises (69), which may be important for reducing knee valgus that is prevalent in females during dynamic tasks (35, 66). Furthermore, greater strength in the hip external rotators can help reduce PFPS (9), which is prevalent in young females. Split stance exercises have been reported to increase hamstring activation in comparison to bilateral exercises (3). Considering that females are more quadriceps-dominant (31), exercises that result in increased hamstring recruitment may be vital for injury prevention, especially to reduce the risk of ACL injury (28).

While it may be suitable to programme an equal balance in training volume between the upper- and lower-body in boys, girls may warrant additional focus on developing their upper-body musculature, as men have significantly more upper-body muscle mass than females (50). Considering the utilization of upper-body strength in a number of sports, developing strength in this area is key for all female athletes. Introducing girls to a variety of pushing and pulling exercises in both the horizontal and vertical plane is essential in order to build upper-body strength. Many girls do not enjoy upper-body strength training, usually due to the fact they find it difficult or are afraid of developing too much muscle mass. Therefore, the strength and conditioning coach may need to use a range of equipment and different pedagogical methods to create athlete buy-in and promote education. The use of upper-body gymnastic supports, suspension training, resistance bands and medicine balls can all be used to complement the traditional dumbbell and barbell training methods to develop upper-body strength.

Plyometric training may improve landing mechanics (reduce valgus stress and strain), improve eccentric muscle control, and increase hamstrings activity, which may help minimize the heightened risk of ACL injuries in females (21, 47). A recent meta-analysis demonstrated that plyometric training improves physical performance in female athletes regardless of age, type of sport and competition level (96). Tall girls, and those experiencing peak height velocity (PHV), are likely to find jumping and landing tasks more challenging, therefore technical competency should be prioritized when programming plyometric exercises. Teaching basic jumping and landing mechanics to girls at an early age should have benefits both from a performance and injury prevention point of view.

Designing strength and conditioning training programmes will be based primarily on technical competency, with consideration given to other variables, including stage of maturation, training experience, sex of the individual, and priority of the training block. In an attempt to determine how training sessions may differ when working with youth athletes of differing abilities, Tables 7.1 and 7.2 present examples of training sessions for novice and experienced females respectively. Transitioning from Table 7.1 to 7.2, it is evident that while a number of AMSCs are present in both sessions, the technical difficulty of the exercises, volumes and relative loads, and rest periods are altered.

Warm Up			
Exercise	Volume	Load	
Arch to Dish Shapes	2 x 10	BW	
Straddle to Shoulder Stand	2 x 10	BW	
Spiderman	2 x 6 E.L	BW	
Inchworm	2 x 6	BW	
Mini-band walks	2 x 8 E.L	Light mini-band	
Bear Crawl	2 x 10m	BW	
Low Box Jumps	2 x 6	BW	
Main Session			
Exercise	Volume	Load	Rest
Goblet Squat	3 x 10	8kg	60s
KB Deadlift	3 x 8	8kg	60s
Rear foot elevated split squat	3 x 6 E.L	BW	60s
Incline press up	3 x 8	BW	60s
Inverse Row	3 x 8	BW	60s
Single Arm KB Press	3 x 6 E.A	4kg	60s

Table 7.1 Example training session for a novice female athlete.

SUMMARY

Research clearly shows that strength and conditioning offers young female athletes multiple benefits for physical performance, injury risk reduction and general health and wellbeing. Specifically, data has shown:

- From a developmental perspective, developmentally appropriate training appears to facilitate healthy growth and development.
- Well-designed training can induce a 'neuromuscular spurt' that young female athletes may not experience through natural development.
- All fitness components are trainable in young female athletes irrespective of stage of maturation.
- Effective training can reduce the relative risk of injury for young female athletes, especially for knee injuries.
- The risks of young athletes experiencing the female athlete triad syndrome can be alleviated by well-planned and carefully monitored training processes, recovery strategies and nutritional intake.

Warm Up			
Exercise	**Volume**	**Load**	
Deadbugs	2 x 8 E.S	BW	
Glute Bridge	2 x 10	BW	
Hamstring bridge	2 x 10	BW	
Squat to Stand	2 x 10	BW	
Mini-band walks	2 x 8 E.S	Light mini-band	
Overhead Walking Lunge	2 x 6 E.L	BW	
Lateral Bear Crawl	2 x 10m	BW	
Box Jumps	2 x 6	BW	
Main Session			
Exercise	**Volume**	**Load**	**Rest**
Hang Clean	3 x 4	85% 1RM	180s
Back Squat	3 x 5	80% 1RM	120s
RDL	3 x 6	78% 1RM	120s
Reverse Lunge	3 x 6 E.L	75% 1RM	120s
DB Bench Press	3 x 8	70% 1RM	120s
Bent Over Row	3 x 8	70% 1RM	120s
Jammer Press	3 x 6 E.A	70% 1RM	120s

Table 7.2 Example training session for an experienced female athlete.

REFERENCES

1. Alentorn-Geli, E., Myer, G.D., Silvers, H.J., Samitier, G., Romero, D., Lazaro-Haro, C. and Cugat, R. (2009) Prevention of non-contact anterior cruciate ligament injuries in soccer players. Part 1: Mechanisms of injury and underlying risk factors. *Knee Surgery, Sports Traumatology, Arthroscopy*, 17, 705–729.

2. Alleyne, J. and Bennell, K. (2012) Women and activity-related issues across the lifespan, in: *Brukner and Khan's Clinical Sports Medicine*. P. Brukner, K.M. Khan, R. Bahr, S.N. Blair, J. Cook, K. Crossley, J. McConnell, P. McCrory, T. Noakes, (eds.) NSW: Australia: McGraw-Hill Australia Pty Ltd, pp.910–935.

3. Andersen, V., Fimland, M.S., Brennset, O., Haslestad, L.R., Lundteigen, M.S., Skalleberg, K. and Saeterbakken, A.H. (2014) Muscle activation and strength in squat and Bulgarian squat on stable and unstable surface. *International Journal of Sports Medicine*, 35, 1196–1202.

4. Armstrong, N. and Baker, A.R. (2011) Endurance training and elite young athletes. *Medicine and Sports Science*, 56: 59–83.

5. Armstrong, N., Barker, A.R. and McManus, A.M. (2015) Muscle metabolism changes with age and maturation: How do they relate to youth sport performance? *British Journal of Sports Medicine*, 49, 860–864.

6. Baquet, G., Berthoin, S., Dupont, G., Blondel, N., Fabre, C. and van Praagh, E. (2002) Effects of high intensity intermittent training on peak VO(2) in prepubertal children. *International Journal of Sports Medicine*, 23, 439–444.

7. Baquet, G., van Praagh, E. and Berthoin,

S. (2003) Endurance training and aerobic fitness in young people. *Sports Medicine*, 33, 1127–1143.

8. Barrack, M.T., Gibbs, J.C., De Souza, M.J., Williams, N.I., Nichols, J.F., Rauh, M.J. and Nattiv, A. (2014) Higher incidence of bone stress injuries with increasing female athlete triad-related risk factors: a prospective multisite study of exercising girls and women. *American Journal of Sports Medicine*. 42, 949–958.

9. Barton, C.J., Lack, S., Malliaras, P. and Morrissey, D. (2013) Gluteal muscle activity and patellofemoral pain syndrome: a systematic review. *British Journal of Sports Medicine*, 47, 207–214.

10. Baumgarten, S. and Pagnano-Richardson, K. (2010) Educational gymnastics: enhancing children's physical literacy. *Journal of Physical Education, Recreation and Dance*, 81, 18–25.

11. Baxter-Jones, A.D.G., Eisenmann, J.C. and Sherar, L.B. (2005) Controlling for maturation in pediatric exercise science. *Pediatric Exercise Science*, 17, 18–30.

12. Behm, D. and Colado, J.C. (2012) The effectiveness of resistance training using unstable surfaces and devices for rehabilitation. *International Journal of Sports Physical Therapy*, 7, 226–241.

13. Behringer, M., Vom Heede, A., Yue, Z. and Mester, J. (2010) Effects of resistance training in children and adolescents: a meta-analysis. *Pediatrics*, 126, e1199–1210.

14. Bergeron, M.F., Mountjoy, M., Armstrong, N., Chia, M., Cote, J., Emery, C.A., Faigenbaum, A., Hall, G. Jr., Kriemler, S., Leglise, M., Malina, R.M., Pensgaard, A.M., Sanchez, A., Soligard, T., Sundgot-Borgen, J., van Mechelen, W., Weissensteiner, J.R. and Engebretsen, L. (2015) International Olympic Committee consensus statement on youth athletic development. *British Journal of Sports Medicine*, 49, 843–851.

15. Beunen, G.P. and Malina, R.M. (2008) Growth and biological maturation: relevance to athletic performance, in: *The Young Athlete*. H. Hebestreit, O. Bar-Or, (eds.) Oxford: Blackwell Publishing, pp.3–17.

16. Boden, B.P., Torg, J.S., Knowles, S.B. and Hewett, T.E. (2009) Video analysis of anterior cruciate ligament injury: abnormalities in hip and ankle kinematics. *American Journal of Sports Medicine*, 37, 252–259.

17. Boisseau, N. and Delamarche, P. (2000) Metabolic and hormonal responses to exercise in children and adolescents. *Sports Medicine*, 30, 405–422.

18. Borms, J. (1986) The child and exercise: an overview. *Journal of Sports Science*, 4, 3–20.

19. Branta, C., Haubenstricker, J. and Seefeldt, V. (1984) Age changes in motor skills during childhood and adolescence. *Exercise and Sport Science Review*, 12, 467–520.

20. Catley, M.J. and Tomkinson, G.R. (2013) Normative health-related fitness values for children: analysis of 85,347 test results on 9–17-year-old Australians since 1985. *British Journal of Sports Medicine*, 47, 98–108.

21. Chimera, N.J., Swanik, K.A., Swanik, C.B. and Straub, S.J. (2004) Effects of Plyometric Training on Muscle-Activation Strategies and Performance in Female Athletes. *Journal of Athletic Training*, 39, 24–31.

22. Cohen, D.D., Voss, C., Taylor, M.J., Delextrat, A., Ogunleye, A.A. and Sandercock, G.R. (2011) Ten-year secular changes in muscular fitness in English children. *Acta Paediatrica*, 100, e175–177.

23. Cumming, S.P., Sherar, L.B., Pindus, D.M., Coelho-e-Silva, M.J., Malina, R.M. and Jardine, P.R. (2012) A biocultural model of maturity-associated variance in adolescent physical activity. *International Review of Sport Exercise Psychology*, 5, 23–43.

24. D'Hondt, E., Deforche, B., Gentier, I., Verstuyf, J., Vaeyens, R., De Bourdeaudhuij, I., Philippaerts, R. and Lenoir, M. (2014) A longitudinal study of gross motor coordination and weight status in children. *Obesity (Silver Spring)*

22, 1505–1511.

25. De Souza, M.J., Nattiv, A., Joy, E., Misra, M., Williams, N.I., Mallinson, R.J., Gibbs, J.C., Olmsted, M., Goolsby, M. and Matheson, G. (2014) Female Athlete Triad Coalition, American College of Sports Medicine, American Medical Society for Sports Medicine, and American Bone Health Association. 2014 Female Athlete Triad Coalition consensus statement on treatment and return to play of the female athlete triad: 1st International Conference held in San Francisco, CA, May 2012, and 2nd International Conference held in Indianapolis, IN, May 2013. *Clinical Journal of Sport Medicine*, 24, 96–119.

26. De Ste Croix, M.B., Armstrong, N., Welsman, J.R. and Sharpe, P. (2002) Longitudinal changes in isokinetic leg strength in 10–14-year-olds. *Annals of Human Biology*, 29, 50–62.

27. De Ste Croix, M.B., Priestley, A.M., Lloyd, R.S. and Oliver, J.L. (2014) ACL injury risk in elite female youth soccer: Changes in neuromuscular control of the knee following soccer-specific fatigue. *Scandinavian Journal of Medicine and Science in Sports*, 25, e531–538.

28. DeMorat, G., Weinhold, P., Blackburn, T., Chudik, S. and Garrett, W. (2004) Aggressive quadriceps loading can induce noncontact anterior cruciate ligament injury. *American Journal of Sports Medicine*, 32, 477–483.

29. DiFiori, J.P., Benjamin, H.J., Brenner, J., Gregory, A., Jayanthi, N., Landry, G.L. and Luke, A. (2014) Overuse injuries and burnout in youth sports: a position statement from the American Medical Society for Sports Medicine. *Clinical Journal of Sport Medicine*, 24, 3–20.

30. Dotan, R., Mitchell, C., Cohen, R., Klentrou, P., Gabriel, D. and Falk, B. (2012) Child-adult differences in muscle activation – a review. *Pediatric Exercise Science*, 24, 2–21.

31. Ebben, W.P., Fauth, M.L., Petushek, E.J., Garceau, L.R., Hsu, B.E., Lutsch, B.N. and Feldmann, C.R. (2010) Gender-based analysis of hamstring and quadriceps muscle activation during jump landings and cutting. *Journal of Strength and Conditioning Research*, 24, 408–415.

32. Engeser, S. and Rheinberg, F. (2008) Flow, performance and moderators of challenge-skill balance. *Motivation and Emotion*, 32, 158–172.

33. Faigenbaum, A.D., Lloyd, R.S., MacDonald, J. and Myer, G.D. (2016) Citius, Altius, Fortius: beneficial effects of resistance training for young athletes: narrative review. *British Journal of Sports Medicine*, 50, 3–7.

34. Falk, B. and Dotan, R. (2006) Child-adult differences in the recovery from high-intensity exercise. *Exercise and Sport Science Review*, 34, 107–112.

35. Ford, K.R., Myer, G.D. and Hewett, T.E. (2003) Valgus knee motion during landing in high school female and male basketball players. *Medicine and Science in Sports and Exercise*, 35, 1745–1750.

36. Ford, K.R., Shapiro, R., Myer, G.D., Van Den Bogert, A.J. and Hewett, T.E. (2010) Longitudinal sex differences during landing in knee abduction in young athletes. *Medicine and Science in Sports and Exercise*, 42, 1923–1931.

37. Glenmark, B., Hedberg, G. and Jansson, E. (1992) Changes in muscle fibre type from adolescence to adulthood in women and men. *Acta Physiologica Scandinavica*, 146, 251–259.

38. Gogtay, N., Giedd, J.N., Lusk, L., Hayashi, K.M., Greenstein, D., Vaituzis, A.C., Nugent, T.F. 3rd, Herman, D.H., Clasen, L.S., Toga, A.W., Rapoport, J.L. and Thompson, P.M. (2004) Dynamic mapping of human cortical development during childhood through early adulthood. *Proceedings of the National Academy of Sciences*, USA, 101, 8174–8179.

39. Granacher, U., Lesinski, M., Busch, D., Muehlbauer, T., Prieske, O., Puta, C., Gollhofer, A. and Behm, D.G. (2016) Effects of Resistance Training in Youth Athletes on Muscular Fitness and Athletic Performance: A Conceptual Model for Long-Term Athlete Development.

Frontiers in Physiology, 7, 164.

40. Hall, R., Barber Foss, K., Hewett, T.E. and Myer, G.D. (2015) Sport specialization's association with an increased risk of developing anterior knee pain in adolescent female athletes. *Journal of Sport Rehabilitation*, 24, 31–35.

41. Hanrahan, S.J. and Cerin, E. (2009) Gender, level of participation, and type of sport: differences in achievement goal orientation and attributional style. *Journal of Science and Medicine in Sport*, 12, 508–512.

42. Hardy, L.L., Reinten-Reynolds, T., Espinel, P., Zask, A. and Okely, A.D. (2012) Prevalence and correlates of low fundamental movement skill competency in children. *Pediatrics*, 130, e390–398.

43. Herring, S.A., Bergfeld, J.A., Bernhardt, D.T., Boyajian-O'Neil, L., Gregory, A., Indelicato, P.A., Jaffe, R., Joy, S.M., Kibler, W.B., Lowe, W. and Putukian, M. (2008) Selected issues for the adolescent athlete and the team physician: a consensus statement. *Medicine and Science in Sports Exercise*, 40, 1997–2012.

44. Hewett, T.E., Lindenfeld, T.N., Riccobene, J.V. and Noyes, F.R. (1999) The effect of neuromuscular training on the incidence of knee injury in female athletes. A prospective study. *American Journal of Sports Medicine*, 27, 699–706.

45. Hewett, T.E., Myer, G.D. and Ford, K.R. (2004) Decrease in neuromuscular control about the knee with maturation in female athletes. *Journal of Bone and Joint Surgery – American Volume*, 86-A, 1601–1608.

46. Hewett, T.E., Myer, G.D., Ford, K.R., Heidt, R.S. Jr., Colosimo, A.J., McLean, S.G., van den Bogert, A.J., Paterno, M.V. and Succop, P. (2005) Biomechanical measures of neuromuscular control and valgus loading of the knee predict anterior cruciate ligament injury risk in female athletes: a prospective study. *American Journal of Sports Medicine*, 33, 492–501.

47. Hewett, T.E., Stroupe, A.L., Nance, T.A. and Noyes, F.R. (1996) Plyometric training in female athletes. Decreased impact forces and increased hamstring torques. *American Journal of Sports Medicine*, 24, 765–773.

48. Hoch, A.Z., Pajewski, N.M., Moraski, L., Carrera, G.F., Wilson, C.R., Hoffmann, R.G., Schimke, J.E. and Gutterman, D.D. (2009) Prevalence of the female athlete triad in high school athletes and sedentary students. *Clinical Journal of Sport Medicine*, 19, 421–428.

49. Ivkovic, A., Franic, M., Bojanic, I. and Pecina, M. (2007) Overuse injuries in female athletes. *Croatian Medical Journal*, 48, 767–778.

50. Janssen, I., Heymsfield, S.B., Wang, Z.M. and Ross, R. (2000) Skeletal muscle mass and distribution in 468 men and women aged 18–88 yrs. *Journal of Applied Physiology* (1985) 89, 81–88.

51. Jayanthi, N., Pinkham, C., Dugas, L., Patrick, B. and LaBella, C. (2013) Sports specialization in young athletes: evidence-based recommendations. *Sports Health*, 5, 251–257.

52. Jayanthi, N., LaBella, C., Fischer, D., Pasulka, J. and Dugas, L.R. (2015) Sports-specialized intensive training and the risk of injury in young athletes: a clinical case-control study. *American Journal of Sports Medicine*, 43, 794–801.

53. Johnston, F.E. and Malina, R.M. (1966) Age changes in the composition of the upper arm in Philadelphia children. *Human Biology*, 38, 1–21.

54. Kemper, H.C. and Verschuur, R. (1981) Maximal aerobic power in 13- and 14-year-old teenagers in relation to biologic age. *International Journal of Sports Medicine*, 2, 97–100.

55. Kemper, H.C.G. (2000) Skeletal development during childhood and adolescence and the effects of physical activity. *Pediatric Exercise Science*, 12, 198–216.

56. Kristianslund, E., Faul, O., Bahr, R., Myklebust, G. and Krosshaug, T. (2014) Sidestep cutting technique and knee abduction loading: implications for ACL prevention exercises. *British Journal of*

Sports Medicine, 48, 779–783.

57. Lesinski, M., Prieske, O. and Granacher, U. (2016) Effects and dose-response relationships of resistance training on physical performance in youth athletes: a systematic review and meta-analysis. *British Journal of Sports Medicine*, 50, 781-795.

58. Lirgg, C.D. (1991) Gender differences in self-confidence in physical activity: a meta-analysis of recent studies. *Journal of Sport and Exercise Psychology*, 13, 294–310.

59. Lloyd, R.S., Cronin, J.B., Faigenbaum, A.D., Haff, G.G., Howard, R., Kraemer, W.J., Micheli, L.J., Myer, G.D. and Oliver, J.L. (2016) National Strength and Conditioning Association Position Statement on Long-Term Athletic Development. *Journal of Strength and Conditioning Research*, 30, 1491–1509.

60. Lloyd, R.S., Faigenbaum, A.D., Stone, M.H., Oliver, J.L., Jeffreys, I., Moody, J.A., Brewer, C., Pierce, K.C., McCambridge, T.M., Howard, R., Herrington, L., Hainline, B., Micheli, L.J., Jaques, R., Kraemer, W.J., McBride, M.G., Best, T.M., Chu, D.A., Alvar, B.A. and Myer, G.D. (2014) Position statement on youth resistance training: the 2014 International Consensus. *British Journal of Sports Medicine*, 48, 498–505.

61. Lloyd, R.S. and Oliver, J.L. (2012) The youth physical development model: a new approach to long-term athletic development. *Strength and Conditioning Journal*, 34, 61–72.

62. Lloyd, R.S. and Oliver, J.L. (2014) The Developing Athlete, in: High Performance Sports Conditioning. D. Joyce, D. Lewindon, (eds). Champaign, IL: *Human Kinetics*, pp.15–28.

63. Lloyd, R.S., Oliver, J.L., Faigenbaum, A.D., Howard, R., De Ste Croix, M.B., Williams, C.A., Best, T.M., Alvar, B.A., Micheli, L.J., Thomas, D.P., Hatfield, D.L., Cronin, J.B. and Myer, G.D. (2015) Long-term athletic development – part 1: a pathway for all youth. *Journal of Strength and Conditioning Research*, 29, 1439–1450.

64. Mahon, A.D. (2008) Aerobic training, in: *Paediatric Exercise Science and Medicine*. N. Armstrong, W. van Mechelen, (eds.) Oxford: Oxford University Press, pp.273–286.

65. Malina, R.M.B., Bouchard, C. and Bar-Or, O. (2004) *Growth, Maturation and Physical Activity*. Champaign, IL: Human Kinetics.

66. Malinzak, R.A., Colby, S.M., Kirkendall, D.T., Yu, B. and Garrett, W.E. (2001) A comparison of knee joint motion patterns between men and women in selected athletic tasks. *Clinical Biomechanics* (Bristol, Avon) 16, 438–445.

67. Mathisen, G.E. and Pettersen, S.A. (2015) The effect of speed training on sprint and agility performance in female youth. *Journal of Physical Education and Sport*, 15, 395–399.

68. Matos, N. and Winsley, R.J. (2007) Trainability of young athletes and overtraining. *Journal of Sports Science and Medicine*, 6, 353–367.

69. McCurdy, K., O'Kelley, E., Kutz, M., Langford, G., Ernest, J. and Torres, M. (2010) Comparison of lower extremity EMG between the 2-leg squat and modified single-leg squat in female athletes. *Journal of Sport Rehabilitation*, 19, 57–70.

70. McLean, S.G., Borotikar, B. and Lucey, S.M. (2010) Lower limb muscle pre-motor time measures during a choice reaction task associate with knee abduction loads during dynamic single leg landings. *Clinical Biomechanics* (Bristol, Avon), 25, 563–569.

71. McManus, A.M., Armstrong, N. and Williams, C.A. (1997) Effect of training on the aerobic power and anaerobic performance of prepubertal girls. *Acta Paediatrica*, 86, 456–459.

72. Melin, A., Tornberg, A.B., Skouby, S., Moller, S.S., Sundgot-Borgen, J., Faber, J., Sidelmann, J.J., Aziz, M. and Sjodin, A. (2015) Energy availability and the female athlete triad in elite endurance athletes. *Scandinavian Journal of Medicine and Science in Sports*, 25, 610–622.

73. Moliner-Urdiales, D., Ruiz, J.R., Ortega,

F.B., Jimenez-Pavon, D., Vicente-Rodriguez, G., Rey-Lopez, J.P., Martinez-Gomez, D., Casajus, J.A., Mesana, M.I., Marcos, A., Noriega-Borge, M.J., Sjostrom, M., Castillo, M.J. and Moreno, L.A. (2010) Avena, and Groups HS. Secular trends in health-related physical fitness in Spanish adolescents: the AVENA and HELENA studies. *Journal of Science and Medicine in Sport*, 13, 584–588.

74. Myer, G.D., Faigenbaum, A.D., Edwards, N.M., Clark, J.F., Best, T.M. and Sallis, R.E. (2015) Sixty minutes of what? A developing brain perspective for activating children with an integrative exercise approach. *British Journal of Sports Medicine*, 49, 1510-1516.

75. Myer, G.D., Ford, K.R., Di Stasi, S.L., Foss, K.D., Micheli, L.J. and Hewett, T.E. (2015) High knee abduction moments are common risk factors for patellofemoral pain (PFP) and anterior cruciate ligament (ACL) injury in girls: is PFP itself a predictor for subsequent ACL injury? *British Journal of Sports Medicine*, 49, 118–122.

76. Myer, G.D., Ford, K.R. and Hewett, T.E. (2005) The effects of gender on quadriceps muscle activation strategies during a maneuver that mimics a high ACL injury risk position. *Journal of Electromyography and Kinesiology*, 15, 181–189.

77. Myer, G.D., Ford, K.R., Palumbo, J.P. and Hewett, T.E. (2005) Neuromuscular training improves performance and lower-extremity biomechanics in female athletes. *Journal of Strength Conditioning Research*, 19, 51–60.

78. Myer, G.D., Jayanthi, N., DiFiori, J.P., Faigenbaum, A.D., Kiefer, A.W., Logerstedt, D. and Micheli, L.J. (2016) Sports Specialization, Part II: Alternative Solutions to Early Sport Specialization in Youth Athletes. *Sports Health*, 8, 65–73.

79. Myer, G.D., Kushner, A.M., Faigenbaum, A.D., Kiefer, A., Kashikar-Zuck, S. and Clark, J.F. (2013) Training the developing brain, part I: cognitive developmental considerations for training youth. *Current Sports Medicine Reports*, 12, 304–310.

80. Myer, G.D., Sugimoto, D., Thomas, S. and Hewett, T.E. (2013) The influence of age on the effectiveness of neuromuscular training to reduce anterior cruciate ligament injury in female athletes: a meta-analysis. *American Journal of Sports Medicine*, 41, 203–215.

81. Nattiv, A., Loucks, A.B., Manore, M.M., Sanborn, C.F., Sundgot-Borgen, J., Warren, M.P. and American College of Sports Medicine. (2007) American College of Sports Medicine position stand. The female athlete triad. *Medicine and Science in Sports and Exercise*, 39, 1867–1882.

82. Obert, P., Mandigout, M., Vinet, A. and Courteix, D. (2001) Effect of a 13-week aerobic training programme on the maximal power developed during a force–velocity test in prepubertal boys and girls. *International Journal of Sports Medicine*, 22, 442–446.

83. Ogden, C.L., Carroll, M.D., Kit, B.K. and Flegal, K.M. (2012) Prevalence of obesity and trends in body mass index among US children and adolescents, 1999–2010. *JAMA* 307, 483–490.

84. Olsen, S.J. 2nd, Fleisig, G.S., Dun, S., Loftice, J. and Andrews, J.R. (2006) Risk factors for shoulder and elbow injuries in adolescent baseball pitchers. *American Journal of Sports Medicine*, 34, 905–912.

85. Ortega, F.B., Konstabel, K., Pasquali, E., Ruiz, J.R., Hurtig-Wennlof, A., Maestu, J., Lof, M., Harro, J., Bellocco, R., Labayen, I., Veidebaum, T. and Sjostrom, M. (2013) Objectively measured physical activity and sedentary time during childhood, adolescence and young adulthood: a cohort study. *PLoS One* 8: e60871.

86. Parker, D.F., Round, J.M., Sacco, P. and Jones, D.A. (1990) A cross-sectional survey of upper and lower limb strength in boys and girls during childhood and adolescence. *Annals of Human Biology*, 17, 199–211.

87. Poiss, C.C., Sullivan, P.A., Paup, D.C. and Westerman, B.J. (2004) Perceived importance of weight training to selected

NCAA Division III men and women student-athletes. *Journal of Strength and Conditioning Research*, 18, 108–114.

88. Powers, C.M. (2003) The influence of altered lower-extremity kinematics on patellofemoral joint dysfunction: a theoretical perspective. *Journal of Orthopaedic and Sports Physical Therapy*, 33: 639–646.

89. Ramos, E., Frontera, W.R., Llopart, A. and Feliciano, D. (1998) Muscle strength and hormonal levels in adolescents: gender related differences. *International Journal of Sports Medicine*, 19, 526–531.

90. Renstrom, P., Ljungqvist, A., Arendt, E., Beynnon, B., Fukubayashi, T., Garrett, W., Georgoulis, T., Hewett, T.E., Johnson, R., Krosshaug, T., Mandelbaum, B., Micheli, L., Myklebust, G., Roos, E., Roos, H., Schamasch, P., Shultz, S., Werner, S., Wojtys, E. and Engebretsen, L. (2008) Non-contact ACL injuries in female athletes: an International Olympic Committee current concepts statement. *British Journal of Sports Medicine*, 42, 394–412.

91. Round, J.M., Jones, D.A., Honour, J.W. and Nevill, A.M. (1999) Hormonal factors in the development of differences in strength between boys and girls during adolescence: a longitudinal study. *Annals of Human Biology*, 26, 49–62.

92. Runhaar, J., Collard, D.C., Singh, A.S., Kemper, H.C., van Mechelen, W. and Chinapaw, M. (2010) Motor fitness in Dutch youth: differences over a 26-year period (1980–2006). *Journal of Science and Medicine in Sport*, 13, 323–328.

93. Scofield, K.L. and Hecht, S. (2012) Bone health in endurance athletes: runners, cyclists, and swimmers. *Current Sports Medicine Reports*, 11, 328–334.

94. Sherar, L.B., Mirwald, R.L., Baxter-Jones, A.D. and Thomis, M. (2005) Prediction of adult height using maturity-based cumulative height velocity curves. *Journal of Pediatrics*, 147, 508–514.

95. Sport_England. Active People Survey: Once a week participation in sport. *Sport England*, 2016, pp.1–3.

96. Stojanovic, E., Ristic, V., McMaster, D.T. and Milanovic, Z. (2017) Effect of Plyometric Training on Vertical Jump Performance in Female Athletes: A Systematic Review and Meta-Analysis. *Sports Medicine*, 47, 975-986.

97. Stracciolini, A., Hanson, E., Kiefer, A.W., Myer, G.D. and Faigenbaum, A.D. (2016) Resistance Training for Pediatric Female Dancers. *Journal of Dance Medical Science*, 20, 64–71.

98. Sundgot-Borgen, J. (1994) Risk and trigger factors for the development of eating disorders in female elite athletes. *Medicine and Science in Sports and Exercise*, 26, 414–419.

99. Tammelin, T., Nayha, S., Laitinen, J., Rintamaki, H. and Jarvelin, M.R. (2003) Physical activity and social status in adolescence as predictors of physical inactivity in adulthood. *Preventive Medicine*, 37, 375–381.

100. Telama, R., Yang, X., Viikari, J., Valimaki, I., Wanne, O. and Raitakari, O. (2005) Physical activity from childhood to adulthood: a 21-year tracking study. *American Journal of Preventive Medicine*, 28, 267–273.

101. Torstveit, M.K. and Sundgot-Borgen, J. (2005) The female athlete triad exists in both elite athletes and controls. *Medicine and Science in Sports and Exercise*, 37, 1449–1459.

102. Tyler, T.F., Nicholas, S.J., Mullaney, M.J. and McHugh, M.P. (2006) The role of hip muscle function in the treatment of patellofemoral pain syndrome. *American Journal of Sports Medicine*, 34, 630–636.

103. Weiss Kelly, A.K. and Hecht, S., (2016) Council On Sports Medicine and Fitness. The Female Athlete Triad. *Pediatrics*, 138.

104. Yan, X., Zhu, M.J., Dodson, M.V. and Du, M. (2013) Developmental programming of fetal skeletal muscle and adipose tissue development. *Journal of Genomics*, 1, 29–38.

105. Yu, B. and Garrett, W.E. (2007) Mechanisms of non-contact ACL injuries. *British Journal of Sports Medicine*, 41 Suppl 1, i47–51.

CHAPTER 8
THE MENSTRUAL CYCLE, EXERCISE AND PERFORMANCE

Keith Barker MSc, ASCC

Due to the complexity of hormonal interaction and individual differences, the influence of menstruation on exercise, training, adaptation and sports performance is not well evidenced, with guidance often being contradictory within sports science research. Despite the lack of clarity in this area, an individual female athlete should take her menstrual cycle into consideration when designing a training plan and attempting to optimize performance. The phases of the menstrual cycle present female athletes with hormonal fluctuations and symptoms that differ significantly between individuals. The exercise performance of some athletes may not be noticeably affected, while others frequently experience performance decreases at specific points during their cycle. Athletes experiencing premenstrual syndrome (PMS) symptoms or severe period pain will find their training and/or competitive performance particularly impacted upon.

Variations in hormone levels throughout the cycle (typically twenty-eight days) may affect exercise performance in a number of relatively subtle ways such as abnormal body temperature regulation and how the body processes carbohydrates, protein and fat. Injury risk may also be elevated during specific phases of the cycle due to factors such as increased joint laxity or a reduction in reactive strength. Individual athletes should therefore be well aware of their own states and responses in relation to the menstrual cycle in order to enable positive adaptive responses to training stimuli and perform successfully in their sport.

After providing a basic outline of key aspects of the menstrual cycle, this chapter will offer best practice guidance regarding programming and training that may be applied by individual athletes to enable optimal training and competition performance.

ANATOMICAL/PHYSIOLOGICAL OVERVIEW

Menstruation occurs in fertile women in cycles that range from twenty-four to thirty-five days and refers to the physiological changes that are experienced. Each cycle comprises three phases: menstrual phase (menses), pre-ovulatory (follicular) phase and post-ovulatory (luteal) phase.

As represented in Fig. 8.1, the menstrual cycle involves significant modulation of hormones that may affect physical performance, recovery and adaptation to training stimuli. The two most influential hormones in this context are likely to be oestrogen and progesterone, with fluctuations in follicle stimulating hormone (FSH), and luteinizing hormone (LH) also potentially significant.

Female hormone levels impact significantly upon substrate (carbohydrate, fat, and protein) metabolism, plasma volume levels, and thermoregulation. Oestrogen is known to reduce carbohydrate oxidation and increase free fatty acid utilization. This means that when oestrogen levels are high, the bodies of female athletes will tend towards conserving glycogen stores and more readily utilize fat as

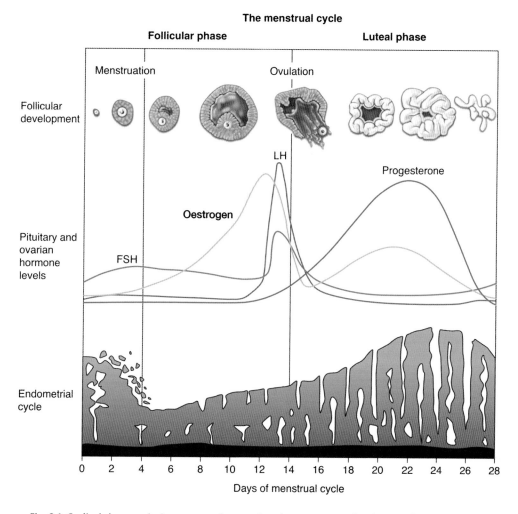

Fig. 8.1 Cyclical changes during a woman's normal ovulatory menstrual cycle, Encyclopædia Britannica Online. (Accessed 15 June 2015)

a fuel. This could be potentially beneficial for extended endurance activities performed at moderate intensities. The defaulting to glycogen-sparing during this phase may well be a disadvantage when training or competition requires the athlete to exercise at high intensities.

Progesterone antagonizes several of the actions of oestrogen, with levels being relatively high during the luteal phase of the menstrual cycle. Progesterone promotes protein breakdown and high levels have also been shown to increase core body temperature and minute ventilation (VE) (Reilly, 2000). Elevated progesterone during the luteal phase has been associated with elevated VE response to exercise and a higher rating of perceived exertion (Frankovich and Lebrun, 2000).

Where the maintenance of an athletic body composition is relevant to performance, it is important for female athletes to have at least a basic understanding of how fluctuations in oestrogen and progesterone due to the menstrual cycle impact upon the potential for fat gain or loss through direct biochemical factors and their more subtle influences over other hormones.

In very general terms – for optimal exercise performance, female athletes are likely to be set up to perform best whilst in a low hormone phase. This could be either just prior to menstruation or at the very start of menstruation. It is however appropriate for individual athletes to consider that menstrual bleeding can be extremely inconvenient during training and/or competition. Their premenstrual symptoms immediately preceding this phase may well also contribute to a state that is sub-optimal for performance both mentally and physically.

Menses

The first day of the cycle is determined by the first day of menses after the unfertilized egg causes the uterus lining to break down. This menstrual phase involves the discharge of blood (usually 25ml–65ml), tissue and associated fluid. This periodic bleeding normally lasts for approximately three to seven days.

Typically the decrease in haemoglobin and iron levels due to bleeding is not significant enough to affect exercise performance (Janse de Jonge, 2003). If an athlete experiences high blood loss, it may be appropriate to increase iron and ferritin intake during this time either through manipulation of dietary intake or supplementation.

Around the second day of bleeding, oestrogen and progesterone reduce to their lowest levels, with FSH and LH also being low at this time. This favourable hormonal state should enable positive exercise performance. That is of course if the athlete doesn't suffer too badly from the physical symptoms of period pains or any negative psychological

effects during this time. Regular exercise may well help reduce the severity of period pains as chemicals released by the womb are more rapidly dispersed via increased blood flow and the movement of abdominal muscles can ease cramping. Exercise also stimulates the production of endorphins, which can alleviate symptoms. Famously, Paula Radcliffe set her first marathon world record, at the 2002 Chicago Marathon, on the day her period started. Whether this is an optimal time for all female athletes to perform is very much dependent upon individual symptoms and responses.

Follicular Phase

The time between the start of menses and ovulation is called the 'follicular phase' (roughly days one to fourteen of the cycle). During this stage the female egg matures under the influence of follicle stimulating hormone (FSH). This phase is characterized by increasing oestrogen levels, relatively low progesterone levels, and normally regulated body temperature. Initially being low, oestrogen levels rise to peak at approximately day twelve. This oestrogen peak coupled with a luteinizing hormone (LH) surge causes ovulation. Ovulation occurs when the ovary releases an egg. At this point, oestrogen increases, while progesterone and body temperature remain stable.

The follicular phase is associated with increased insulin sensitivity, an increase in pain tolerance (Price et al., 1998) and increased levels of endurance for athletes (Fischetto and Sax, A., 2013). Low hormone levels (particularly progesterone) during the follicular phase will limit pre-exercise carbohydrate storage as the athlete is primed for utilizing carbohydrates as a fuel source. Other possible positive symptoms of the early follicular phase may include increases in responsiveness to strength training and recovery rate from heavy exercise bouts. The athlete may also be more resistant to the catabolic effects of prolonged endurance exercise and muscle damage aiding the retention of lean muscle mass and recovery between training sessions or competitive events (Roupas and Georgopoulos, 2011).

Overall the early and mid-follicular phases of the menstrual cycle are a time when the female athlete is often well positioned to tolerate and positively adapt to high-intensity training. The mid-follicular phase of the menstrual cycle may well be a good time to focus on high-intensity anaerobic conditioning and strength- and power-training activities. Depending upon the demands of their sport, the optimal window of athletic performance for most women is probably around days six to twelve of the cycle after bleeding has finished and energy levels have normalized.

Luteal Phase

The time between ovulation and the start of menses again is called the luteal phase (LP). Ovulation occurs around the mid-point of the menstrual cycle (approximately days twelve to sixteen). During ovulation, elevated oestrogen levels may mean female athletes are more prone to injury due to increased joint laxity and impaired reactive strength. Chapter 10 of this book contains detailed guidance relating to gender-specific injury risk. Upon ovulation, oestrogen levels have peaked and now begin to decline, while progesterone levels increase to prepare the lining of the uterus for egg implantation. The luteal phase may be characterized by relatively high levels of oestrogen and particularly high progesterone. During this phase, levels of both oestrogen and progesterone rise to their highest level around days twenty to twenty-six of the cycle. This is often the time in the menstrual cycle when premenstrual symptoms become evident. If there is no egg implanted, progesterone levels fall, the lining of the uterus is broken down and the cycle recommences.

Hormonal levels during the luteal phase trigger several physiological changes that can affect exercise performance and nutrient utilization. Training and competition performance may be compromised predominantly due to critical changes in thermoregulation, ventilation rate and metabolism. During the luteal phase, an increase in oestrogen promotes fat utilization as fuel, with the body sparing glycogen. For endurance athletes, this glycogen-sparing function along with greater use of free fatty acids during the luteal phase could possibly support the performance of prolonged submaximal exercise (Reilly, 2000). Elevated oestrogen and progesterone levels during the luteal phase cause a drop in plasma volume meaning blood becomes thickened. Thickened blood concentration results in slower blood flow between muscles. As a consequence, recovery time between high-intensity bouts of exercise will be extended due to restricted oxygen delivery and removal of waste products. The lower residual levels of fluid and electrolytes in the blood also mean that hydration takes on increased significance during the luteal phase of the menstrual cycle (Sims et al., 2007).

High levels of progesterone during the luteal phase of the menstrual cycle may elicit a slightly elevated core body temperature. Decreased plasma volume also contributes to a change in thermoregulation as lower plasma volumes mean a delay in the athlete beginning to sweat, therefore body temperature will rise. The threshold where vasodilation is initiated in order to shed heat is altered. Heat tolerance is therefore reduced, which could lead to earlier onset of fatigue. Increased cardiovascular strain may also be experienced by athletes exercising in hot and humid conditions with an elevated body temperature. For athletes preparing to perform in hot environments, heat acclimatization and adequate fluid intake take on increased value during the luteal phase. Athletes may also experience an accelerated ventilation rate triggered by the progesterone peak a few days post-ovulation which adds increased levels of perceived exertion and the other negative physiological changes during this time (Kolka and Stephenson, 1997 and Stachenfeld, Keefe and Palter, 2001).

Premenstrual syndrome (PMS) is the name given to the physical, psychological and behavioural symptoms that can occur during the late luteal phase due to the rapid drop in oestrogen levels. In the days preceeding menstruation, most women of childbearing age will experience some premenstrual symptoms. The symptoms of PMS may well impinge upon training and competition performance, but vary significantly between individuals. The classic PMS symptoms include water retention and bloating, irritability, breast pain, strong cravings and fluctuations in pain tolerance, as well as reduction in energy levels. Regular exercise can suppress the negative symptoms of PMS and they should normally improve with the onset of menstruation. Acute magnesium supplementation a few days before PMS symptoms usually start, up until menstruation, may also redress calcium-magnesium balance and alleviate symptoms of headaches and cramping. PMS may also be associated with increased appetite and cravings. Increasing the proportion of dietary carbohydrates may improve these symptoms.

There are several (sometimes contradictory) effects created by the hormone levels experienced by female athletes during the luteal phase. On balance the mid and late luteal phases of the menstrual cycle may well be a time when athletes should focus upon lower intensity training activities rather than expecting to achieve optimal performance or undertaking high-intensity training involving complex movements. Modified thermoregulation, fluid and fuel utilization characteristics during the second half of the menstrual cycle mean that female athletes may be more predisposed to overtraining or inadequate recovery.

CONTRACEPTION AND EXERCISE PERFORMANCE

Any individual considering the use of any birth control measures should only do so following careful consideration and consultation with their doctor.

Contraceptives are utilized for a variety of reasons, with their primary function being the prevention of pregnancy. Given the significant alternation to natural function and health provoked by contraceptive intake, the use of contraception to improve exercise performance and training should only be considered if the abilities of professional or elite level athletes are chronically impaired by symptoms of their menstrual cycle.

Some professional female athletes may choose to modulate their menstrual cycle through the use of oral contraceptives in order to prevent bleeding on the day(s) of key competition events, reduce pre-menstrual and/or menstrual symptoms or to reduce variability in performance and recovery between the follicular and luteal phases. Athletes preparing for a single major competitive goal may utilize oral contraceptives for brief timescales in order to manage the sychronization of positive phases of their menstrual cycle with their competition date(s). Not all women will respond to oral contraception in the same way, for example some may experience increased water retention and more pronounced mood swings. Competitive athletes beginning a course of contraception should therefore do so at least six months prior to any major competition as it may take time to establish a formula that works well for their body. This approach is less relevant to athletes who have extended competition seasons and therefore need to perform at their best for weeks at a time, multiple times a year, making such scheduling impractical.

IRREGULAR CYCLES OR CESSATION OF THE MENSTRUAL CYCLE

Female athletes engaging in chronically high training loads increase the chances of changes to their menstrual cycle. These include irregular cycles (oligomenorrhea) or complete cessation of the cycle (amenorrhea). This elevated chance of interrupted menstruation may be attributed to one or more factors such as extremely heavy training loads, high levels of stress around training, family life and competition or chronically low body fat.

Very heavy training loads coupled with very low body fat and poor nutrition may prevent menstruating (athletic amenorrhea). Female athletes should avoid excessive restrictions of energy and nutrient intake, extreme body fat reduction regimes, and other unhealthy approaches that can lead to missing a menstruation cycle. In essence, the human survival instinct dictates that the body responds to this state of deprivation and physiological stress by deeming menstruation to be unnecessary and not vital for survival.

Chronic training overload and malnutrition may also lead to an increased risk of osteoporosis and fertility problems. Amenorrhea is also linked to reduction in the body's capacity to absorb calcium, decreases bone density and increases the risk of musculoskeletal injury (Soleimany *et al.*, 2012).

Athletes experiencing irregular or infrequent menstrual cycles should consult their doctor as this may lead to significant health issues if left unresolved.

MONITORING OF THE MENSTRUAL CYCLE AND EXERCISE PERFORMANCE

Given the range of individual athlete experiences and responses to their own menstrual cycle and the range of advice available, it can be key to successful performance in both training and competition that each athlete develops an understanding of how their own menstrual cycle specifically affects them on an ongoing basis rather than simply attempting to apply generic advice to how they go about their training, nutrition and competing. There certainly isn't sufficient consistency of evidence relating to the menstrual cycle and exercise performance to provide all female athletes with meaningful generic guidance.

Daily wellness monitoring using a simple scale along with an associated training/performance diary can be an inexpensive and effective means of charting how the phases of the cycle are linked to an individual athlete performing well or poorly in training and competition. The key to the effectiveness of this type of monitoring intervention is the frequent and consistent use of objective measures of wellness and performance. Paper notation, word processed records or one of the commercially available smartphone applications may all be effectively utilized to record sleep, macronutrient consumption, exercise intensity, training load, energy levels and perceived exertion ratings for training sessions. It is then possible to track the menstrual cycle (by recording the first day of menstruation for each cycle) against performance or wellbeing measures and predict the expected dates of the worst symptoms.

It may be that an individual female athlete consistently performs (and feels) poorly at one specific stage in their cycle that doesn't seem to fit in with established norms, their menstrual cycle is consistently longer than the typical four to five weeks, or their performance could seem largely unaffected by their menstrual cycle. What is important is that an athlete is aware of how their menstrual cycle affects them so that training (and possibly competitions) may be planned appropriately around largely predictable positive and negative points within the cycle.

THE ORGANIZATION OF TRAINING AND THE MENSTRUAL CYCLE

The application of traditional models of periodization is often based around three- to six-week blocks (mesocycles) of strategic stimulus application, loading and unloading in order to obtain medium- to long-term physical adaptation(s) and performance improvement. These training plans are normally designed so that the athlete can be in an optimal physical state for significant competition events. Traditional patterns of training and regeneration are based upon sound underpinning principles of physical development. Any strategic training plan should adhere to the fundamentals of 'progressive overload', 'specific adaptation to imposed demands' and 'supercompensation' in some form or other.

For those female athletes who don't suffer too badly from PMS symptoms or heavy bleeding during menstruation, traditional periodization approaches with only minor modifications may well be most appropriate for the optimization of performance. For athletes whose exercise performance is significantly affected by different phases of their menstrual cycle, or those who are involved in high-intensity jumping or agility-based sports, it may be appropriate to organize training around different stages of their cycle. All athletes need to continue training during their luteal phase, but it may well be that female athletes are able to push a bit harder during the first two weeks of their cycle (including menstruation).

In general, female athletes tend to experience a higher RPE at any given exercise intensity, elevated heart rate and cardiovascular strain, and decreased efficiency during the luteal phase. It may therefore be advisable to avoid planning high training activities in hot, humid conditions during the luteal phase, as body temperature is already slightly elevated.

In all likelihood, maximal force production (strength) capability won't vary significantly over the different phases of the menstrual cycle for most athletes. If an athlete is able to complete a sustained block of strength training stimulus with appropriate intensity, frequency and volume, the associated adaptations are likely to be largely independent of menstruation or the use of contraceptives. The main challenge for some individuals who suffer from severe PMS symptoms or heavy bleeding during menstruation is being able to sustain sufficient consistency of training.

Some female athletes are able to develop strength more effectively during the follicular phase. In the low hormone state of the FP athletes may benefit from decreased muscle damage and more efficient recovery between exercise bouts (Sarwar, Niclos and Rutherford, 1996). It is possible for strength training programmes to be effectively structured around an athlete's menstrual cycle. As shown in Table 8.1 below, strength development programmes that take into account these cyclical hormonal fluctuations could utilize highest intensities of loading during the mid follicular and early luteal phases. Lower intensity strength endurance stimuli will then be applied during the early follicular, late follicular and mid luteal phases. The late luteal phase and possibly the first couple of days of menstruation are then the time for de-loading and recovery activities.

High oestrogen peaks during the late follicular phase just prior to ovulation and the mid luteal phase can tend to decrease spatial abilities and coordination slightly. A secondary symptom of high oestrogen levels is slightly increased joint and ligament laxity so potential

Week	Day	Phase	Hormone Levels	Physiological/Psychological State	Training Advice	Focus	Intensity
1	1–2	Early follicular (menses)	Oestrogen, progesterone & testosterone all low	Increased stress, poor reaction times and perception of exertion. Immune depression	Avoid complex movements. Reduce training stress and volume	Recovery	Light
	3–5				Include strength & power training along with anaerobic conditioning activities	Conditioning	Moderate
	6–8	Mid-follicular	Oestrogen rises, progesterone low, growth hormone high	Increase in glycogen storage & uptake	Include high intensity, low volume, complex tasks. Strength & power development and intensity tolerance conditioning	Strength & high tolerance conditioning	Moderate
2	9–13	Late follicular	Oestrogen peak	Increased glycogen, fat, protein & electrolyte storage	Include low intensity – high volume aerobic training. Emphasize non-weight bearing training modes	Endurance & injury prevention work	Moderate – high
	14	Ovulation	Testosterone peak	Possible behavioural changes	Strength & power training		
3	15–20	Early luteal	Progesterone rises	Increased glycogen storage in liver & muscle. Increase in total energy and fat intake. Lowered blood lactate levels. Greatest retention of water, sodium chloride and potassium	Include high intensity, low volume, complex tasks. Strength & power development and intensity tolerance conditioning	Max strength / power	Very high
4	21–24	Mid-luteal	Oestrogen and progesterone high	Increased protein breakdown. Muscular endurance low. Increased glycogen, fat and protein, water and electrolyte stores	Include low intensity – high volume aerobic training. Emphasize non-weight bearing training modes	Endurance & injury prevention work	Moderate
5	25–31	Late luteal	Oestrogen, progesterone & testosterone all low	Increased stress, poor reaction times and perception of exertion. Immune depression	Avoid complex movements. Reduce training stress and volume. Include strength & power training along with anaerobic conditioning activities. Possible recovery week	Varied recovery activities.	Light

Table 8.1 Example of periodization guidance based around the menstrual cycle. (Modified from Hamilton, 2012)

197

for joint injury may be a higher risk at these times for athletes involved in sports and training that include multi-directional agility, cutting and landing manoeuvres or plyometric activities. Where this is applicable to the training process, it would be prudent to reduce the volume, intensity and frequency of these training modalities during the times of the two oestrogen peaks within the cycle.

The time of maximum training and performance effectiveness and efficiency for many athletes involved in a wide range of sports may well be pre-ovulation and post-ovulation. For those experiencing a thirty-one-day menstrual cycle, that approximates to days fifteen to twenty. For many athletes this section of the cycle may be characterized by a higher tolerance for pain, the highest maximum voluntary force generation capacity and peak levels of endurance. In these hormonal conditions the body will also be more prone to utilizing muscle glycogen to fuel exercise facilitating high-intensity exercise performance. High-intensity training activities should be the focus of most training programmes during the pre- and post-ovulation sections of the cycle.

For many athletes, tolerance for pain can be higher during the mid and late follicular phases of the cycle, once menstruation has taken place. If metabolic conditioning activities are being planned around the athlete's menstrual cycle, this is therefore a relevant time to undertake relatively high-intensity tolerance interval sessions. These sessions may also effectively target the energy production of the glycolytic system.

During the mid and late luteal phases, with body temperature higher than normal, athletes often experience higher cardiovascular strain and decreased time to exhaustion when undertaking endurance-based activities. In addition to this, increased water retention and the associated weight gains during the mid and late luteal phases may also significantly affect exercise performance, particularly if the training or competition activities include running or jumping modalities. This increased mass can lead to elevated perception of exertion (and actual exertion) during exercise. This stage may therefore be well suited to moderate or light training activities emphasizing non-weight bearing modalities.

During the early follicular (menses) phase, testosterone, oestrogen and progesterone concentrations are low with evidence that female athletes may be more vulnerable to errors and incidence of injuries (Reilly, 2000). Therefore training at this time could focus upon regeneration and moderate intensity activities. Through the mid follicular phase the athlete's body may be well positioned to focus upon increased intensity of training stimulus involving strength and high-intensity endurance training. Placing greater emphasis on thorough warm-ups, including frequent recovery sessions, monitoring and awareness of fatigue and the insistence on technical excellence when performing training activities rather than intensity or function in a fatigued state are all appropriate actions at this stage.

At ovulation and during the early luteal phase, heavier strength training of high intensity and low volume should be prioritized as oestrogen and overall strength is peaked. This is the optimal time in the cycle to really push the intensity of loading in heavy compound exercises involving the largest muscle groups and highest force production such as squats and deadlifts. This is also an excellent time to develop performance through complex exercises such as Olympic or combination lifts.

During the mid luteal phase the body is more prone to utilize fat as a fuel source for exercise rather than muscle glycogen. This stage in the cycle is therefore well suited to submaximal exercise of long duration and low intensity that can effectively utilize fat as fuel. The hormonal context during this time is well set for utilizing lower-intensity aerobic exercise coupled with moderate intensity strength endurance training. For those athletes suffering from extreme fatigue and discomfort from PMS symptoms, the urge to miss training should be resisted as mixed non-weight bearing aerobic base-type exercise can significantly ease these symptoms. For athletes who are targeting fat loss over the medium to long term, long duration moderate intensity aerobic endurance training should be emphasized during the mid and late luteal phase. When targeting medium to long-term strength development, the luteal phase is not ideal for really high intensity loading and an athlete may perform less well in activities requiring rapid and/or high force production compared to their capabilities at other times in the cycle. This is the time of the phase to plan things like steady state runs, bike or elliptical training sessions, easy swims or other activities that are fuelled predominantly by the aerobic system.

Finally, during the late luteal phase, characterized by testosterone, oestrogen and progesterone concentrations returning to lower levels, it might be best to reduce training intensity and volume and focus on assistance, supplementary and recovery activities (similar to the first couple of days of menstruation).

ATHLETIC NUTRITION AND THE MENSTRUAL CYCLE

Ongoing healthy eating and lifestyle habits coupled with purposeful nutritional interventions can help an athlete to optimize their training and competition performance throughout their menstrual cycle. When an athlete is familiar with the phases of their cycle and the impact that it has on key factors influencing their exercise performance and body composition, it is possible to utilize strategic nutritional interventions to minimize the negative effects.

Female athletes may need to be more mindful of their calorie intake during the luteal phase (when progesterone is high) than during the follicular phase because of a natural urge to eat more. The elevated progesterone levels

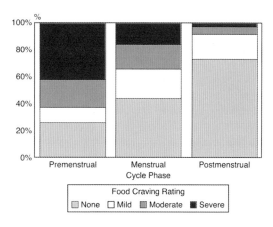

Fig. 8.2 Percentage of subjects reporting food cravings (varying degrees of severity) at three stages of the menstrual cycle (Dye & Blundell, 1997).

during the luteal phase also increase body temperature, metabolic rate and energy expenditure, at least partially compensating for increased energy intake. Overeating during the luteal phase can be problematic for those needing to maintain lean athletic body composition as progesterone independently promotes fat storage via its effects on lipoprotein lipase in fat tissue, and decreases fatty acid concentrations in the blood, which can increase cravings for fatty foods. As indicated in Fig. 8.2, during the luteal phase athletes may experience cravings for any or every macronutrient (protein, carbohydrates, and fat), probably reflecting personal preferences and just a general increase in appetite.

Examples of Nutritional Approaches Based Around the Menstrual Cycle

- Maintaining consistent overall calorie intake whilst increasing the proportion of dietary carbohydrate can help suppress

199

cravings during the luteal phase and decrease PMS symptoms.

- Carbohydrate supplementation can be very important during the mid-luteal (high hormone) phase in order to adequately fuel the high-intensity exercise performance that could be performed without such supplementation during the low hormone follicular phase.
- Elevated progesterone during the luteal phase opposes the action of oestrogen and may make the body more insulin-resistant resulting in a greater propensity to store fat and lose muscle (Isacco *et al.*, 2012). Athletes who have body composition goals should bear this in mind.
- Pre-loading with a sodium-based drink prior to exercise may well have a significant positive impact upon training and performance during the luteal phase.
- Acute magnesium supplementation leading up to and during the pre-menstrual days may help ease cramps by decreasing vascular spasms and nerve hyper-excitability.
- There are many supplements designed specifically to moderate PMS symptoms that might have a positive impact for individuals at this stage in their cycle. It may be a case of trial and error before an athlete finds the most effective blend of supplementation for them around their pre-menstrual phase.
- During the low hormone follicular phase (the first two weeks of the menstrual cycle), the body is pre-disposed to readily use, rather than spare, glycogen and blood glucose to fuel exercise. Carbohydrate loading approaches within the twenty-four hours before endurance competition could therefore be more important for female endurance athletes at this time.

Rather than attempting to maintain consistent energy intake throughout the month, some athletes may successfully manage their nutrition and body composition by significantly lowering calorie intake during the two weeks immediately after menstruation when hunger levels are lower and cravings less frequent. Calorie intake may then be increased, returning to a maintenance level during the week before and during menstruation. This move to higher energy consumption may mitigate the natural increase in appetite post-menstruation and regulate the metabolism.

As with anything relating to the menstrual cycle and exercise performance, optimal nutrition strategies need to be individualized and best fit to the individual athlete's needs, patterns of performance and recovery and PMS symptoms. Ongoing healthy nutrition and lifestyle always supersedes supplementation of the diet. In order to reach a situation where nutrition best supports an athlete's training and performance, it is likely that a sustained trial and error approach to discover the most successful blend of nutrients, energy intake and supplementation is required.

SUMMARY

In order for relatively trained athletes to be successful in most sports performance contexts, it is necessary to consistently adhere to a structured programme incorporating strategic non-linear loading. In many sports, the accumulation of a high volume of relevant training activity over several years is also necessary. For some female athletes most physiological parameters related to performance (such as strength, endurance and anaerobic capacity) can be largely unaffected by the menstrual cycle or taking hormonal contraceptives.

Female athletes should respect, rather than try to ignore, their menstrual cycle and respond to how the phases of the cycle affect their body. Many female athletes experience exercise performance variations associated with specific phases of their menstrual cycle. These variations are often more a function of PMS/menstrual symptoms including motivation, concentration, and lethargy than changes in physiological variables.

Finally, it is important to remember that the evidence and knowledge around the menstrual cycle, exercise performance and adaptation is largely inconclusive or contradictory overall. The optimal structure or pattern of planning training and competition around different phases of the menstrual cycle must be developed specifically for individual athletes. The fundamental underpinning principles of physical development must be adhered to if relatively trained athletes are to effectively progress. It is though entirely possible to do this around specific phases of the menstrual cycle. A combination of basic principles applied through an understanding of an athlete's menstrual cycle and how it impacts upon their exercise performance can enable extremely effective physical development and may also moderate injury risk. Athletes themselves must develop strategies over time to manage the complex combination of symptoms associated with the menstrual cycle without compromising their training or their performance. For elite female athletes, there can't be any excuses when it comes to performing in key competitions.

REFERENCES

Cardinale, M. and Stone M. H. (2006) Is T influencing sports performance? *Journal of Strength and Conditioning Research*, 20(1), 103–107.

Casey, E., Hameed, F. and Dhahe, Y. (2014) The Muscle Stretch Reflex throughout the Menstrual Cycle. Medicine & Science in Sports & Exercise; 46(3),: 600–610.

Cook, C.J. *et al.* (2012) Comparison of baseline vs. free testosterone and cortisol concentrations between elite and non-elite female athletes. *American Journal of Human Biology*, 24, 856–858.

Davidsen, L. *et al.* (2007) Impact of the Menstrual Cycle on Determinants of Energy Balance: A putative role in weight loss attempts. *International Journal of Obesity*, 31, 887–890.

Dye, L. and Blundell, J.E. (1997) Menstrual cycle and appetite control: implications for weight regulation. https://www.ncbi.nlm.nih.gov/pubmed/9221991, 12(6), 1142–51.

Encyclopaedia Britannica Online. (2017) Cyclical changes during a woman's normal ovulatory menstrual cycle. *Encyclopædia Britannica*, Inc. Web. [accessed 15 June 2017] https://www.britannica.com/science/menstruation#ref607154

Fischetto, G. and Sax, A. (2013) The Menstrual Cycle and Sport Performance. *New Studies in Athletics*, 28:3/4, 57–69.

Frankovich, R.J. and Lebrun, C.M. (2000) Menstrual cycle, contraception, and performance. *Clinics in Sports Medicine*, 19, 251–271.

Gordon, D. *et al.* (2013) The effects of menstrual cycle phase on the development of peak torque under isokinetic conditions. *Isokinetics and Exercise Science*, 21, 285–291.

Hamilton, D. (2012) *The Impact of Monitoring Strategies on a Team Sport Through an Olympiad: Physical Development, Taper and Recovery*. UKSCA Annual Conference. Lecture conducted from Royal Holloway University, Egham, London.

Hansen, M. *et al.* (2013) Impact of oral contraceptive use and menstrual phases on patellar tendon morphology, biochemical composition, and biomechanical properties in female athletes. *Journal of Applied Physiology*, 114, 998–1008.

Hoeger, M.K. *et al.* (2009) The role of the menstrual cycle phase in pain perception before and after isometric fatiguing contraction. *European Journal of Applied Physiology*, 106, 105–112.

Holloway, J.B. and Baechle, T.R. (1990) Strength training for female athletes. *Sports Medicine*, 9, 216–228.

Isacco, L. *et al.* (2012) Influence of hormonal status on substrate utilisation at rest and during exercise in the female population. *Sports Medicine*, 42(4), 327–342.

Janse De Jonge, X.A.K. *et al.* (2001) The influence of menstrual cycle phase on skeletal muscle contractile characteristics in humans. *The Journal of Physiology*, 530, 161–166.

Janse De Jonge, X.A.K. (2003) Effects of the menstrual cycle on exercise performance. https://www.ncbi.nlm.nih.gov/pubmed/12959622, 33(11), 833–51.

Janse De Jonge, X.A.K. *et al.* (2012) Exercise Performance over the Menstrual Cycle in Temperate and Hot, Humid Conditions. *Medicine and Science in Sports and Exercise*, 44(11), 2190–2198.

Julian, R., Hecksteden, A., Fullagar, H.H.K. and Meyer, T. (2017) *The effects of menstrual cycle phase on physical performance in female soccer players.* PLoS One, 12(3).

Kolka, M.A. and Stephenson, L.A. (1997) Effect of luteal phase elevation in core temperature on forearm blood flow during exercise. *Journal of Applied Physiology*, 82, 1079–1083.

Lagowska, K. *et al.* (2014) Effects of dietary intervention in young female athletes with menstrual disorders. *Journal of the International Society of Sports Nutrition*, 11, 21.

Markofski, M.M. and Braun, W.A. (2014) Influence of menstrual cycle on indices of contraction-induced muscle damage. *Journal of Strength and Conditioning Research*, 28(9), 2649–2656.

Oosthuyse, T. and Bosch, A.N. (2010) The effect of the menstrual cycle on exercise metabolism: implications for exercise performance in eumenorrheic women. *Sports Medicine*, 40(3), 207–227.

Phillips S.K. *et al.* (1996) Changes in maximal voluntary force of human adductor pollicis muscle during the menstrual cycle. *The Journal of Physiology*, 496: 551–557.

Price, D. *et al.* (1998). A meta-analytic review of pain perception across the menstrual cycle. *Journal of the International Association for the Study of Pain*, 81(3), 225–235.

Reilly, T. (2000) The Menstrual Cycle and Human Performance: An Overview. *Biological Rhythm Research*, 31, 29–40.

Roupas, N.D. and Georgopoulos, N.A. (2011). *Menstrual function in sports.* Hormones, 10, 104–116.

Sarwar R., Niclos B.B., and Rutherford O.M. (1996) Changes in muscle strength, relaxation rate and fatiguability during the human menstrual cycle. *The Journal of Physiology*, 493, 267–272.

Šimić, N. and Ravlić, A. (2013) *Changes In Body Temperature And Reaction Times During Menstrual Cycle.* Arh Hig Rada Toksikol, 64, 99–106.

Sims, S.T., Rehrer, N.J., Bell, M.L. and Cotter, J.D. (2007) Pre-exercise sodium loading aids fluid balance and endurance for women exercising in the heat. *Journal of Applied Physiology*, 103, 534–541.

Soleimany, G. *et al.* (2012) Bone Mineral Changes and Cardiovascular Effects among Female Athletes with Chronic Menstrual Dysfunction. *Asian Journal of Sports Medicine*, 3(1), 53–58. Stachenfeld, NS., Keefe. D.L. and Palter, S.F. (2001) Estrogen and progesterone effects on transcapillary fluid dynamics. *American Journal of Physiology, Regulatory Integrative and Comparative Physiology*, 281, 1319–1329.

Tsampoukos, A. *et al.* (2010) Effect of menstrual cycle phase on sprinting performance. *European Journal of Applied Physiology*, 109, 659–667.

Williams, T. (1997) Menstrual Cycle Phase and Running Economy. *Medicine and Science in Sports and Exercise*, 29(12), 1609–1618.

Wojtys, E.M. *et al.* (2014) Athletic Activity and Hormone Concentrations in High School Female Athletes. *Journal of Athletic Training*, 49(3).

CHAPTER 9
TRAINING DURING PREGNANCY AND FOLLOWING CHILDBIRTH

Keith Barker MSc, ASCC

Pregnancy is a time when significant hormonal, metabolic, blood sugar and body mass changes in the female athlete's body mean that additional care must be taken when planning and undertaking exercise. An individual's body, physical condition, abilities, preferences and training history all play a role in what is best for mother and developing foetus.

There are many positive health and wellbeing benefits of exercise during pregnancy for both mother and baby but pregnant athletes must be aware of contraindications to exercises and 'red flag' symptoms that indicate exercise must cease. Strength training in particular may result in positive outcomes through pregnancy and beyond. By following sensible guidelines, utilizing familiar training modes and exercises and focusing upon excellent form, female athletes can safely engage in a comprehensive training programme during pregnancy. Pregnant athletes must be guided by the advice of their medical professionals/maternity team and continue to heed their advice throughout pregnancy and the postpartum phase.

In most cases, pregnant athletes can continue training up until relatively close to the date when the baby is due. After giving birth, women should return to gentle exercise as soon as they feel able but there is a very specific progression of exercises that should begin with pelvic floor and lower abdominal strengthening and walking. Through pregnancy and childbirth the female athlete undergoes tremendous changes. The postpartum return to training must take these changes into account and allow time to return to the training undertaken before becoming pregnant.

This chapter will outline key clinical advice and summarize the potential benefits and risks associated with a range of modalities and intensities of maternal exercise before presenting recommended exercises and programme examples. The training activities provided have been developed based upon current scientific guidance and practical experience in order to enable pregnant and postpartum athletes to exercise safely and effectively.

CLINICAL ADVICE FOR MATERNAL EXERCISE

If pregnant athletes have any questions about their health or activities during pregnancy they should consult their doctor, specialist or maternity team. Best practice clinical advice has evolved significantly as the understanding of exercise, physiology and their interaction with mother and unborn baby improves. In the UK, the National Health Service (NHS) provides online guidance for exercise during pregnancy at http://www.nhs.uk/conditions/pregnancy-and-baby/pages/pregnancy-exercise.aspx [accessed 15 Jan. 2017]. Key messages from this NHS exercise guidance are outlined below:

- *Keep up your normal daily physical activity or exercise... for as long as you feel comfortable.*
- *Don't exhaust yourself. You may need to slow down as your pregnancy progresses or if your maternity team advises you to. If in doubt, consult your maternity team. As a general rule, you should be able to hold a conversation as you exercise when pregnant. If you become breathless as you talk, then you're probably exercising too strenuously.*
- *If you weren't active before you got pregnant, don't suddenly take up strenuous exercise. If you start an aerobic exercise programme... tell the instructor that you're pregnant and begin with no more than fifteen minutes of continuous exercise, three times a week. Increase this gradually to at least four thirty-minute sessions a week. Remember that exercise doesn't have to be strenuous to be beneficial.*

Exercise tips when you're pregnant:
- *Always warm up before exercising, and cool down afterwards.*
- *Try to keep active on a daily basis: half an hour of walking each day can be enough, but if you can't manage that, any amount is better than nothing.*
- *Avoid any strenuous exercise in hot weather.*
- *Drink plenty of water and other fluids.*
- *If you go to exercise classes, make sure your teacher is properly qualified, and knows that you're pregnant as well as how many weeks pregnant you are.*
- *You might like to try swimming because the water will support your increased weight. Some local swimming pools provide aquanatal classes with qualified instructors.*
- *Exercises that have a risk of falling, such as horse riding, downhill skiing, ice hockey, gymnastics and cycling, should only be done with caution. Falls may risk damage to the baby.*

Exercises to avoid in pregnancy:
- *Don't lie flat on your back, particularly after sixteen weeks, because the weight of your bump presses on the main blood vessel bringing blood back to your heart and this can make you feel faint.*
- *Don't take part in contact sports where there's a risk of being hit, such as kickboxing, judo or squash.*
- *Don't go scuba diving, because the baby has no protection against decompression sickness and gas embolism (gas bubbles in the bloodstream).*
- *Don't exercise at heights over 2,500m above sea level until you have acclimatized: this is because you and your baby are at risk of http://www.nhs.uk/ conditions/altitude-sickness/ pages/introduction.aspx*

This NHS advice outlines a rational approach to maternal exercise as applicable to the general public rather than being specifically targeted at the athletic population. This guidance should be factored into the development of a training programme appropriate for a pregnant athlete, but as with any training programme it must be individualized to match the athlete's physical state. The subsequent sections of this chapter will expand upon this generic guidance and provide examples of training activities that can be both safe and effective for pregnant athletes.

CONTRAINDICATIONS TO EXERCISE DURING PREGNANCY

Pregnancy places the female athlete in a relatively vulnerable state and precautions need to be taken to ensure that exercise stresses do not have a deleterious impact. During pregnancy, symptoms may either pre-exist or develop that mean the athlete should stop exercising. Athletes need to be aware of the circumstances that require the cessation of exercise and a medical evaluation. These 'red flag' symptoms include vaginal bleeding, breathlessness at rest or out of proportion to the effort, dizziness, headaches, chest pain, racing heart rate, muscle weakness, significant swelling in feet or legs, uterine contractions that occur more than 30 minutes after exercise, decreased foetal movement, pelvic, hip, or worsening back pain, chronic fatigue and the leakage of fluids.

Within Table 9.1, the American College of Obstetricians and Gynecologists (2009) outlines a summary of contraindications to maternal exercise and symptoms that must be acted upon by the immediate cessation of exercise and contacting a relevant medical professional.

FUNDAMENTAL CONSIDERATIONS FOR EXERCISE DURING PREGNANCY AND POSTPARTUM

The continuation of structured training through pregnancy can help maintain strength and fitness qualities and provide female athletes with several significant health benefits. These positive effects may include:

- Lower incidence of backaches and less severe headaches (Garshasbi, A. and Faghih Zadeh, S., 2005)
- Moderated weight gain and enhanced body image (Boscaglia, N., Skouteris, H., and Wertheim, E.H., 2003)
- Feelings of wellbeing and positive mood state (Poudevigne, M.S. and O'Connor, P.J., 2006)

Absolute Contraindications to Exercise	Warning Signs to Stop Exercising
Hemodynamically significant heart disease	Vaginal bleeding
Restrictive lung disease	Dyspnea (shortness of breath) prior to exertion
Incompetant cervix/cerclage	Dizziness
Multiple gestation at risk for premature labor	Headache
Persistent 2nd or 3rd trimester bleeding	Chest pain
Placenta previa after 26 weeks	Muscle weakness
Premature labor during current pregnancy	Calf pain or swelling
Ruptured membranes	Preterm labor
Preeclampsia/pregnancy-induced hypertension	Decreased fetal movement
	Amniotic fluid leakage

Table 9.1 Contraindications to maternal exercise. Source: American College of Obstetricians and Gynecologists (2009).

- Maintenance of energy levels, flexibility and aerobic capacity (Downs, D.S. *et al.*, 2012)
- Greater muscle strength and coordination, which helps with adjusting to increased bodyweight and changes in balance during pregnancy along with enhanced postpartum recovery and return to training (White, E., Pivarnik, J. and Pfeiffer, K., 2014)
- Reduced risk of gestational diabetes (Dye, T.D. *et al.*, 1997)
- Fewer problems experienced during childbirth (Hall, D.C. and Kaufman, D.A., 1987).

Much of the existing research evidence and associated guidance relating to exercise during pregnancy is difficult for athletes to interpret and apply as it is extremely generic and doesn't differentiate between different modalities, energy system development activities or training goals, rather it just refers to physical activity in general and is aimed at women in the general population who are often relatively sedentary, rather than those who routinely undertake high volumes or intensities of training.

During pregnancy a woman undergoes significant physiological, psychological and morphological changes throughout the term. These changes must be accounted for within programme design and any evidence of contraindication to exercise must be immediately acted upon with the cessation of training and medical support sought. As is the case when planning a training programme for any individual athlete, there is no one-size-fits-all pre-natal fitness paradigm. Health status,

> With the long-term health of mother and unborn baby being a far greater priority that any athletic success, it is essential that pregnant athletes follow any medical advice that they receive as this clearly supersedes any training or exercise goal.

> The aim of any training activities undertaken during pregnancy should be to maintain current levels of fitness rather than attempting to hit new peaks in performance. Pregnant athletes should not undertake any activity that is particularly new or novel or where impact risk is elevated.

physical state, training history before becoming pregnant, which trimester and how the athlete is feeling should all guide the programming of exercise during pregnancy.

In general terms, most pregnant athletes are able to continue something close to their usual training regime during the first trimester. Exercise intensity should not exceed pre-pregnancy levels. It is therefore essential that each individual athlete reads the signs from their body and modifies their exercise accordingly.

Moderate intensity exercise during pregnancy can help athletes avoid excessive gestational weight gain, strengthen the body ready for childbirth and potentially accelerate recovery after giving birth.

Few pregnancies go exactly as planned; it is therefore important that any training programme undertaken during pregnancy is open and flexible, having the objective of maintaining physical qualities rather than seeking significant performance improvement. On becoming pregnant, athletes should shift their training plan to one that moderates detraining and enables a more efficient return to normal training post-childbirth.

During the first trimester of pregnancy, rapid foetal development occurs accompanied by significant physiological changes but relatively minor anthropometric changes for the pregnant athlete. Blood volume increases and the uterus enlarges and maternal weight gain is normally moderate. Many exercises are therefore fine to continue during the first trimester. Athletes experiencing sickness or excessive fatigue during the first trimester should adopt a cautious approach to their training and modify exercise intensity accordingly (Downs, D.S. *et al.*, 2012).

Through the second and third trimesters of pregnancy, the athlete undergoes significant morphological changes. Significant weight gain centred around the mid-section alters posture. Breathing can also become more difficult due to the foetus inhibiting the function of the diaphragm. When training beyond the first trimester, athletes should avoid exercises performed in the supine position as well as those requiring significant trunk flexion. Overhead lifting should also be avoided after the first trimester as the postural changes that have occurred elevate the risk of damaging stress on the lower back (Schoenfeld, B., 2011).

Elevated levels of oestrogen and relaxin during trimester three trigger the remodelling of soft tissues, cartilage and ligaments, as well as an increase in the laxity of skeletal joints, particularly around the pelvis. This can lead to biomechanical changes in movement strategies, running gait, discomfort and an increased risk for falls and injury. Ballistic and high-intensity plyometric exercises should be avoided, as injury risk would be unacceptably elevated (Stevenson, L., 1997).

It is generally recommended that an athlete wait six to eight weeks after labour and delivery to return to their usual training regimen. Some athletes will bounce back much sooner and a rationally graduated return to training can be undertaken. It is essential for each individual to listen to their body and advice from their health practitioner in terms of readiness for exercise and return to training postpartum.

STRENGTH TRAINING DURING PREGNANCY

The changes associated with pregnancy can cause a number of problems for the child-bearer. Many of these problems are related to a weakened musculature as a result of reduced activity levels or inactivity coupled with the additional stress placed upon the body as a result of pregnancy-related weight gain.

> Before beginning a strength-training programme during pregnancy, athletes should always have medical clearance from their doctor and confirmation that no contraindications exist.

Exercise in general, and structured strength training in particular, can help maintain the function of supporting muscles, postural integrity and lessen the back pain and overall muscle and joint weakness often associated with pregnancy. The objective of a maternal strength programme should be to mitigate strength losses rather than chasing new elevated strength levels.

The use of free weights, resistance machines or resistance bands can be safe and extremely valuable during pregnancy for those athletes that usually include strength training within their programme. Resistance training and maintaining strength levels during pregnancy can aid preparation for childbirth and the lifting and pushing activities required after the child is born. Once given medical clearance, strength training can effectively form a key part of the maternal exercise programme (White, E., Pivarnik, J. and Pfeiffer, K., 2014).

Elevated secretion of the hormone relaxin during pregnancy promotes soft tissues such as ligaments and tendons to become more lax and flexible, which is necessary to carry a baby full term and prepare for labour/delivery. This increased range of movement leads to decreased joint stability. This stabilization function might be the greatest argument for maternal strength training, with the postural muscles of the trunk being of particular importance.

A light to moderate progressive warm-up routine of at least 10 minutes should be completed prior to any strength session with a similar cool-down post-session also being valuable in order to avoid acute spikes in heart rate during the strength training session. Strengthening movements such as squatting and bridging can encourage movement, strength, control and positioning through the pelvis, while helping to increase stability through the lower back. Proper abdominal and trunk training is important during pregnancy because of the changing posture and additional weight being added to the anterior (front) side of the body, coupled with increased spinal ligament laxity.

STRENGTH TRAINING ACTIVITIES TO BE AVOIDED DURING PREGNANCY

Heavy weightlifting, time-constrained weightlifting formats and crossfit-type challenges should generally be avoided during pregnancy. Olympic lifts where the barbell makes contact with the body through the transition and travels rapidly up past the trunk also represent an unacceptable risk. Heavy pulls, upright row, and so on where the barbell may contact the stomach should therefore be avoided for the same reason. High-intensity compound exercises, for example heavy squatting where the athlete utilizes the valsalva manoeuvre, or the holding of breath should also be avoided during pregnancy as significant increase in intra-abdominal pressure can result in a decreased up-flow of blood and nutrients to the foetus. A natural rhythmical breathing rate should be maintained whilst exercising when pregnant (Bø, K. et al., 2016).

Throughout pregnancy, when using resistance machines, athletes must avoid machines where a pad presses against the stomach, such as some seated row and abdominal crunch machines. Beyond the first trimester of pregnancy (after twelve weeks), there are several further considerations for strength exercises that should be avoided, with modified loading or positioning being utilized instead:

- Heavy overhead barbell presses behind the neck should be avoided due to the stability and postural challenge presented by this exercise.
- Exercises such as weighted crunches and abdominal rotations should also not be performed after twelve weeks due to the nature of the stress placed up the abdomen.
- Athletes in the second and third trimesters of pregnancy should avoid exercising or lifting in a supine position; exercises where the athlete maintains either an inclined or upright position should be carried out instead.
- Any exercise that involves lying on the front (prone) should not form part of the training programme beyond the first trimester, as this will place pressure on the abdomen and may cause pain. Instead, exercises should focus upon the postural strength and the function of muscle groups that will undergo significant pregnancy related stress.

PRENATAL STRENGTH PROGRAMMING GUIDANCE

Given that the emphasis of the prenatal strength programme should be the maintenance of strength qualities rather than seeking significant performance gains, two to three sessions per week performed at least forty-eight hours apart is sufficient frequency for most athletes. With this session frequency in mind, whole body sessions should be undertaken rather than split routines, with posture and the trunk musculature being a possible focus for multiple exercises within each session. The weight used for each exercise should be scaled down from the loads utilized prior to pregnancy with the focus on form being prioritized. Technical excellence is more important than ever when strength training during pregnancy. Strength training with poor technique during pregnancy may exacerbate low back pain and other aches and pains, while lifting with good form on a regular basis may help prevent both back pain and sciatica.

Athletes who were relatively strength trained prior to pregnancy can utilize a varied programme that involves two to four sets of each exercise with at least two minutes inter-set recoveries to allow the heart rate and body temperature to normalize before beginning the next set. Given the changes to joint mobility and heart rate during pregnancy, it is advised that strength training involves lower intensity than used in normal conditions. Rather than sets of three to five repetitions that might be utilized for strength development prior to pregnancy, athletes should now complete sets of at least ten repetitions at approximate loads of less than 75 per cent of one repetition maximum for each exercise. Sets should not be continued until exhaustion or failure but should be somewhat hard with the capacity to complete two or three further repetitions being held in reserve. Timed isometric holds should similarly be performed to a challenging duration but never to the point of failure (Schoenfeld, B., 2011).

An example strength programme that could be utilized effectively during pregnancy is outlined in Table 9.2. This programme is provided just as an example of how guidelines for strength training during pregnancy may be applied in practice. The programme includes two strength-training sessions. The first session may be used during the first trimester

Trimester 1 Strength Session (can be completed up to 3 times per week)				
FOCUS	**EXERCISE**	**SETS**	**REPS**	
Lower Body	Alternate leg barbell lunge	2-4	10-16	
Upper Body Push	Dumbbell Bench Press	2-4	10-15	RPE 7-8 out of 10 for
Upper Body Pull	Dumbbell Single Arm Row	2-4	10-12 each arm	the set ie. could
Trunk	Dead Bug	2-4	5-8 each side	complete 2 or 3 more
Posterior Chain	Stiff-Legged Deadlift	2-4	10-15	repetitions. Rest at
Upper Body Push	Seated Machine Shoulder Press	2-4	10-15	least 2 minutes
Upper Body Pull	Lat Pull Down	2-4	10-15	between sets.
Trunk	Side Plank Leg Raise	2-4	6-10 each side	
Trimester 2 & 3 Strength Session (can be completed up to 3 times per week)				
FOCUS	**EXERCISE**	**SETS**	**REPS**	
Lower Body	Dumbbell Squat	2-3	10-15	
Upper Body Push	Seated Machine Chest Press	2-3	10-15	RPE 6-7 out of 10 for
Upper Body Pull	Standing Single Arm Cable Row	2-3	10-12 each arm	the set ie. could
Trunk	Bird Dog	2-3	5-8 each side	complete 3 or 4 more
Lower Body	Dumbbell Split Squat	2-3	10-12 each leg	repetitions. Rest at
Shoulders	Dumbbell Lateral Raise	2-3	10-12	least 2 minutes
Posterior Chain	Standing Kick Back (with support)	2-3	10-12 each leg	between sets.
Trunk	Side Plank Hip Lift	2-3	6-10 each side	

Table 9.2 Example Maternal Strength Programme. (Modified from Schoenfeld, 2011)

and repeated three times per week. The second session can be utilized during the second and third trimesters and again may be repeated up to three times per week, reflecting the changes in training guidance for these times during the pregnancy. The programme is meant as a guide only. Athletes should always follow strength-training programmes that are well matched to their training history and physical state, so it could be appropriate to modify the example provided to create a best-fit programme for them.

ENDURANCE EXERCISE DURING PREGNANCY

Aerobic endurance activities undertaken during pregnancy can make an extremely positive contribution to the health of both the athlete and unborn baby. A range of exercise modalities performed at moderate intensity can be utilized with either steady state, fartlek or interval protocol being performed. As with any training during pregnancy, the athlete's training history should be considered when planning endurance training. Whatever endurance training the athlete was accustomed to before pregnancy can be maintained to a moderate level. All pregnant athletes must also be fully aware of proper hydration, the additional nutritional requirements of pregnancy and exercise, and the dangers of heat stress (Artal, R. and O'Toole, M., 2003). Even for experienced endurance athletes, the intensity of training should remain below 80 per cent of maximal throughout pregnancy although it is always important to base judgements of intensity upon the athlete's individual physical state (Hall, D.C. and Kaufman, D.A., 1987).

> It must be emphasized that there is no generic 'safe' upper limit applicable to all athletes. Pregnant athletes should not begin new or novel training interventions when pregnant.

In the early phases of pregnancy in particular, it is essential to maintain a stable core temperature of less than 39°C. Exercising in hot environments must therefore be avoided and it is advised that exercise intensity remains at approximately 60 per cent–70 per cent of maximum for a duration of less than 60 minutes.

The massive (approximately 50 per cent) increase in blood volume experienced during pregnancy can actually help to maintain endurance capabilities. Heart rate increases during pregnancy (normally by 15–20bpm) as does cardiac output, meaning heart rate-based training activities are affected with the heart rate response to any given exercise intensity not being comparable with those before pregnancy. Varied endurance training within moderate ranges of intensity is the most appropriate approach when planning the programme.

Athletes with a history of running regularly will find it safe and healthy to continue running during pregnancy, as long as no ill effects are felt. The unborn baby will not be harmed by the impacts or movement created. The running motion and ground contacts may actually comfort the unborn baby. If the training programme doesn't normally include running, then pregnancy isn't the time to start. With overheating being of increased concern during pregnancy, hydration and cool clothing will be key pieces of equipment for running sessions. Running in hot conditions should be avoided, particularly in the first twelve weeks of pregnancy. The intensity of work intervals along with associated responses should be closely monitored, with appropriate modifications being made. Athletes who run during pregnancy should run over even ground or on a treadmill rather than hill or trail running, in order to minimize the risk of falling. As the bump grows and the athlete gets heavier into the third trimester, pacing of training runs will slow.

Many athletes continue running during

pregnancy until it becomes too uncomfortable to do so. When this occurs, athletes should consider switching to non-weight bearing modalities, such as pool running or swimming. During pregnancy, runners may find it effective to train for a defined duration rather than a specified distance in order to manage the inevitable slowing of pace. Perceived exertion rather than pace to manage intensity may also work well. As perceived exertion can be elevated during pregnancy, it is appropriate to vary the sessions within a programme in an attempt to maintain engagement and enjoyment.

Athletes who utilized cycling as an endurance training modality prior to becoming pregnant can continue to do so effectively in the absence of any contraindications and in a safe environment. As the pregnancy progresses and the bump grows, however, balance is affected which could increase the likelihood of a fall. Experienced cyclists will be safe to continue until they begin to feel less stable than usual. At this point it may be advised to switch to using a static exercise bike, which should be safe throughout the term.

Swimming can be a great mode of maternal exercise as the water provides support to the bump, eases muscular tension and limits the stress on joints and connective tissue. Swimming can be used effectively to maintain aerobic endurance during pregnancy. Ideally athletes who continue swimming through pregnancy should aim to avoid busy times at the pool in order to minimize the chance of

Sedentary Prior to Pregnancy			
TYPE	INTENSITY	DURATION	FREQUENCY
Low impact eg. walking, static cycling, swimming, and other aqua exercise.	Moderately hard: RPE 5–6 out of 10.	Progress up to 30 minutes.	Begin 3 times per week, progress up to 5 times per week.
Recreational Endurance Athlete			
TYPE	INTENSITY	DURATION	FREQUENCY
Low impact eg. walking, static cycling, swimming and other aqua exercise plus prior training activities such as running.	Moderately hard to hard: Up to RPE 6–8 out of 10.	30–60 minutes.	3–5 times per week.
Elite Endurance Athlete			
TYPE	INTENSITY	DURATION	FREQUENCY
Low impact eg. walking, static cycling, swimming and other aqua exercise plus prior training activities such as running and cycling depending on gestational age.	Moderately hard to hard: Up to RPE 6–8 out of 10.	60–90 minutes	4–6 times per week

Table 9.3 Example framework for endurance exercise during pregnancy.

being bumped around by other pool users. Swimming may also be utilized more frequently in the second and third trimesters as a low-impact comfortable exercise mode to replace higher impact modalities during the later stages of pregnancy. Swimming with goggles is advisable as it enables a more comfortable posture, with the athlete's head down and spine in a more neutral alignment. A stroke that is comfortable, pain-free and avoids violent twisting of the trunk should be used (Stan, E.A., 2014). As with any other maternal exercise, pregnant athletes should ensure that they take a water bottle to the pool and shouldn't swim in water that is particularly warm (above 32°C).

If taking part in organized exercise classes, athletes should always inform the instructor that they are pregnant and if there are any related medical complications. During pregnancy it becomes more important than ever to monitor the intensity and perceived exertion of exercise intervals carefully, err on the side of caution and cease exercise if feeling unwell or in the presence of any adverse symptoms. In addition to planned training, pregnant athletes should aim to maintain relatively active daily habits. Low intensity activities such as walking can be an important supplement to planned training and should be utilized frequently during all phases of pregnancy.

Table 9.3 outlines a simple framework for the prescription of endurance exercise during pregnancy and could be effectively used as a basis for athletes and coaches to prescribe endurance-training activities based upon activity levels prior to pregnancy. This is meant purely as an initial guide, as the athlete must be guided by how they feel and respond to exercise.

FLEXIBILITY TRAINING DURING PREGNANCY

Any flexibility training undertaken during pregnancy should aim to improve stability, strength and movement quality throughout the athlete's normal range of motion rather than seeking any new or additional range. As the foetus grows, the abdominal muscles naturally become stretched and weakened and this can cause the lower back muscles to shorten. Along with the maintenance of mobility around all joints, maternal flexibility exercises should focus upon additional stretching of the hip-flexors and muscles of the lower back in order to prevent exacerbating the lordotic condition.

Forms of yoga or Pilates may be valuable training activities when aiming to maintain flexibility, stability and strength through ranges of movement and postural integrity throughout pregnancy. As with all maternal exercise, the activity should be stopped if any pain is experienced. Pregnant athletes who attend yoga classes should ensure that the instructor is appropriately trained and is informed of the pregnancy and any related conditions. There are plenty of yoga sessions and classes designed specifically for pregnant women that could be safely undertaken. The breathing techniques incorporated in these classes can aid relaxation, which may well be valuable for the mother-to-be. In general, when undertaking yoga or Pilates, pregnant athletes should avoid novel or advanced poses and Bikram or hot yoga classes. As the term progresses, it may well be relevant to move to more gentle yoga formats such as Hatha and move more slowly between poses.

SPEED/AGILITY TRAINING DURING PREGNANCY

Pregnancy is not an appropriate time for athletes to focus upon the development of running-based speed or agility. As a high-intensity (fast) stimulus is required in order to elicit positive adaptations in speed characteristics, it is not likely that pregnant athletes will be able to undertake effective training, particularly as the pregnancy progresses. Speed athletes should instead use pregnancy as a time to focus upon strength and postural maintenance, as these qualities will enable a more efficient return to speed training postpartum. The shift in centre of mass associated with pregnancy (due to baby bump) coupled with increased joint laxity mean that high-impact and/or multi-directional agility tasks are associated with a significantly elevated injury risk. High-intensity speed-agility exercises should therefore be removed from the training programme during pregnancy and replaced with modalities that enable the safe continuation of training.

MONITORING EXERCISE INTENSITY DURING PREGNANCY

In the first few weeks of pregnancy, resting heart rate naturally rises and this continues into the third trimester (may rise by approximately 15–20bpm). Blood volume and cardiac output also increase during pregnancy. These cardiorespiratory changes coupled with significant hormonal shifts lead to a reduction in exercise capacity for the athlete. Heart rate monitoring is therefore not an effective indicator of exercise intensity during pregnancy. Perceived exertion is likely to be the best parameter for exercise intensity monitoring under these altered physiological conditions.

Pregnant athletes should perform the bulk of their training at or below moderate exercise intensity. Exercising at a very high intensity above 90 per cent of their own peak heart rate, or 9 out of 10 on an RPE scale for any sustained periods may compromise blood flow to the foetus and potentially negatively impact upon foetal wellbeing in some cases (Salvesen, K. et al., 2012). That isn't a risk worth taking in the pursuit of a training goal. For the same reasons, exercising to exhaustion or failure should not form part of the maternal exercise regimen.

Using a rating of perceived exertion (RPE) scale to guide maternal exercise can be an extremely effective means of managing training intensity. Commonly applied RPE scales may be based upon either the 6–20 'Borg Scale', originally developed by Gunnar Borg, (Borg, G., 1998), or a 1–10 scale such as the 'Adult OMNI scale of Perceived Exertion for Walking/Running Exercise' (Utter, A.C. et al., 2004). The perceived exertion score indicated by an athlete should reflect how heavy and strenuous the exercise feels to the individual, combining all sensations and feelings of physical stress, effort, and fatigue. As pictured in Fig. 9.1, the Borg RPE scale ranges from 6 to

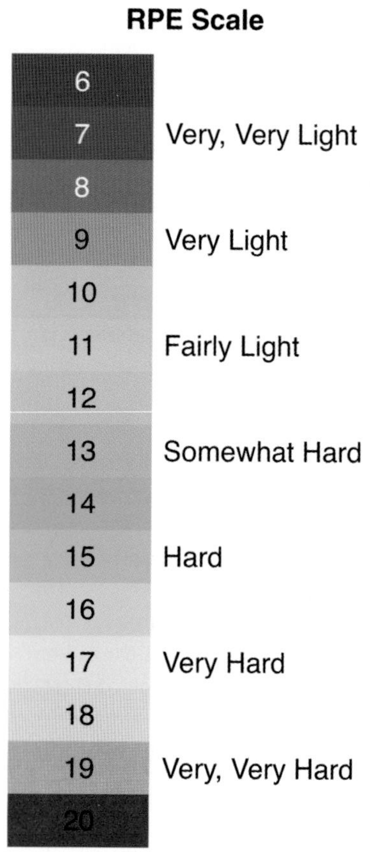

RPE Scale

Fig. 9.1 Borg Scale of Perceived Exertion (Borg, 1998).

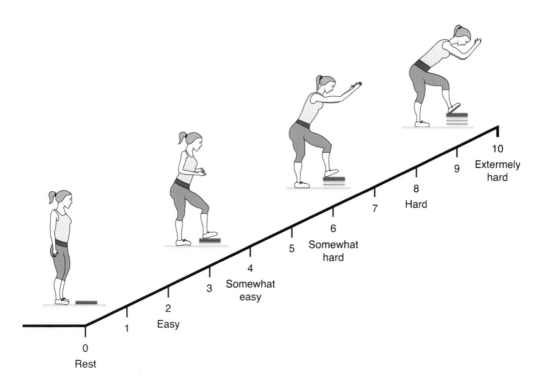

Fig. 9.2 OMNI bench stepping scale of perceived exertion (Krause *et al.*, 2012).

20, where 6 refers to 'no exertion at all' and 20 means 'maximal exertion'. This scale was developed to correspond to approximate heart rate, so a score of 9 corresponds to approximately 90bpm. Due to the specific conditions of pregnancy, this correlation between heart rate and perceived exertion does not hold true for prenatal exercise. Broadly speaking, pregnant athletes should aim to exercise at intensities no greater than 14–16 (hard) on the Borg Scale.

When applying a 10-point scale such as the 'OMNI bench stepping scale of perceived exertion' (Fig. 9.2) to their training, pregnant athletes aim for exercise intensities of 8 (hard) or below. Pregnancy is definitely a time when female athletes should listen to their bodies and not be afraid to back off exercise intensity if they experience feeling unwell or any adverse symptoms. If the athlete feels great, is being appropriately challenged, breathing hard but not out of breath, and allowing ample recovery during and between workouts, then they are striking the right balance. Any evidence of contraindications when exercising should always mean that the athlete ceases exercising immediately and contacts their doctor or maternity support staff.

PELVIC FLOOR EXERCISES

Pregnancy and birth weaken the pelvic floor muscles. These muscles are located within the pelvis and run from the pubic bone at the front to the base of the spine. The pelvic floor muscles support the bowels, womb and bladder during running, jumping and lifting

Exercise	Description	Sets / Reps
Isometric holds	In either sitting or standing with knees slightly apart, squeeze the pelvic floor as if trying not to pass wind and squeeze the muscles as if trying not to pass urine. Then squeeze both together and hold for as long as possible. Initially the duration of hold may just be 2-3 seconds, this should be gradually increased as the athlete is able up to approximately 10 second holds. Rest for approx. 10 seconds between each squeeze.	Work up to 10 repetitions.
On-off contractions	Use the same techniques as described for the isometric holds but rather than continuing to hold, release the tension immediately then repeat the squeezing action.	Work up to 3x10 repetitions.
Kegel exercises	Squeeze and hold the vaginal muscles for 10 seconds and then slowly release. Squeeze again and release quickly.	Work up to 10-20 repetitions.

Table 9.4 Example pelvic floor exercise routine.

activities amongst other things and control the passage of urine. They are also utilized during the second stage of labour to push the baby out during vaginal delivery. In order to maintain the function of the pelvic floor muscles during pregnancy and after childbirth, it is important to exercise them frequently throughout the pregnancy on at least a daily basis. Reduced function of these muscles may lead to postnatal incontinence problems. Low-level pelvic floor strengthening exercises should be performed with high frequency to fit around daily activities rather than planning separate designated pelvic floor training sessions.

These low-level exercises should be performed very frequently throughout pregnancy and after giving birth. During pregnancy, completing the routine three to five times per day is advisable. After giving birth and having recovered bladder control, it would be good practice to continue the routine once a day indefinitely. A member of the maternity support team can carry out an assessment of pelvic floor function and provide more detailed individualized advice.

ACTIVITIES TO AVOID DURING PREGNANCY

For athletes exercising during pregnancy, there are a number of training activities that should be either avoided or significantly modified. Contact sports where there is significant risk of being hit such as taekwondo, judo, kickboxing, rugby, hockey, and so on should be avoided throughout pregnancy. It is advised that pregnant athletes refrain from moderate- to high-intensity training at altitude greater than 1,500–2,000metres. The relative hypoxia in these environments means that the unborn baby will receive a reduced oxygen supply (Entin, P.L. and Coffin, L., 2004). Scuba diving is also not a safe activity during pregnancy as it is possible that nitrogen gas bubbles may pass across the placenta. The unborn baby has no protection against decompression sickness.

Intense exercise in extremely hot and/or humid environments should be avoided. Pregnant athletes must ensure they stay well hydrated and adjust fluid intake based upon the intensity and duration of training sessions, so they should always have a water bottle with them. Dehydration during pregnancy may cause preterm uterine contractions and in extreme cases preterm labour. If pregnant athletes experience any unusual symptoms during exercise, the exercise should be stopped immediately and the doctor or maternity team contacted.

Particular caution should be taken when engaging in any activities where losing your balance could result in significant impact, for example horse riding, skiing or cycling, as the growing bump alters the body's centre of mass making a loss of balance more likely. For athletes who engage in multi-directional running and agility tasks within their training and competition, increased joint laxity and a changed centre of mass during pregnancy mean that these activities need to be either significantly moderated, modified or removed from the training programme. Rapid changes of direction and aggressive decelerations should not be included in the maternal training programme. High-intensity plyometric activities are also not advised after the first trimester.

Beyond the first trimester of pregnancy, it is not advisable to exercise in a supine (flat on your back) position as the weight of the baby may restrict the blood flow to the heart, reducing blood pressure and causing dizziness. It is therefore advised that pregnant athletes do not exercise in this position.

Some abdominal conditioning exercises may exacerbate abdominal separation (diastasis recti) in some individuals. After the first trimester and immediately postpartum, abdominal flexion exercises such as sit-ups, crunches and oblique twists should be removed from the training programme. Isometric 'pillar' trunk strength and postural strengthening exercises should instead be the focus of abdominal conditioning exercise. Extended holds in a front-lying plank position may also lead to the weight of the foetus pressing against the abdominal wall; extended holds in this position should therefore be avoided after the first trimester of pregnancy.

ABDOMINAL MUSCLE SEPARATION (DIASTASIS RECTI)

Every woman's abdominal muscles widen and stretch during pregnancy. This is a perfectly normal process. The rectus abdominis muscles run down the centre of the belly. The left and right side of these muscles are joined together by the linea alba (connective tissue). Commonly, pregnant women may develop a gap between the two parts of the outermost abdominal muscle layer (rectus abdominis) during the third trimester as the linea alba becomes very thin and soft. The medical term for this phenomenon is 'diastasis recti'. The risk of developing diastasis recti is elevated for women who are beyond thirty-five years old, are carrying a baby with high birth weight, carrying multiple babies, have weak abdominal muscles, or who already have children. This separation is created by increased pressure against the abdominal wall from the growing uterus, coupled with biomechanical changes through pregnancy. This space in the abdominal musculature is not a separation of the muscle itself but a stretching of the connective tissue (linea alba) of the abdominal midline.

Regular exercise throughout pregnancy reduces the risk of diastasis recti. Integrating pelvic alignment exercises into the maternal training programme can significantly reduce the pressure that the uterus creates on the abdominal wall and mitigate the risk of diastasis recti. Performing transverse abdominal-focused exercises while pregnant can also reduce the risk of diastasis recti postpartum.

The long-term maintenance of postural integrity, spinal and pelvic alignment, strength, back health, appearance and athletic performance require that this space in the abdominal midline is closed as soon as possible. The gap in the abdominal midline may not always close immediately after giving birth. For those athletes who experience diastasis recti, the gap will usually close naturally six to eight weeks postpartum and should definitely have closed by three to four months postpartum at the latest. If it does not, then the athlete should seek treatment from their doctor.

RETURNING TO TRAINING AFTER CHILDBIRTH

When returning to training and eventually competition after childbirth, it is important that the athlete is patient and realistic about the type, intensity and volume of training undertaken.

Postnatal exercise should be deferred until bleeding has stopped. Warning signs to ease off on postnatal exercise should be strictly heeded. Any colour changes to lochia (postpartum vaginal flow) to pink or red, heavier lochia flow, or if lochia starts flowing again after it had stopped, indicate that the athlete should rest until these symptoms desist. If symptoms do not improve immediately then medical advice should be sought. Once symptoms have cleared up, low-intensity training and load with gradual progression may recommence.

After childbirth it is important to strengthen the pelvic floor muscles that will have become stretched. It is normally safe to commence very

> All athletes should consult with their doctor or midwife before starting any postnatal exercise programme and may be advised to wait or adapt exercises.

gentle exercises of this nature three to five days after childbirth. Following caesarean section, women are normally safe to start exercise once the incision is properly healed. The pelvic floor exercise routine that was performed during pregnancy (Table 9.4) should again be performed several times a day as soon as the individual feels able. New mums should also start walking as soon as they feel able, starting with a ten-minute walk and gradually building up the duration of daily walks.

Ligaments and joints will normally remain relatively lax for three to six months after giving birth due to the continued presence of the hormone relaxine. Activities that place stress on the unstable pelvic floor, pelvis and hip joints should be deferred until strength and stability have improved. High-impact exercises or sports that require rapid direction changes should be avoided for this period. Aggressive stretching to increase range of movement should also be avoided until joint stability and pelvic floor function are fully re-established. Recommended exercises for the initial period after childbirth include: brisk walking, swimming, yoga, Pilates, light resistance training and static cycling.

If an athlete has had significant abdominal separation during pregnancy, they should ensure that the abdominal muscles have healed properly before undertaking any exercises involving vigorous movement of the trunk, such as crunches. For all athletes returning to exercise after childbirth, the abdominal muscles should be challenged through functional positions and movements such as squats, split squats and so on, rather than isolated abdominal exercises. In the initial stages of returning to these exercises, athletes should gently pull in the abdominal muscles prior to bending or lifting. The lower abdominal muscles should initially be strengthened whilst lying on the side or back then progress to seated and plank type positions.

Light to moderate resistance exercise should

initially involve exercises that improve posture and strengthen the muscles required for everyday life and baby care before addressing any sports performance objectives. The exercises should be performed at a controlled tempo throughout with a focus upon technical excellence and movement quality, under gradually increasing loading. As is the case during pregnancy, athletes undertaking post-natal exercise must ensure good hydration through the frequent intake of fluids. This is particularly important if breastfeeding. Athletes should ensure they have a water bottle with them when doing any form of exercise.

Postnatal stretching should initially aim to lengthen muscles that have tightened and shortened during pregnancy. Anterior hip, chest and calf muscles in particular should be the focus of flexibility training to help correct postural changes and reduce muscular tension.

Every woman's experience of pregnancy and childbirth is different, as is their recovery after giving birth, so it is essential that the post-natal exercise programme is individualized, realistic and progressed based upon the individual response to a progressive application of exercise stimulus.

SUMMARY

Female athletes should not view pregnancy as something that hinders their performance, but

> **Pregnant athletes must be guided by the advice of their medical professionals or maternity team and continue to heed their advice throughout pregnancy and the postpartum phase.**

something that can be managed, exercised through and they will be able to return to high intensity, volume and performance afterwards. The health of mother and baby are paramount throughout pregnancy and must be prioritized over any physical performance goals. For many athletes this requires a change of mind-set, making decisions on a daily basis based upon a combination of medical advice and how they feel.

An athlete's training plan throughout pregnancy must be very flexible and predominantly utilize familiar exercises and training modalities; this is not the time to experiment with novel training interventions. Pregnant athletes should not feel an obligation to constantly push hard in training. This is a time for the athlete to enjoy training without any concerns about hitting prescribed or predicted training loads or objectives.

After giving birth, the return to exercise and training must be progressively managed and will largely depend upon what happened during the birth and any associated physical implications.

REFERENCES

American College of Obstetricians and Gynecologists. (2009) Exercise during pregnancy and the postpartum period (ACOG Committee Opinion No. 267). *Obstetrics & Gynecology*, 99, 171–173.

Artal, R. and O'Toole, M. (2003) Guidelines of the American College of Obstetricians and Gynecologists for Exercise during Pregnancy and the Postpartum Period. *Exercise in Pregnancy*. Web [accessed 20 Apr. 2014] http://bjsm.bmj.com/content/37/1/6.long.

Barakat, R. et al. (2014) Exercise Throughout Pregnancy Does not Cause Preterm Delivery: A Randomized, Controlled Trial. *Journal of Physical Activity and Health*, 11, 1012–1017.

Bø, K. et al. (2016) Exercise and pregnancy in recreational and elite athletes: 2016 evidence summary from the IOC expert group meeting, Lausane. Part 1 – exercise in women planning pregnancy and those who are pregnant. *British Journal of Sports Medicine*, 50, 571–589.

Borg, G. (1998) *Borg's Perceived Exertion and Pain Scales*. Champaign, IL: Human Kinetics.

Boscaglia, N., Skouteris, H. and Wertheim, E.H. (2003) Changes in body image satisfaction during pregnancy: A comparison of high exercising and low exercising women. Aust. NZ. *Obstetrics & Gynaecology*, 43, 41–45.

Downs, D.S. et al. (2012) Physical Activity and Pregnancy: Past and Present Evidence and Future Recommendations. *Research Quarterly for Exercise and Sport*, 83(4), 485–502.

Dye, T.D. et al. (1997) Physical activity, obesity and diabetes in pregnancy. American Journal of Epidemiology, 146, 961–965.

Entin, P.L. and Coffin, L. (2004) Physiological basis for recommendations regarding exercise during pregnancy at high altitude. *High Altitude Medicine & Biology*, 5, 321–34.

Evenson, K.R. et al. (2014) Guidelines for Physical Activity during Pregnancy: Comparisons From Around the World. *American Journal of Lifestyle Medicine*, 8(2), 102–121.

Fieril et al. (2014) Experiences of Exercise During Pregnancy Among Women Who Perform Regular Resistance Training: A Qualitative Study. *Physical Therapy*, 94(8).

Garshasbi, A. and Faghih, Zadeh, S. (2005) The effect of exercise on low back pain in pregnant women. *International Journal of Gynaecology and Obstetrics*, 88, 271–275.

Hall, D.C. and Kaufman, D.A. (1987) Effects of aerobic and strength conditioning on pregnancy outcomes. *American Journal of Obstetrics and Gynecology*, 157, 1199–1203.

Jensen, D. et al. (2008) Mechanical ventilatory constraints during incremental cycle exercise in human pregnancy: implications for respiratory sensation. *Journal of Physiology*, 586, 19, 4735–4750.

Kardel, K.R. (2005) Effects of intense training during and after pregnancy in top-level athletes. *Journal of Medicine and Science in Sports*, 15, 79–86.

Krause, M.P. et al. (2012) Concurrent validity of an OMNI rating of perceived exertion scale for bench stepping exercise. *Journal of Strength and Conditioning Research*, 26(2), 506–512.

Lamina, S. and Agbanusi, E.C. (2013) Effect of Aerobic Exercise Training on Maternal Weight Gain In Pregnancy: A Meta-Analysis Of Randomized Controlled Trials. *Ethiopian Journal of Health Sciences*, 23(1), 59–64.

NHS England. (2017) Exercise in Pregnancy. Web [accessed 15 Jan. 2017] http://www.nhs.uk/conditions/pregnancy-and-baby/pages/pregnancy-exercise.aspx.

Paisley, T.S. (2003) Exercise During Pregnancy: A Practical Approach. *Current Sports Medicine Reports*, 2, 325–330.

Penney, D.S. (2008) http://www.sciencedirect.com/science/article/pii/S1526952307005454. *Journal of Midwifery and Women's Health*, 53(2), 155–159.

Poudevigne, M.S. and O'Connor, P.J. (2006) A review of physical activity patterns in pregnant women and their relationship to psychological health. *Sports Medicine*, 36, 19–38, 2006.

Runge, S.B. *et al.* (2013) http://oem.bmj.com/content/early/2013/07/08/oemed-2012-101173.abstract. *Occupational and Environmental Medicine*, oemed-21012.

Salvesen, K. *et al.* (2012) http://bjsm.bmj.com/content/46/4/279.abstract. *British Journal of Sports Medicine*, 46(4), 279–283.

Schoenfeld, B. (2011) Resistance Training During Pregnancy: Safe and Effective Program design. *Strength and Conditioning Journal*, 33(5), 67–75.

Stan, E.A. (2014) Pregnancy and Aquatic Aerobic Activity. *Sport and Society*, 14, 260–268.

Stevenson, L. (1997) Exercise in pregnancy. Part 1: Update on pathophysiology. *Canadian Family Physician*, 43, 97–104.

Szymanski, L.M. and Satin, A.J. (2012) Exercise During Pregnancy: Fetal Responses to Current Public Health Guidelines. *Obstetrics & Gynecology*, 119(3), 603–610.

Tomic, V. *et al.* (2013) The effect of maternal exercise during pregnancy on abnormal fetal growth. *Croatian Medical Journal*, 54, 362–368.

Utter, A.C. *et al.* (2004) Validation of the Adult OMNI scale of Perceived Exertion for Walking/Running Exercise. *Medicine and Science in Sports and Exercise*, 36(10), 1776–1780.

Vladutio, C.J. *et al.* (2010) http://www.scopus.com/record/display.url?eid=2-s2.0-78549262152andorigin=inwardandtxGid=2D6A5497306AE21C2E15DA407752B899.fM4vPBipdL1BpirDq5CCw%3a2. *Journal of Physical Activity and Health*, 7(6), 761–769.

White, E., Pivarnik, J. and Pfeiffer, K. (2014) Resistance Training During Pregnancy and Perinatal Outcomes. *Journal of Physical Activity and Health*, 11, 1141–1148.

Chapter 10

GENDER SPECIFIC LOWER LIMB INJURIES; IDENTIFICATION OF RISK FACTORS AND MANAGEMENT STRATEGIES

Dr Lee Herrington PhD MCSP

Senior Lecturer in Sports Rehabilitation, University of Salford, UK

Technical Lead Physiotherapist (lower limb injury rehabilitation), English Institute of Sport.

The last three decades have witnessed a tremendous increase in female sports participation at all levels. However, increased female sports participation has also increased the incidence of sport-related injuries, both of the acute traumatic type and the non-contact overuse ones. Any internet literature search would, at first look, appear to indicate females are at far greater risk than males of getting sports-related injuries. As with most things to do with the internet, it is too grand and sweeping a statement to state females are injured more, in fact retrospective analysis of injury data (Ristolainen *et al.*, 2009; Sallis *et al.*, 2001) would indicate that there is very little difference in the overall rate of sports injuries between male and female athletes. What seems to be happening is that there are gender-specific clusters of particular injuries often in specific sports. This chapter aims to identify the most significant injuries in the lower limbs of female athletes, then discuss why these injuries might be occurring and in so doing identify the predominant risk factors. Once the most significant modifiable risk factors have been highlighted, then methods to identify these risk factors in the female athlete and means to manage them will be discussed.

GENDER SPECIFIC INJURIES IN THE LOWER LIMB: WHAT DO FEMALES INJURE MORE?

One of the major areas of gender disparity in sports injury rates is injuries to the knee, specifically injuries to the anterior cruciate ligament (ACL) and the patellofemoral joint (PFJ). Though other injuries show gender bias, for instance ankle ligament injuries, these tend to only occur in specific sports such as basketball (Beynnon *et al.*, 2005). An athlete who has an ACL injury can expect a prolonged period of rehabilitation often lasting six to twelve months before returning to sport. Athletes sustaining PFJ problems often suffer from regular interruptions and restrictions to training once they develop this problem, as it remains a difficult one to treat and often reoccurs.

The increased incidence of ACL injury in females is around 3 times higher across all comparable sports activity exposure (Joseph *et al.* 2013; Moses *et al.*, 2012). In specific sports the increased risk can range from 2 times higher in soccer (Walden *et al.*, 2011), 4 times higher in basketball (Joseph *et al.*, 2013) to 5.3 in rugby (Peck *et al.*, 2013). The prevalence of patellofemoral pain (PFP) is also higher in females and ranges between 13 per cent and 27 per cent higher incidence (McCarthy and

Strickland, 2013). This appears to be particularly significant in the adolescent group where girls potentially have pain 2–10 times more frequently than similar-aged males (Myer et al., 2010) and the presence of PFP may then predispose the female athlete to future ACL injury (Myer et al., 2015). Evidence is lacking for injury rates in the older female athlete, but anecdotally, age does not seem to mitigate these elevated levels of risk; this may be because the same risk factors are present in all of these female athletes regardless of age.

GENDER SPECIFIC RISK FACTORS FOR INJURY: WHY DO FEMALES HAVE THESE INJURIES MORE?

When assessing risk factors, the literature typically defines these as either modifiable or non-modifiable. This delineation is important as non-modifiable factors, though not changeable, need to be considered within the profile of the athlete, as they often act as an amplifier for the modifiable risk factors. The classification of risk factors into modifiable and non-modifiable may be expanded upon further by considering if the individual risk factor is either an extrinsic or intrinsic one. Intrinsic variables include those inherent to the individual athlete, such as sex, hormonal milieu, genetic factors, neuromuscular and cognitive function, anatomic variables (for example knee joint geometry, lower extremity alignment, body mass index), and previous injury to the knee or the lower extremity. Extrinsic factors are external to the athlete and may include level and type of activity, type of playing surface and environmental conditions, as well as equipment used. Listing risk factors in this manner may allow the practitioner to start to be able to prioritize factors, which can be modified for the individual to reduce overall risk of injury.

For the female athlete there are a number of apparent intrinsic non-modifiable risk factors for both ACL injury and PFP related specifically to their gender. These include: hormonal milieu, anatomical factors (pelvis width and femoral angle, ACL size, trochlear notch size and depth) and their greater propensity for hypermobility and generalized laxity. All these factors are likely to amplify the impact of the presence of modifiable factors such as neuromuscular function, which will be discussed next.

Female athletes, when they land and cut (change direction), have a tendency to do so with increased hip adduction and internal rotation, decreased knee flexion and increased knee valgus (see Fig. 10.1). This movement pattern has been associated with increased risk of ACL injury and stress on the PFJ (Myer et al., 2015). Females when they run have been shown to have a tendency to demonstrate increased contralateral pelvic drop, hip adduction and internal rotation, and knee valgus which have all been linked with increased stress on the PFJ and the development of PFP (Myer et al., 2010).

The movement patterns highlighted above have been globally termed 'valgus collapse'. This movement pattern of increased hip adduction (often with simultaneous contralateral pelvic drop), hip internal rotation and knee valgus, with the concurrent increase in corresponding external joint moments has been associated with weakness and a failure of muscle recruitment of the gluteal muscles (gluteus maximus and medius) and the quadriceps muscles (McCarthy and Strickland, 2013). The most significant intrinsic modifiable risk factor for the female athlete for the knee injuries of PFP and ACL rupture would therefore appear to be the presence of valgus collapse during functional tasks and the presence of weakness in the gluteal and quadriceps muscles. This had led to the development of strengthening programmes for these muscles and neuromuscular control training programmes in an attempt to reduce

223

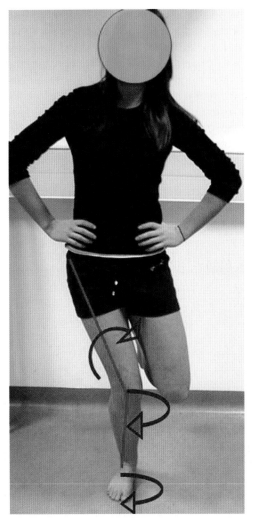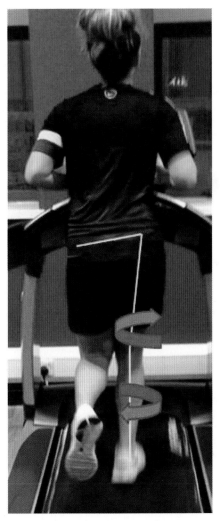

Fig. 10.1 Valgus collapse during squatting and running. Subjects showing typical valgus collapse during squat and running, note the opposite pelvic drop, increased hip adduction and internal rotation, knee valgus, tibial external rotation and foot pronation.

the injury risk from these factors. What follows is a brief discussion of the impact of these programmes on reducing the risk of injury through valgus collapse, preceded by a description of commonly used screening tests to identify poor neuromuscular control, especially 'valgus collapse'.

Screening for Neuromuscular Control

There are a large number of screening tools that have been used to assess for sub-optimal movement strategies, which may predispose female athletes to injury. Presented below are a few of the most commonly used, which are easiest to undertake in the field as opposed to the laboratory.

Landing error scoring system (LESS)

The landing error scoring system (LESS) is a clinical movement-assessment tool, which can be used to assess for suboptimal movement strategies whilst undertaking the bilateral drop jump-landing task. The LESS has been shown to be both reliable and valid (Padua *et al.*, 2009). Padua *et al.* (2011) devised a modified version of the test (LESS-RT), which involves all participants performing four trials of a standardized drop jump-landing task. This involves participants jumping forward from a 30cm-high box, which is placed at a distance of 50 per cent of their height away from the target landing area; land in the target landing area; and immediately rebound by jumping to maximal vertical height on landing. A successful jump was defined as one where both feet simultaneously left the box; the participant jumping forward off the box, without a large upward motion after take-off, to reach the target landing area; and

LESS-RT item	Operational definition	Score item	Score
Stance width	If the subject lands with a wide or narrow stance when viewed from the front they receive an error (+1)	Narrow (1) Wide (1) Normal (0)	
Maximum foot rotation position	If subject's feet are moderately externally rotated (turned out) or slightly internally rotated (turned in) at any point during the landing they receive an error (+1)	Foot turned out (1) Foot turned in (1) Normal (0)	
Initial foot contact symmetry	If 1 foot lands before the other or if foot lands heel to toe & other lands toe to heel, subject receives an error (+1)	Symmetrical (0) Non symmetrical (1)	
Maximum knee valgus angle	If subject has small amount knee valgus receives error (+1), if subject has large amount knee valgus (+2)	None (0) Small (1) Large (2)	
Amount of lateral trunk flexion	If the subject's trunk is leaning to side (not vertical) on landing they receive an error (+1)	None (0) Trunk lean (1)	
Initial landing of feet	If subject lands heel to toe or with a flat foot on landing they receive an error (+1)	Toe to heel (0) Heel to toe (1) Flat foot (1)	
Amount of knee flexion displacement	If subject goes through a small (+2) or moderate (+1) amount of knee bending on landing they receive an error	Large (0) Moderate (1) Small (2)	
Amount of trunk flexion displacement	If the subject goes through a small (+2) or moderate (+1) amount of trunk flexion on landing they receive an error	Large (0) Moderate (1) Small (2)	
Total joint displacement	If subject goes through large displacement of trunk & knees, then score soft (0), moderate amount (1), small amount then score stiff (2)	Large (0) Moderate (1) Small (2)	
Overall impression	Excellent (0) if subjects displays soft landing, no frontal plane motion of knee, poor (+2) if has stiff landing with large frontal plane knee motion, all other landings are average (+1)	Excellent (0) Average (1) Poor (2)	
		Total (out of 15)	

Table 10.1 LESS-RT score for drop jump landing. (Padua *et al*, 2011)

completing the task in a fluid motion (no pause in movement after making contact with the ground until takeoff for subsequent jump). Both lower extremities are assessed during the initial landing off the box onto the target landing area. If one lower extremity demonstrates an error (for example if the foot was externally rotated) and the other lower extremity did not (the toes pointed forward), this specific item is scored as an error. Each participant receives a final composite score, which was calculated by summing all the items on the LESS-RT score sheet. Table 10.1 shows the scoring system, with Fig. 10.2 giving an example of a score.

Qualitative assessment of single leg squat (QASLS)

The two assessment tools above both involve bilateral landing and jumping; the QASLS tool assesses the subject's ability to single leg squat. This test has been validated against 3D motion capture (Herrington and Munro, 2014) and has excellent inter-tester reliability (Almangoush et al., 2013). The scoring system looks at the strategies adopted from the arms down to the feet with optimal behaviour involving minimal deviation or body movement from that prescribed, that is arms do not move; trunk is slightly flexed, but held still; pelvis stays in mid position with minimal tilt; thighs stay parallel and approximately vertically oriented; patellae point towards middle of foot and foot demonstrates minimal wobble. If the participant deviates at all from the optimal behaviour across the five repetitions of the test, then the error is scored on the sheet (see Table 10.2 and Fig. 10.3).

Tuck jump test

The tuck jump test is another example of a bilateral clinical movement-assessment tool, which can be used to assess for suboptimal movement strategies whilst undertaking multiple tuck jumps. The test was originally reported by Myer et al. (2011) with reliability shown by Herrington et al. (2013). The test involves the subject undertaking ten consecutive tuck jumps attempting to stay on the same spot and lift the knees above the level of the hips. The subject is scored across three areas: the knee and thigh motion; the foot position during landing and the plyometric technique. If an error is made in the particular domain at any point across the ten repetitions, then an error score of one is given. Each participant receives a final composite score, calculated by summing all the items giving a score out of ten. Fig. 10.4 shows the scoring criteria.

TRAINING OPTIONS TO IMPROVE NEUROMUSCULAR CONTROL

As discussed above, the most significant intrinsic modifiable risk factor in the female athlete for the knee injuries of PFP and ACL rupture would appear to be the presence of valgus collapse during functional tasks. This had led to the development of a variety of neuromuscular control training programmes to modify this risk factor. A recent systematic review (Noyes and Barber-Westin, 2012) found fifty-seven studies describing forty-two different ACL injury-prevention training programmes. The two programmes they (Noyes and Barber-Westin, 2012) found significantly reduced ACL injury rates and improved athletic performance tests were the Sportsmetrics and the Prevent Injury and Enhance Performance (PEP) programme. Alongside these two, considerable work has been done supported by FIFA on the FIFA 11+ programme, which is a more soccer-specific injury prevention programme. These programmes have all focused on the reduction of ACL injuries rates, but as the movement and loading patterns are common also to PFP these programmes are likely to have a positive impact on PFP risk as well (Myer et al., 2015). This next section will discuss these three

LESS-RT item	Score item	Score
Stance width	Narrow (1) Wide (1) Normal (0)	1
Maximum foot rotation position	Foot turned out (1) Foot turned in (1) Normal (0)	1
Initial foot contact symmetry	Symmetrical (0) Non symmetrical (1)	0
Maximum knee valgus angle	None (0) Small (1) Large (2)	2
Amount of lateral trunk flexion	None (0) Trunk lean (1)	0
Initial landing of feet	Toe to heel (0) Heel to toe (1) Flat foot (1)	0
Amount of knee flexion displacement	Large (0) Moderate (1) Small (2)	1
Amount of trunk flexion displacement	Large (0) Moderate (1) Small (2)	1
Total joint displacement	Large (0) Moderate (1) Small (2)	1
Overall impression	Excellent (0) Average (1) Poor (2)	1
Total (out of 15)		8

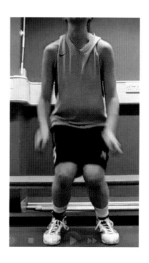

Fig. 10.2 An example of LESS-RT scoring

QASIS		Left	Right
Arm Strategy	Excessive arm movement to balance		
Trunk Alignment	Leaning in any direction		
Pelvic plane	Loss of horizonal plane		
	Excessive tilt or roatation		
Thigh motion	WB thigh moves into hip adduction		
	NWB thigh not held in neutral		
Knee position	Patella pointing towards 2nd toe (noticable valgus)		
Steady stance	Touches down with NWB foot		

Table 10.2

Optimal	Sub-optimal	Optimal	Sub-optimal
Arm strategy Goal: arm stays relaxed by side	Excessive arm movement to balance		
Trunk alignment Goal: trunk remains in neutral or slightly flexed position	Leaning in any direction		
Pelvic plane Goal: pelvis maintains horizontal position, doesn't rotate relative to thigh	Loss of horizontal plane		
	Excessive tilt or rotation		
Thigh motion Goal: WB thigh remains in neutral position. NWB thigh remains parallel with WB thigh	WB thigh moves into hip adduction		

	NWB thigh not held in neutral	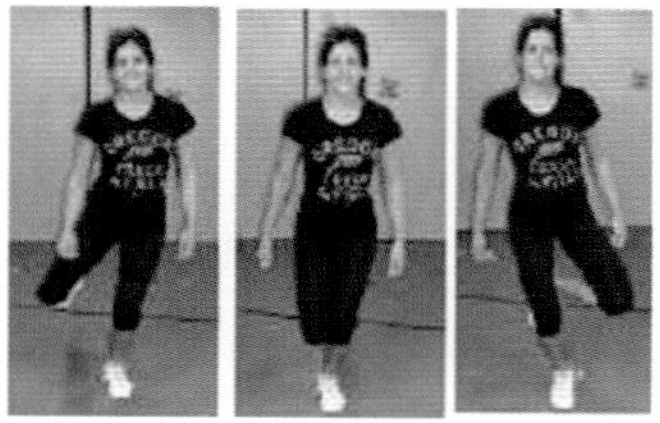
Knee position Goal: patella stays aligned over middle of foot	Patella pointing towards 2nd toe (noticeable valgus)	Patella pointing past inside of foot (significant valgus)
Steady stance Goal: stance leg is held still for three seconds, NWB doesn't touch down	Touches down with NWB foot	Stance leg wobbles noticeably
Total		

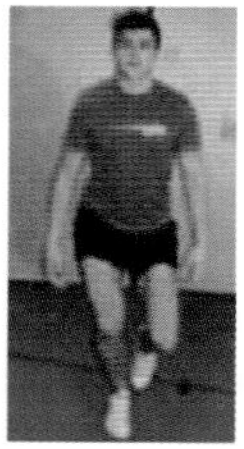

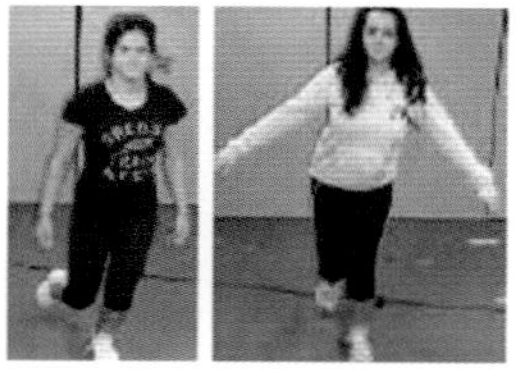

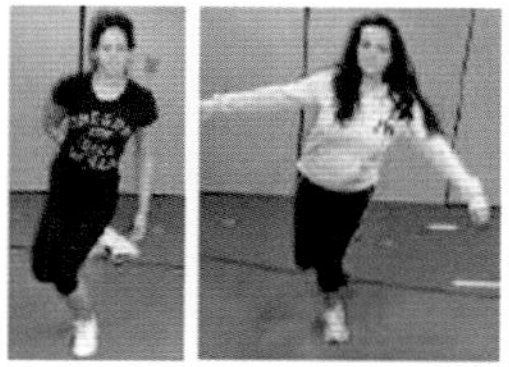

Fig. 10.3 Qualitative assessment of single leg squat (QASLS).

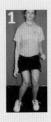 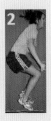 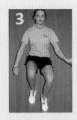 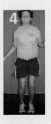 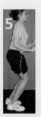 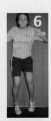

Knee and thigh motion

1. Presence of knee valgus on landing. Hip, knee and foot remain aligned with no collapse of the knee inwards
2. Thighs not reaching parallel at the peak of the jump
3. Thighs not equal side to side during the flight phase

Foot position during landing

4. Foot placement is not shoulder width apart (either more or less)
5. Foot placement not parallel (front to back)
6. Foot contact timing not symmetrical (landing asymmetrical)
7. Does not land in the same point consistently
8. Excessive landing contact noise

Scoring sheet	
Name:	**Score**
Knee and thigh motion	
1. Knee valgus on landing	
2. Thighs not reaching parallel (peak of jump)	
3. Thighs not equal side to side (during flight)	
Foot position during landing	
4. Foot placement not shoulder width apart	
5. Foot placement not parallel (front to back)	
6. Foot contact timing not equal	
7. Does not land in same foot print	
8. Excessive landing contact noise	
Plyometric technique	
9. Pause between jumps	
10. Technique declines prior to 10 seconds	
Total Score	

Fig. 10.4 Tuck Jump Test scoring criteria. Marking criteria: If the participant fails to meet the criteria below then they score a (1) for each item they fail on, if they meet the criteria then they score (0) for the respective category.

programmes along with an abridged jump-landing programme.

Sportsmetrics programme
http://sportsmetrics.org/
The Sportsmetrics programme was devised by researchers and clinicians from the Cincinnati Sports Medicine Centre and the Cincinnati Children's Hospital. The programme involves a combination of activities including strengthening, mobility-stretching and a progressive jump-landing training programme. This programme has been shown to both reduce ACL injury rates and improve athletic performance (Noyes and Barber-Westin, 2012). The programme takes approximately one hour to complete and it is recommended to be undertaken two to three times per week in the preseason period (six to eight weeks).

Prevent Injury and Enhance Performance (PEP) programme
http://smsmf.org/files/PEP_Program_0412201 1.pdf
The Prevent Injury and Enhance Performance (PEP) programme was devised by researchers and clinicians from the Santa Monica Sports Medicine Research Foundation. The programme comprises a combination of running agility drills, body weight exercises, jump-landing activities and mobility-stretching exercises. This programme has been shown to both reduce ACL injury rates and improve athletic performance (Gilchrist et al., 2008; Noyes and Barber-Westin, 2012). The programme takes 15–20 minutes to complete and it is recommended that it should be done prior to training as a modified warm-up activity.

FIFA 11+
http://www.f-marc.com/downloads /cards/11pluscards_e.pdf
The FIFA 11+ injury prevention programme was devised by the FIFA Medical Assessment and Research Centre (F-MARC), as a development of the PEP programme. The programme comprises a combination of running agility drills, body weight exercises, jump-landing activities and mobility-stretching exercises. This programme has been shown to reduce both ACL injury rates and general injury rates, and improve athletic performance (Bizzini and Dvorak, 2015). The programme takes 15–20 minutes to complete and it is recommended that it should be done prior to training as a modified warm-up activity at least twice per week.

Abridged 'jump' programme (Herrington, 2010)
The programmes outlined above involve combinations of running and agility drills, plyometric 'jump-landing', strength and flexibility training; they take at least fifteen to twenty minutes, if not longer, to complete and were recommended to be done at least two to three times per week (Voskanian, 2013). It is unclear which elements of these multimodal exercise programmes bring about the changes in neuromuscular control seen, as some elements such as the strength training elements would appear not to strengthen, as often only body weight load is used. There may therefore be some redundancy amongst the large number of exercises used. Alongside this, poor compliance when undertaking these programmes has been reported as a major problem; this has been attributed to the length of time the programmes require (Dai et al., 2014). With the issues of programme duration and content in mind, Herrington (2010) proposed an abridged jump-landing training programme, which took under fifteen minutes to complete and incorporated only progressive jumping (plyometric) and landing tasks. This programme was shown to significantly improve neuromuscular control on landing (Herrington et al., 2015; Herrington, 2010), it also brought about changes in performance markers (Herrington

Table 10.3 Jump training programme.

Preparation phase (3 sessions)	
Exercise	
Assisted jump	3x10
Vertical jump	3x10
Assisted hop	3x10
Lunge walk	10

Jump training phase (12 sessions)	
Session 1: Exercises	*Duration*
Board jump (stick landing)	5x3 jumps
Squat jumps	5x3 jumps
Forward jumps (barrier)	5x3 jumps
180° jumps	10 jumps
Lunge walk	10
Session 2: Exercises	*Duration*
Board jump (stick landing)	5x3 jumps
Squat jumps	5x3 jumps
Forward jumps (barrier)	5x3 jumps
180° jumps	10 jumps
Lunge walk	10
Session 3: Exercises	*Duration*
Board jump (stick landing)	5x5 jumps
Squat jumps	5x5 jumps
Forward jumps (barrier)	7x3 jumps
180° jumps	5 jumps
Lunge walk	10
Session 4: Exercises	*Duration*
Board jump (stick landing)	5x5 jumps
Squat jumps	5x7 jumps
Forward jumps (barrier)	7x3 jumps
180° jumps	7 jumps
Lunge walk	10

Session 5: Exercises	*Duration*
Board jump (stick landing) distance	5x3 jumps
Jump, jump, vertical	5x3 jumps
Side jumps (barrier)	7x3 jumps
180° jumps	10 jumps
Split lunge	3x4 jumps
Session 6: Exercises	*Duration*
Board jump (stick landing) distance	5x5 jumps
Jump, jump, vertical	5x5 jumps
Side jumps (barrier)	7x3 jumps
180° jumps	10 jumps
Split lunge	2x6 jumps
Session 7: Exercises	*Duration*
Hop	5x3 jumps
Jump, jump, vertical (180°)	5x3 jumps
Forward hops (barrier)	5x3 jumps
180° jumps	3x5 jumps
Split lunge	2x 6 jumps
Session 8: Exercises	*Duration*
Hop	5x3 jumps
Jump, jump, vertical (180°)	5x5 jumps
Forward hops (barrier)	7x3 jumps
90° hops	6 jumps (3 each way)
Split lunge	2x 8 jumps
Session 9: Exercises	*Duration*
Hop	5x5 jumps
Jump, jump, single land	5x1 jumps
Side hops (barrier)	5x3 jumps
90° hops	10 jumps (3 each way)
Split lunge	2x 8 jumps

Session 10: Exercises	Duration
Hop	6x5 jumps
Jump, jump, single land	7x1 jumps
Side hops (barrier)	7x3 jumps
90° hops	10 jumps (3 each way)
Split lunge	2x8 jumps

Session 11: Exercises	Duration
Crossover hop (4 hops)	6x1 jumps
Jump, jump, single land	10x1 jumps cont.
Side hops (barrier)	7x3 jumps
180° hops	6 jumps (3 each way)
Split lunge	4x5 jumps

Session 12: Exercises	Duration
Crossover hop (4 hops)	6x1 jumps
Jump, jump, single land	10x1 jumps
Side hops (barrier)	7x3 jumps
180° hops	6 jumps (3 each way)
Split lunge 180°	4x5 jumps

2010). In Table 10.3 this jump landing programme is presented in full.

The Future of ACL-PFP Prevention Programmes

How much the ability to execute an appropriate landing strategy tranfers into a sporting context remains an unknown factor in rehabilitation and performance scenarios. There are no current studies that assess the transfer of appropriate landing and cutting strategies into sport-specific skills. Current training practices have a reliance on closed-skill activities carried out in a block order; typically, this involves repeated practices of the closed skill (same-movement tasks in stable, predictable environments most often carried out at a pace defined by the participant). To more appropriately reflect the motor skill requirements of sports, especially team sports, the programmes need to have progressively increasing complexity where more open-skill (non-planned skills/tasks) elements become incorporated in a more and more random training environment, once the closed skill tasks have been mastered (Herrington and Comfort, 2013). Using this motor skill learning approach would then lead to practices that are initially controlled and self-paced, allowing the participant to understand and learn the specifics of the appropriate movement patterns in environments that are predictable and static to allow them to plan their movements in advance (closed skill practice), which is essentially what current programmes do. The practices would then need to progress to incorporate more random elements, where the environment is unpredictable and changing so that the performer needs to adapt their movements in response (open-skill practice).

SUMMARY

- Female athletes appear to be more susceptible to specific injuries than males.
- Female athletes have elevated risk of rupturing their ACL and injuring their patellofemoral joint.
- Numerous risk factors exist to explain the elevated incidence of knee injuries in female athletes; one of the most significant modifiable factors is poor neuromuscular control of the leg during landing and cutting.
- Specific training addressing neuromuscular control during landing and cutting tasks appears to reduce risk of injury.
- The amount of transference of neuromuscular control from these quite constrained training tasks to sport-specific tasks is still unclear.

REFERENCES

Almangoush, A., Herrington, L. and Jones, R. (2014) A preliminary reliability study of a qualitative scoring system of limb alignment during single leg squat. *Physical Therapy and Rehabilitation*, 1;2, http://dx.doi.org/10.7243/2055-2386-1-2

Attar, A., Soomro, N., Pappas, E., Sinclair, P. and Sanders, R. (2015) How effective are F-MARC injury prevention programmes for soccer players? A systematic review and meta-analysis. *Sports Medicine*, (Epub ahead of print).

Beynnon, B., Vacek, P., Murphy, D., Alosa, D. and Paller, D. (2005) First time inversion ankle ligament trauma: the effects of sex, level of competition, and sport on incidence of injury. *American Journal of Sports Medicine*, 33, 1485–1491.

Bizzini, M. and Dvorak, J. (2015) FIFA 11+: an effective programme to prevent football injuries in various player groups worldwide – a narrative review. *British Journal of Sports Medicine*, 49, 577–579.

Dai, B., Mao, D., Garrett, W. and Yu, B. (2014) Anterior Cruciate ligament injuries in soccer: loading mechanisms, risk factors and prevention programs. *Journal of Sport and Health Science*, 3, 299–306.

Gilchrist, J., Mandelbaum, B., Melancon, H. and Silvers, H. (2008) A randomized controlled trial to prevent noncontact anterior cruciate ligament injury in female collegiate soccer players. *American Journal of Sports Medicine*. 36, 1476–83.

Herrington, L. (2010) The effects of four weeks of jump training on landing knee valgus and cross over hop performance in female basketball players. *Journal of Strength and Conditioning Research*, 24, 3427–3432.

Herrington, L. and Comfort, P. (2013) Training for prevention ACL injury: incorporation landing skill challenges into a program. *Strength and Conditioning Journal*, 35, 59–65.

Herrington, L. and Munro, A. (2014) A preliminary investigation to establish the criterion validity of a qualitative scoring system of limb alignment during single leg squat and landing. *Journal of Exercise, Sports and Orthopedics*, 1, 1–6. DOI: http://dx.doi.org/10.15226/2374-6904/1/2/00113.

Herrington, L., Munro, A. and Comfort, P. (2015) The effect of jumping-landing training and strength training on frontal plane projection angle. *Manual Therapy* (in press), doi: 10.1016/j.math.2015. 04.009

Herrington, L., Myer, G. and Munro, A. (2013) Intra and inter-tester reliability of the Tuck jump assessment. *Physical Therapy in Sport*, 14, 152–155.

Joseph, A., Collins, C., Henke, N., Yard, E., Fields, S. and Comstock, D. (2013) A multisport epidemiologic comparison of Anterior Cruciate Ligament injuries in high school athletes. *Journal of Athletic Training*, 48, 810–817.

McCarthy, M. and Strickland, S. (2013) Patellofemoral pain: an update on diagnostic and treatment options. *Current Reviews in Musculoskeletal Medicine*, 6, 188–194.

Michaelidis, M. and Koumantakis, G. (2014) Effects of knee injury primary prevention programs on anterior cruciate ligament injury rates in female athletes in different sports: a systematic review. *Physical Therapy in Sport*, 15, 200–210.

Moses, B. and Orchard, J. (2012) Systematic review: annual incidence of ACL injury and surgery in various populations. *Research in Sports Medicine*, 20, 157–179.

Myer, G., Ford, K. and Barber Foss, K. (2010) The incidence and potential pathomechanics of patellofemoral pain in female athletes. *Clinical Biomechanics*, 25, 700–707.

Myer, G., Brent, J., Ford, K. and Hewett, T. (2011) Real-time assessment and neuromuscular training feedback techniques to prevent ACL injury in female athletes. *Strength and Conditioning*, J 33, 21–35.

Myer, G., Ford, K., Di Stasi, S., Foss, K., Micheli, L. and Hewett, T. (2015) High knee abduction moments are common risk factors for patellofemoral pain and anterior cruciate ligament injury in girls: is PFP itself a predictor for subsequent ACL injury? *British Journal of Sports Medicine*, 49, 118–122.

Noyes, F. and Barber-Westin, S. (2012) Anterior Cruciate ligament injury prevention training in female athletes: a systematic review of injury reduction and results of athletic performance tests. *Sports Health*, 4, 36–46.

Padua, D., Marshall, S., Boling, M., Thigpen, C., Garret, W. and Beutler, A. (2009) The landing error scoring system (LESS) is a valid and reliable clinical assessment tool of jump-landing biomechanics: the JUMP-ACL study. *American Journal of Sports Medicine*, 37, 1996–2002.

Padua, D., Boling, M., DiStefano, L., Onate, J., Beutler, A. and Marshall, S. (2011) Reliability of the landing error scoring system-real time, a clinical assessment tool of jump landing biomechanics. *Journal of Sports Rehabilitation*, 20, 145–156.

Peck, K., Johnston, D., Owens, B. and Cameron, K. (2013) The incidence of injury among male and female intercollegiate rugby players. *Sports Health*, 5, 327–333.

Ristolainen, L., Heinonen, A., Waller, B., Kujala, U. and Kettunen, J. (2009) Gender differences in sport injury risk and types of injuries: a retrospective 12 month study on cross country skiers, swimmers, long distance runners and soccer players. *Journal of Sports Science and Medicine*, 8, 443–451.

Sallis, R., Jones, K., Sunshine, S., Smith, G. and Simon, L. (2001) Comparing sports injuries in men and women. *International Journal of Sports Medicine*, 22, 420–423.

Walden, M., Hagglund, M., Werner, J. and Ekstrand, J. (2011) The epidemiology of anterior cruciate ligament injury in football (soccer): a review of the literature from a gender-related perspective. *Knee Surgery, Sports Traumatology, Arthroscopy*, 19, 3–10.

Voskanian, N. (2013) ACL injury prevention in female athletes: a review of the literature and practical considerations in implementing an ACL prevention program. *Current Reviews in Musculoskeletal Medicine*, 6, 158–163.

CHAPTER 11
COACHING FEMALE ATHLETES

Debby Sargent, MSc, PGDipl, ASCC1
University of Gloucestershire, UK

The principle of individualization necessitates that the strength and conditioning (S&C) coach consider *'the athlete's abilities, potential, and learning characteristics and the demands of the athlete's sport, regardless of the performance level. Each athlete has physiological and psychological attributes that need to be considered when developing a training plan'* (Bompa and Haff, 2009, p.38). Gender differences play a key role in the individualization process (Bompa and Haff, 2009, p.40) since there are maturational (Lloyd *et al.*, 2015; Ford *et al.*, 2011), physiological and psychological (sports coach UK, b, no date) differences between males and females. However, when it comes to the literature on coaching effectiveness, leadership and expertise, researchers typically generalize 'how to coach' with no specific recommendations made for coaching female athletes. In other words, the female athletic population is not considered a 'special population' group that requires specific attention or modifications to the more general coaching recommendations. Therefore, it is up to you as the coach to interpret and adapt these findings to suit the specific context in which you are working.

An alternative belief held by some S&C coaches is that males and females are sufficiently different that some broad variation in approaches to coaching can be justified between different sex athletes to optimize coaching effectiveness. Anecdotal evidence to support this lies in the comments made by some S&C and sport-specific coaches that claim that they are unable to coach female athletes on the basis that 'they do not have a psychology degree'!

There is also the concept of gender which is defined as the state of being male or female and typically refers to social and cultural differences rather than biological ones (sex differences) (Cambridge English Dictionary, 2017). Masculine stereotypes reinforced in the media include traits such as being dominant, independent, aggressive, active and courageous, whereas female traits typically include being affectionate, emotional, dependent, submissive and sexy (Rose *et al.*, 2012). As a coach, it is entirely possible that you work with some male athletes who display female traits and female athletes that display strong tendency for masculine traits. Both 'sex' (Beilock and McConnell, 2004; Jones and Greer, 2011; Krendl *et al.*, 2012; Hively and Alayli, 2014) and 'gender' (Rose *et al*, 2012) stereotyping do exist in the media, and within sport (Rose *et al.*, 2012; Chalabaev *et al.*, 2013). An interesting question worthy of consideration is whether we, either consciously or subconsciously, coach individuals differently because of these sex/gender stereotypes and, if yes, are we doing our athletes a disservice in doing so? Female athletes recognize that they are different to their male counterparts and that these differences should inform the planning and decision-making process when it comes to training and programming, but they typically see themselves as athletes first and women second. As such they want to be provided with the same opportunities and driven by the same high expectations that any S&C would expect from male athletes (sports coach UK, a, no date). This should come as no surprise, with exceptional elite performers often being described as being obsessed with achieving success (Mallett and Hanrahan, 2004). Intuitively this means when working with female athletes there will be some 'gender neutral' elements of good practice that will be relevant for all athletes, but perhaps there are also windows of opportunity that allow us to hone in on the specific needs and requirements of the female athletes to further optimize our coaching impact.

The professionalization of sports coaching in the UK has seen an expanding body of research aimed at furthering our understanding of the fundamentals of good quality coaching, including the process of becoming an expert coach (Nash and Sproule, 2009) and the attributes that make a 'great' coach (Becker, 2009; Erickson and Côté, 2016). This body of research is essential considering the fact that coaches, including S&C coaches, are one of the principal determinants of athletes' experiences in sport (Erickson and Côté, 2016) and a primary influence of youth sports participation (Fraser-Thomas et al., 2005).

Both coaching and leadership are complex paradigms (Vella et al., 2010) that are often assumed to be synonymous, to the point that leadership has been reasoned to be 'the essential and indispensable element of coaching practice' (Laios et al., 2003). Not surprising, therefore, is an increased attention in the literature looking at how leadership models complement and enhance coaching practice. Understanding coaching effectiveness has been a key focus in recent years (Côté and Gilbert, 2009; Horn et al., 2008; Nash and Collins, 2006), whilst another emerging area is that of transformational leadership theory (TLT). The latter has been one of the most powerful theories in military (Lowe, Kroeck and Sivasubramaniam, 1996) and business (Antonakis, 2012) settings over the last twenty years that is now being applied successfully to a sports coaching context (transformational coaching). Evidence suggests

that a transformational leadership/coaching style can improve athlete motivation and performance (Arthur et al., 2011, Hodge et al., 2014; Vella et al., 2013; Din and Paskevich, 2013; Amorose and Horn, 2001), athlete wellbeing (Stenling and Tafvelin, 2014), team cohesion and an expectation of excellence (Hodge et al., 2014).

The first part of this chapter will define and explore the concepts of coaching effectiveness, the theory of transformational leadership and the link between them. The second part of the chapter will identify four key coaching behaviours (role modelling, autonomy supportive coaching, reflection and mentoring) and explain how these can have a significant influence on an athlete's development (4 Cs: see definition below), via a manipulation of the four dimensions of transformational leadership/coaching (4 Is) (Kao and Tsai, 2016). Discussions focus on 'how' you can tailor these coaching behaviours to get the most out of your female athletes, although the concepts can equally be applied to male athletes.

COACHES' EXPERT KNOWLEDGE

One of the key attributes of expert coaches is an extensive knowledge base (Côté and Gilbert, 2009, Nash and Collins, 2006; Becker, 2009) that

---

DEFINING COACHING EFFECTIVENESS

Côté and Gilbert (2009) were the first authors to provide an integrated definition of coaching effectiveness based on three broad component parts: coaches' knowledge (specific knowledge in particular contexts), athletes' outcomes (the ability to apply coaching expertise to particular athletes and situations) and coaching contexts (consistent application).
'Coaching effectiveness is the consistent application of integrated professional, interpersonal, and intrapersonal knowledge to improve athletes' competence, confidence, connection and character (4 Cs) in specific sporting contexts.'

can be defined as either 'declarative', which is the explicit knowledge of facts (tactics and training techniques), and the relationship between them, or 'procedural', which is knowledge about how to act, or the steps and actions required to complete a task (Anderson, 1982; Sutton and McIlwain, 2014). An expert S&C coach will possess predominantly three types of knowledge: sport/discipline-specific knowledge; pedagogy (teaching and learning methods), the knowledge of other relevant 'sciences' (such as psychology, kinesiology, sociology, physiology) and this is usually amalgamated to form the more general umbrella term of 'professional knowledge'. Nash and Collins (2006) provided an alternative way of categorizing knowledge as tacit (highly developed procedural knowledge) or explicit (can be readily articulated and verbalized), with tacit knowledge being referred to as the instinctive or intuitive coaching often displayed by more expert coaches.

Strength and conditioning coaches are required to undertake and provide a broad range of services (such as mentor, teacher, parental figure) to athletes and the rest of the support team that go far beyond just being a coach (Becker, 2009). This extends the boundaries and scope of professional practice expected from them, and with that comes a need to develop knowledge and experience in an ever-increasing range of fields. An essential part of an S&C coach's daily role is to *understand, interact with and influence others in the settings in which they work. Central to this is the importance of building functional relationships with athletes and others'* (ICCE and ASOIC, 2012). As such the interpersonal (ability to communicate effectively and appropriately) and intrapersonal (understanding oneself) knowledge is a feature within the definition of coaching effectiveness (Côté and Gilbert, 2009).

ATHLETES' OUTCOMES

The 4 Cs (competence, confidence, connection, character/caring) have been identified as being holistic athletes' development outcomes that should result from successful coach–athlete interactions in any sporting environment (Côté and Gilbert, 2009) and these are summarized in Table 11.1.

COACHING CONTEXTS

Lastly, the performance and development needs of athletes determine the specific coaching context and an understanding of these is critical to the degree of coaching effectiveness because the knowledge and skill set required to meet the athlete's needs can be vastly different. The nature and scope of the work that high performance coaches offer when working with elite athletes is vastly different to that of coaches working more at the participation end of the spectrum (Mallet and Côté, 2006). In a high performance environment, coach-athlete relationships tend to require greater commitment and be more stable in nature, with

Competence	Sport-specific technical and tactical skills, performance skills, improved health and fitness, and healthy training habits.
Confidence	Internal sense of overall positive self-worth.
Connection	Positive bonds and social relationships with people inside and outside of sport.
Character	Respect for the sport and others (morality), integrity, empathy and responsibility.

Table 11.1 Athletes' outcomes that should result from effective coaching.
(Adapted from Côté and Gilbert, 2009)

a greater emphasis on longer-term planning, management, monitoring and control of variables that influence performance (Lyle, 2002; Durand-Bush and Salmela, 2002). Table 11.2 encapsulates the general coaching objectives for developing the 4 Cs in different contexts, based on the developmental athlete needs and the performance level in their sport (Côté and Gilbert, 2009).

For all athletes involved in early specialization sports, such as gymnastics, diving and swimming (Bompa and Haff, 2009, pp.36–37), children and adolescents may experience performance coach set-ups that creates a disparity between their development needs and relevant coaching behaviours to develop the 4 Cs (Fraser-Thomas and Deakin, 2008). Although the performance environment can be tolerated by some children, it can also lead to a greater injury potential and shorter careers (Barreiros et al., 2014) than when children follow a more appropriate long-term athlete development model of progression (Lloyd et al., 2015; Ford et al., 2011).

Effective coaches will align their coaching objectives to the changing needs of athletes across the development spectrum and

Participation Coach for Children
1. Adopt an inclusive focus as opposed to an exclusive selection policy based on performance.
2. Organize a mastery-orientated motivational climate.
3. Set up safe opportunities for athletes to have fun and engage playfully in low-organization games.
4. Teach and assess the development of fundamental movements by focusing on the child first.
5. Promote the social aspect of sport and sampling.
Participation Coach for Adolescents and Adults
1. Provide opportunity for athletes to interact socially.
2. Afford opportunities for athletes to have fun and playfully compete.
3. Promote the development of fitness and health-related physical activities.
4. Teach and assess sport-specific skills in a safe environment for long-term sport involvement.
5. Teach personal and social assets through sport (citizenship).
Performance Coach for Young Adolescents
1. Organize the sport experience to promote a focus on one sport.
2. Teach 'rules of competition'.
3. Offer opportunities for fun with increasingly greater demands for deliberate practice.
4. Teach and assess physical, technical, perceptual, and mental skills in a safe environment.
5. Present positive growth opportunities through sport (i.e., civic engagement responsibility).
Performance Coach for Older Adolescents and Adults
1. Set up training regime grounded in deliberate practice.
2. Allow athletes appropriate mental and physical rest.
3. Prepare athletes for consistent high-level competitive performance.
4. Teach and assess physical, technical, perceptual and mental skills in a safe environment.
5. Provide opportunities for athletes to prepare for 'life after sport'.

Table 11.2 Coaching objectives for developing athletes' outcomes (4Cs) in different contexts. (Adapted from Côté and Gilbert. 2009)

manage their environment accordingly (Sarrazin *et al.*, 2001; Ntoumanis and Biddle, 1999; MacDonald *et al.*, 2011).

COACH LEADERSHIP STYLES (TRANSFORMATIONAL LEADERSHIP THEORY)

One of the basic underpinning assumptions of effective leadership in sport is that *'coach leadership behaviours are used to bring about the desired athlete outcomes of competence, confidence, connection and character'* (the 4 Cs) (Vella *et al.*, 2010). Transformational leadership (TFL) involves coaching behaviours that are 'designed to empower, inspire and challenge followers to enable them to reach their full potential' (Bass and Riggio, 2006), by helping convert followers into leaders of the future (Avolio, 1999). The general term 'followers' refers to those individuals a transformational leader is trying to develop (Turnnidge and Côté, 2016), which in this case would be the female athletes/squads an S&C coach might choose to work with. There are four components parts of TFL (Bass, 1985):

- Idealized influence (leaders demonstrate positive role model behaviours that gain their followers' trust, admiration and respect).
- Inspirational motivation (leaders communicate a clear, aspirational but meaningful vision for the future, demanding a high expectation from the follower, but at the same time demonstrating a strong belief that it can be achieved).
- Intellectual stimulation (leaders empower followers to be innovative and creative, encouraging them to contribute novel ideas).
- Individualized consideration (leaders display a deep understanding of the individual development needs of the follower and show a genuine care

towards their followers).

These 4 Is describe the extent to which an S&C coach is able to motivate and provide incentive to their athletes by the creation of a vision for the future (Vella *et al.*, 2013). A good strength and conditioning coach who uses the transformational leadership/coaching style will align their coaching behaviours to the achievement of the 4 Is.

With a basic understanding and working definition of both coaching effectiveness (Côté and Gilbert, 2009) and TFL/Coaching (Hodge and Smith, 2014; Stenling and Tafvelin, 2014; Vella *et al*, 2013; Turnnidge and Côté, 2016), the remainder of this chapter will explore some key coaching behaviours that can maximize your coaching impact, particularly with female athletes. In essence, these behaviours will provide stepping stones to help you better achieve your key athlete outcomes (4 Cs), by specifically targeting the four component parts (4 Is) of the TFL/coaching model described above.

POSITIVE ROLE MODELLING

A role model has been simply defined in the literature as an individual 'who influences the learners' behaviour simply by way of the learner's exposure to the model' (Bandura and Walters, 1963). If the adoption of the model's behaviours produces favourable outcomes to the learner, it is likely that the learner will be yet further motivated to continue the adopted behaviours (Bandura, 1977) under comparable circumstances. A more recent definition by Gibson (2004) defines a role model *'as a cognitive construction based on the attributes of people in social roles an individual perceives similar to him or herself to some extent and desires to increase perceived similarity by emulating those attributes.'* This suggests that female athletes are likely to selectively search for a number of fitting role models that will encourage behavioural predispositions that already exist within them

(Jung, 1986). For female athletes, other professional female athletes may be an obvious choice for a specific role model whose sporting behaviour on the park may provide a source of inspiration (Fleming *et al.*, 2005). For adolescent athletes there is a wealth of evidence supporting this with some suggestion that the sex of the athletic role model chosen is different between the sexes: boys predominantly only select role models of the same sex, whilst girls had occasionally selected athletic role models of the opposite sex (see review by Mutter and Pawlowski, 2014). On a slightly different level, past studies have also looked at athletes' preferences and attitudes to male and female coaches (Parkhouse and Williams, 1986; Weinberg *et al.*, 1984; Williams and Parkhouse, 1988; Magnusen and Rhea, 2009). The most recent study by Magnusen and Rhea (2009) specifically looked at preference for same-sex or opposite-sex S&C coaches in 275 male and 201 female Division I collegiate football, soccer and volleyball athletes. Female athletes did not demonstrate a gender preference, or display any negative attitudes towards a male strength coach. However, male athletes showed a preference for a same-sex strength coach irrespective of the calibre of the female alternative (p<0.05), reinforcing earlier work with non-S&C-based coaches (Weinberg *et al.*, 1984, Parkhouse and Williams, 1986). The reality is female athletes will give 100 per cent to training regardless of the sex of their strength coach, provided that the coach is knowledgeable about S&C and can specifically tailor programmes to accommodate the needs of the female athlete (Magusen and Rhea, 2009). An additional study exploring the sport-specific coaching experiences of thirty-eight elite female soccer players (Fasting and Pfister, 2000) reported greater satisfaction with female coaches compared to males due to the female coaches providing a better style of communication and a greater knowledge of psychology, or ability to understand their physical and psychological conditions.

Other athletes, both distant (remote geographically, with potentially no direct contact or link) and close (part of the same squad or training environment, with direct contact) (Lyle, 2009) and coaches (including ourselves, as described through idealized influence) can provide relevant and appropriate role models for recreational and competitive female performers as they can inspire behaviour patterns that can be seen to lead to 'success', however that may be defined. However, practically there are a few considerations worth noting. With regards to female athletic role models, a thirty-seven year update on 'Women in Intercollegiate Sport' (Acosta *et al.*, 2014) has reported the highest ever participation rates for female athletes in NCAA programmes, with 9,581 teams found at NCAA schools in 2014, a rise of 307 since 2012. By the same token, the 2012 Olympic Games was proclaimed as the 'Year of the Woman', due to the fact that for the first time 45 per cent of all athletes were women, with every delegation sending a female athlete to take part (Fink, 2015). On the face of it, record numbers of participants and ever increasing levels of performance by female athletes would suggest that female sport-specific role models are increasing their visibility, especially through the increasing use of social media. However, within the traditional sports media there continues to be a salient disproportionate level of coverage for female athletes (Fink, 2015; Bruce, 2016; Eagleman *et al.*, 2014) compared to that of male athletes.

Similarly, excluding a few sports, such as equestrian, netball, gymnastics and swimming, the sports coaching workforce continues to be a largely male-dominated profession (S&C and sports-specific), particularly in head coach positions and in elite sport (Acosta *et al.*, 2014, sportscotland, 2014; sports coach UK, 2015; Burton 2015). Data collected in 2014 on strength and conditioning coaches working specifically within the NCAA system reported that across Division 1, 2 and 3, the percentage of schools that had a female S&C coach was 41.4

per cent, 22.9 per cent and 10.8 per cent respectively (Acosta *et al.*, 2014). Additionally, the percentage of accredited UKSCA (United Kingdom Strength and Conditioning Association) coaches that are female is less than 10 per cent (UKSCA Member data, 2016). What this means is that most female athletes, depending on their sport, are likely to have been coached by both male and female coaches across their lifetime, but it is also possible that some may only have been coached by males.

However, recognizing the importance of relevant and appropriate, positive role models for female athletes and the challenges associated with this, here are some practical steps that S&C coaches can use to maximize the effect of the 'idealized influence' domain of TFL theory.

1. **Be knowledgeable.**
   Female athletes want an S&C coach who is knowledgeable, not just about strength and conditioning, but more specifically about the unique needs and requirements of female athletes. There is a suggestion in the literature (Kavussanu *et al.*, 2008) that education training relating to how best to coach athletes of the opposite sex may be worthy of consideration for sport coaches. So, make sure you commit and engage in a programme of continuous professional development (CPD) in these specific areas, making sure your scope of development is broad to further develop both your declarative and procedural (Sutton and McIlwain, 2014), or tacit and explicit (Nash and Collins, 2006) knowledge of the topic. This way you will not only have more knowledge around 'what' to do, but 'how' to put it into practice. Then demonstrate and evidence your knowledge by sharing it with your female athletes, either individually or as a group. Tell them what you have done and what you have learnt and ask for feedback on how you plan to use this 'new knowledge' to further better planning and training for them. It would

also be beneficial to engage them in the process and get them to think cognitively about what this means to them and their training (intellectual stimulation), and encourage them to think creatively how this may shape future S&C delivery (individualized consideration). Make sure you follow through the outcomes of these decisions/conversations so they are visible to the athlete in the delivery of S&C services. This will keep training sessions fun and varied, which will increase the level of motivation in your female athletes as well as further build positive coach-athlete relationships.

2. **Practise what you preach!**
   Set high expectations (aspirational vision) for yourself and your female athletes ('Inspirational motivation') and communicate these standards and values clearly (for example through your coaching philosophy, shared team values, expected standards of delivery and engagement, athlete interactions), modelling the relevant coaching behaviours, both in and out of the S&C environment. The latter are generally mapped out in a good 'Code of Conduct' (idealized influence). Coach–athlete relationships are deepened by role modelling behaviours when the coach displays high moral and ethical standards, which show an element of self-sacrifice and loyalty towards the vision. Athletes have described 'great' coaches as committed, disciplined and consistent in every aspect of their personality (Becker *et al.*, 2009).

3. **Use and make visible positive female role models where you can in your daily practice.**
   If using case study examples or published research to communicate information, use where possible those that involve female athletes or female subjects. The latter may be difficult considering that there is a

significant under-representation of female athletes as subjects in sports and exercise medicine (Costello *et al.*, 2014), but female athletes will appreciate a coach's effort to apply this where possible. Similarly, if you are using videos or images to aid coaching, attempt to showcase good examples of female athletes.

4. **Training environment.**
    Make the training environment inviting to the female athlete by ensuring that visual images in the training environment and those included in marketing and branding information are proactive in promoting gender equality. Promote female athletes on their athletic capabilities and sporting success, rather than on 'how they look'.

5. **Promote mixed-gender athlete support systems.**
    If you are a male S&C coach, try and ensure that other members of the support team are female (and vice versa) and invite them into your training sessions on a regular basis and from an early stage. Some female athletes may feel more comfortable disclosing some types of information about themselves to another significant female, rather than a male (Officer and Rosenfeld, 1985).

6. **Training partner compatibility.**
    Unless you are coaching female-only groups, training sessions will be mixed, and in some cases can be male dominated. As discussed, female athletes are very accommodating of opposite-sex role models and will happily 'buddy up' to train with male athletes. However, the S&C coaches should manage the environment to make sure these partnerships are compatible. Males typically have a better perception of their athletic ability compared to females (Biddle *et al.*, 2011; Fredricks and

Eccles, 2005; Hilland *et al.*, 2009), Often times, female athletes can also view the S&C environment, at least initially, as a little intimidating, especially when working with younger athletes. Therefore, training 'buddies' of female athletes need to be encouraging by providing just the right amount of challenge to the female athletes (Lyle, 2009). The S&C coach can play a key role in managing who trains with who, to ensure role model compatibility within sessions.

AUTONOMY-SUPPORTIVE COACHING BEHAVIOUR

For an S&C coach, understanding the motivational forces that continually drive athletes to pursue sporting excellence (or not, as the circumstances dictate) is a primary influential factor in how they go about their daily practice. The way in which they plan (such as short- to long-term, from macrocycle through to individual sessions) and structure training, how they choose to make decisions, based on the review process, and the nature of the feedback (quantity and quality) they provide to their athletes are all behaviours that have significant consequences for motivation (Horn, 2002; Mallett and Hanrahan, 2004).

Self-determination theory, SDT (Deci and Ryan, 2000), is a theory of motivation that suggests that the central reasons why people choose to engage, direct effort and persist with an activity can be ordered along a continuum of self-determination (Amorose *et al.*, 2007). Intrinsic motivation, defined as engagement purely *'for the enjoyment inherent in the task and/or because they value the activity'* (Amorose *et al.*, 2007) is at one of the self-determined continuum and is important for personal growth and development (Ahlberg *et al.*, 2008). Amotivation is at the other end of the continuum and reflects a dearth of both intention and motivation (Amorose *et al.*, 2007). Extrinsic, or non-self determining motivation, sits somewhere on the continuum between intrinsic and amotivation and reflects behaviours associated with punishments and rewards, or to avoid feelings of guilt (Mallett and Hanrahan, 2004). Self-determined motivation is a characteristic of elite athletes (Mallett and Hanrahan, 2004), although they often demonstrate strong tendencies for extrinsic motivation (Mageau and Vallerand, 2003), particularly self-determined types such as 'identified' and 'integrated regulation' (Mallett and Hanrahan, 2004; Ryan and Deci, 1985; Vallerand, 2001). The latter refer to extrinsic motives that are adopted through choice because the athlete realizes they are important for their long-term achievement and success (Mageau and Vallerand, 2003).

One of the central beliefs of SDT (Ryan and Deci, 2000) is that self-determined (intrinsic) motivation is affected by the degree of satisfaction and fulfilment of three fundamental psychological needs for human competence (perceptions of adequate ability), autonomy (perceptions of being in control of one's choices and decisions) and relatedness (feeling a secure sense of connection and belonging to others). It is believed by some authors (Sheldon et al., 2003) that SDT provides a rationale to understanding how transformational leaders/coaches are able to positively influence their followers.

Autonomy-supportive interpersonal coaching styles have been shown to positively affect an athlete's overall level of wellbeing, satisfaction, intrinsic and self-determined extrinsic motivation (Iachini, 2013; Mageau and Vallerand, 2003) and these are summarized in Table 11.3.

An S&C coach with a transformational leadership approach will create and communicate an attractive, inspirational vision to athletes, which in itself fosters a need for autonomy (Bass and Riggio, 2006). The vision, by definition, will create 'rules' and 'limits', but in reality there will be multiple approaches with no single 'best way' of getting from point A to point B. The 'vision' or challenge set by the S&C coach may present long- or short-term targets for the athlete or group of athletes to achieve. For example, session objectives (or the vision) can be set for an individual training session, a block of training, or for an entire season (progressively increasing in challenge and complexity). Athletes, either as individuals, or as a group, engage in the problem-solving exercise to establish what might be the best approach to take. Creative and innovative thought are required to achieve the task which may also

1	Provide choice within specific rules and limits.
2	Provide a rationale for tasks and limits.
3	Acknowledge the other person's feelings and perspectives in relations to the tasks and rules set.
4	Provide athletes with opportunities for initiative taking and independent work.
5	Provide non-controlling competence feedback.
6	Avoid controlling behaviours: • overt control (e.g., use and threat of physical power, allocation and withdrawal of resources or privileges, surveillance, psychological control) • criticisms and controlling statements • tangible rewards for interesting tasks
7	Prevent ego-involvement in athletes.

Table 11.3 Coaches' autonomy-supportive behaviours. (Adapted from Mageau and Vallerand, 2003)

challenge and question traditional ways of doing things. The challenge of the task will not only stretch the athletes' cognitive abilities, but will also allow them to demonstrate competency in achieving the task. This will lead to feelings of improved self-confidence. Specific individual athlete requirements may also dictate that different athletes might need to follow a slightly different version of the plan for an optimal outcome. This will not only reinforce the belief that individuals' thoughts have been listened to and understood, but that there is 'a way' that every athlete can meet the expectations of the task or vision. The open communication process between the group or individual, leading to a decision being made, will strengthen the coach-athlete bond (improved relatedness), as well as emphasizing the significance of collective action (Sosik and Godshalk, 2000). This empowerment of the group and accountability to take leadership for achieving success is synonymous with the ethos of TFL.

'Great' S&C coaches are recognized and respected for providing a highly organized structure to training (Becker et al., 2009). For coaches working with elite female athletes they appreciate a degree of autonomy and flexibility in being able to direct their own S&C programme. On the way to reaching a high level of sporting performance they have accumulated a lot of S&C-specific knowledge through practice, as well as a great depth of understanding about what their body needs. They are also greatly driven by personal goals and achievement (Mallett and Hanrahan, 2004) and often times know what they need to do to achieve them. However, engaging athletes in the training process and viewing it as a joint endeavour between coach and athlete should happen irrespective of the age and stage of the performer. Clearly the level of autonomy that you can safely offer a novice athlete will be very different, compared to that of someone with more experience. With the former, the amount of choice options may be limited to choosing five

out of eight exercises in a warm-up for example, with the rest of the session following an orderly prescription with little deviation from that. For experienced athletes, they may take responsibility for writing their own training sessions, with you just offering help and support to enable them to make the right decisions.

Good S&C coaches will naturally explain the rationale and meaning behind tasks, not only because it improves training motivation and intention, but also because it can increase the transferability of S&C training adaptations into actual sports performance. In terms of intellectual function, women have been described as having a 'whole-brain perspective' or 'bigger picture' way, compared to men who are more 'analytical, focused, linear and logical in perspective' (sports coach UK, b, no date). This means that female athletes are more likely to demand information and explanations from the coach to help them understand why they are doing certain tasks and what the outcomes of doing them will be. Coaches need to ensure that they dedicate adequate time, during and outside training sessions, to make sure the female athlete has all the information she needs to justify engaging in the programme. It is good practice to reference the day's training sessions within the context of the annual plan or macrocycle at the start of every training session, so they can clearly see how that session contributes to them achieving longer term plans – a process that can positively impact on the perceived competence of the athlete.

The reality of providing athletes with choice and autonomy is that they may choose a path that the coach does not consider to be the 'smartest' way of achieving the desired outcomes. A true autonomy-supportive coaching style means that unless the decision has adverse consequences, the coach should not provide any form of feedback to the athlete (verbal or non-verbal) (Mageau and Vallerand, 2003) that could be viewed as placing a judgement on the decisions made by the athlete. This is important because female athletes are reported to have 'almost a psychic ability to read faces and tone of voice' (sports coach UK, b, no date), meaning they are very adept at picking up and reading any signs of disapproval that can indirectly control behaviour. It is also important from a learning perspective because we know that failing is a natural part of learning (Dweck, 2016) and we learn from making mistakes.

REFLECTION

The process of reflection is a 'taken for granted' established part of the coaching process that is representative of 'good' educational practice (Cushion, 2016; ICCE and ASOIF, 2012; Mallet, 2004). One definition of reflection is *'a purposeful and complex process that facilitates the examination of experience by questioning the whole self and our agency within the context of practice. This examination transforms experience into learning, which helps us to access, make sense of and develop our knowledge-in-action in order to better understand and/or improve practice and the situation in which it occurs'* (Knowles *et al.*, 2014).

The act of reflection is a highly skilled activity that requires conscious effort and practice. It is essentially about you and involves a process of discovery about who you are, what you do and why you do it. Intrapersonal knowledge is a key ingredient in the working definition of coaching effectiveness (Côté and Gilbert, 2009), the reason being that the more aware we are of 'self', the better able we are to face challenges, choose battles, solve problems, make decisions, and predict the outcome of decisions. A greater understanding of 'you' should lead to a positive change in your behaviours as a coach (Knowles *et al.*, 2014).

Using Reflection to Manage the Female Athlete Training Environment

The effects of an increase in self-awareness on positive athlete-coach relationships is self-evident. However, in relation to working with female athletes there are a few particular points worth highlighting to help the S&C coach.

'Relatedness', or a sense of belonging, is one of the three psychological needs named in SDT, as well as one of the 4 Cs within the coaching effectiveness definition. Generally, when females are in difficult situations, the stress response causes an increase in the hormone oxytocin, which has a calming effect. This is in contrast to males, whose 'flight or fight response' is a greater production of adrenaline and testosterone (sports coach UK, b, no date). Under these circumstances females will respond by reaching out and connecting with other people, with their survival strategy being a 'climate of co-operation' and protection of the group (sports coach UK, b, no date). Therefore, disharmony in a group of female athletes can be very destructive and in my experience, those coaches that have worked with female squads seem to put much greater emphasis and consideration into the planning and management of training camps and competitive ventures to prevent conflicts arising. In addition, the female brain is deeply affected by sex-specific hormones which not only makes them generally more emotional than males, but also emotionally less constant (sports coach UK, b, no date) which can provide additional challenges when trying to understand and manage the training environment. A greater intrapersonal awareness, through reflective practice, will not only help you understand how your behaviours affect the female athletes around you (potentially identifying sources of conflict arising there), but will also help you understand better the relationships and group dynamics within the squads so you can be one step ahead of tensions that may be about to surface. Because of the importance of the 'relatedness' aspect of coaching female athletes, S&C coaches may wish to consider putting a greater emphasis on 'team bonding' sessions (both during training sessions and at times outside sessions) than they would with groups of male athletes. Men typically like competition and thrive in competitive environments, whereas females generally don't (Warner and Dixon, 2015), although this may not necessarily be true for elite-level athletes (Mallett and Vallerand, 2003). We also know from the motivational climate literature (Sarrazin *et al.*, 2001; Ntoumanis and Biddle, 1999; MacDonald *et al.*, 2011) that a 'task'-orientated motivational climate better satisfies the three basic psychological needs of SDT, which leads to an increased level of motivation. Engineering a task-orientated motivational climate in sessions that involve female athletes will foster a feeling of 'co-operation', synonymous with a team-bonding philosophy. It will also empower and encourage members of the group to develop leadership skills and experience, which promotes the philosophy from TFL theory of developing followers into leaders.

Allowing time for social interaction within sessions should feature in the session design/plan if required, so that an emphasis on creating greater team co-operation does not impact on the training outcomes planned for the session. A more harmonious team of athletes will deal with stressful situations more effectively, which may be useful at pressured times of the year, when either the numbers or quality of competitive events is high.

The Power of Shared Reflection

Encouraging the athletes themselves to be reflective, as well as yourself, can be very valuable for both parties. Your athlete may be one of the key people you want to talk to about your reflections and if they have already independently reflected on the same event or similar, the coach-athlete discussion will not only be very fruitful, but will deepen the relationship and understanding between you. For great S&C coaches, athletes will also view you as more than 'just the coach', and will recognize that you are a human being as well (Becker, 2009). Reflection will allow both coaches and athletes to recognize and admit when they

have made mistakes, challenge values and acknowledge and explore gaps in knowledge. It is likely that you will express emotion during the process (good and bad) about how you feel about the related topics and in doing so, will exposure more of your personality. The 'human' side is the part that athletes remember about great coaches; expert knowledge is expected (Becker, 2009). This ability to perceive emotions in others and yourself and being able to manage these relates to the concept of 'emotional intelligence' (Hodge *et al.*, 2009) and has been shown to have a significant relationship with coaching efficacy (Thelwell *et al*, 2008). For female athletes who have an innate interest in people (sports coach UK, a, no date) this can really enhance coach-athlete relations, particularly in relation to trust, honesty and respect. The reflective process ticks all four dimensions of the transformational coaching model, which will again positively influence the 4 Cs of coaching effectiveness.

There have been several suggestions for tools that can aid the reflective process, including mind maps, visual images, personal journals, critical friends, recorded narrative, communities of practice and blogs, to name a few (Knowles *et al.*, 2014). Trial and error using some of these methods will help you discover what combination of these is most useful to this process.

MENTORING

'Behind every successful person, there is one elementary truth; somewhere, somehow, someone cared about their growth and development. This person was their mentor.'

Kaye, 1997

This definition of mentoring resonates particularly well for coaches working with athletes, because fundamentally most athletes will train and perform for you if they believe you care about them. Mentoring allows you to get to know the individual athletes on a one-to-one basis, in an informal and relaxed environment that is usually away from the usual training situation. Your role as a mentor in your athletes' development is summarized in Table 11.4, along with suggestions of how mentoring can help you deliver the 4 Is of transformational coaching. To be effective in this role, the skills that you will need to develop as an S&C coach to enable you to be a good mentor to your athletes include listening, questioning, goals-setting, action-planning, and shared problem-solving. Some of the personal qualities you will need to demonstrate are objectivity, patience and empathy (Jones and Simmons, 2010).

Mentoring allows you to build open and honest relationships with your athletes and makes it possible for you to reinforce not just the 'athlete-centred' approach to your role, but also the 'person-centred' role. Evidence supports the notion that coach-athlete interactions should not be limited to just sport-related matters (Erickson and Côté, 2016), provided professional boundaries are not over-stepped. Understanding what goes on in your athlete's life beyond training and competition and exploring exactly 'what' type of relationship your athlete wants from you is essential. Because of the gender-specific role that females have (family for example), female athletes appreciate the S&C coach knowing what kind of issues they face outside of training because it defines what type of support they may be looking for from you. It may also explain to some extent what happens in the training room or on game day. The amount of time that your athletes demand from you in a mentoring role may be very different – some athletes will require more

individual one-on-one support than others will. For an S&C coach, you have to be mindful and honest about how much time you can dedicate to mentoring and you need to strike a balance between the needs of the individuals and the needs of the group, so that all athletes are treated fairly and equally.

Female athletes often lack confidence in their abilities (Biddle et al., 2011). The mentoring session is an ideal opportunity to provide the athletes with constructive and positive feedback and to verbalize your belief in her as a person and her ability to achieve the desired outcomes. Empowering performance feedback is an effective strategy to use (Hodge et al., 2014), which involves you giving feedback on improving her strengths (things that you have identified that she is already really good at), not just reducing her weakness. Additionally, the use of a 360-degree feedback system can also be constructive. As with any individual athlete, the perceived and actual ability of your female athlete may be very different, so feedback from a number of sources (for example sport-specific coaches, physiotherapist, biomechanist and so on) will complement the monitoring and testing data you collect, to provide a more 'real' and honest picture of where your athlete actually is with regards to performance. Revisiting the goals-setting process is a joint venture that not only reinforces your commitment and belief in the athlete, but also acts to transfer some responsibility and accountability on to the athletes, aligning to the transformational coaching philosophy of developing 'followers'

Athlete Development	Mentor (S & C Coach's role)	Transformational Coaching Dimension
Modelling	Role model, observer	Idealised Influence
Competence	Observer, providing feedback	Inspired Motivation
Reflective/Questioning	Challenger, facilitator	Intellectual Stimulation
Autonomy	Partner in critical enquiry	Individualised Consideration

Table 11.4 The role of the mentor in athlete development.
(Adapted from Jones & Simmons, 2010, to reflect the coach-athlete relationship)

into leaders (Hodge *et al.*, 2014). By adopting a 'listen and ask' tactic rather than a tell approach you will encourage the athlete to develop and discuss their own strategies and ideas about what they need to achieve and how they are going to do it. Whilst you might use your knowledge and experience to help your athletes find solutions to the problems identified (providing choice and promoting autonomy), it is also important to respect professional and personal boundaries and signpost your athlete to additional sources of support if required.

In summary, Table 11.5 provides you with a suggested structure for carrying out your mentoring support to athletes. Although the actual meeting will take time, there is additional preparation and follow-up that is essential to this being an effective process.

SUMMARY

The discussion within this chapter has considered the application of the transformational leadership theory to a strength and conditioning coach's practice. Specific examples have been used throughout to present a rationale for its effectiveness for those coaches working with female athletes, although evidence supports the fact that this approach can be successful for all male athletes as well (Hodge *et al.*, 2014; Stenling and Tafvelin, 2014; Vella *et al.*, 2013; Turnnidge and Côté, 2016). Theoretically, coaching behaviours that tap into the four domains of transformation leadership theory (idealized influence, inspired motivation, intellectual stimulation, individualized consideration) will improve the likelihood of success in achieving the desired successful athlete outcomes as communicated in Côté and Gilbert's (2009) definition of coaching effectiveness (competence, confidence, connection and character).

The quality and degree of closeness of the coach-athlete relationship is a determining factor (Vella *et al.*, 2010) in how successful any partnership is, so the 'human' side to coaching cannot be underestimated. This will be that part of the coach-athlete experience that your athletes will remember long after you have parted company.

The coaching behaviours you display are instrumental in building an effective relationship with your athletes as well as improving your coaching effectiveness (achieving the 4 Cs), through demonstration of the 4 Is from the transformational leadership theory. We have discussed just four coaching behaviours (role modelling, autonomy supportive coaching, reflection and mentoring) that may help you become a better and more successful coach, which will directly have an impact on the wellbeing and satisfaction of your athletes (Bono and Ilies, 2006). These simple strategies can readily be incorporated into your coaching practice. Transformational coaching is more about 'evolution' rather than 'revolution', with small changes making a big difference. Further consideration of the impact of other coaching behaviours on the 4 Is can only further improve the effectiveness of your coaching practice, but small changes applied consistently will serve you well.

Pre-session	Session	Post-session
• Gain a shared understanding of the session. • Clarify expectations. • Establish priorities. • Agree goals.	• Keep the session relaxed and comfortable. • Keep it focused on the agreed priorities. • Agree any actions. • Confirm arrangements for next meeting.	• Reflect on the meeting and actions. • Ensure you follow-up on agreed actions. • Plan your next session.

Table 11.5 Suggested format for conducting your mentoring sessions with your athletes. (Adapted from Simmons and Jones, 2010)

249

REFERENCES

Acosta, R.V. and Carpenter, L.J. (2014) Women in intercollegiate sport: A longitudinal, national study, thirty-seven year update. 1977–2014. Retrieved from http://www.acostacarpenter.org/

Ahlberg, M., Mallett, C.J. and Tinning, R. (2008) Developing autonomy supportive coaching behaviours: An action research approach to coach development. International Journal of Coaching Science, 2(2), 1–20.

Amorose, A.J. and Horn, T.S. (2001) Pre- to post-season changes in the intrinsic motivation of first year college athletes: relationship with coaching behaviour and scholarship status. Journal of Applied Sports Psychology, 13, 355–373.

Amorose, A.J. and Anderson-Butcher, D. (2007) Autonomy-supportive coaching and self-determined motivation in high school and college athletes: A test of self-determination theory. Psychology of Sport and Exercise, 8, 654–670.

Anderson, J. (1982) Acquisition of cognitive skill. Psychological Review, 89, 369–406

Antonakis, J. (2012) Transformational and charismatic leadership. In D.V. Day and J. Antonakis (eds.), The Nature of Leadership (2nd ed.), pp.256–288. Los Angeles, CA: Sage.

Arthur, C.A., Woodman, T., Ong, C., Hardy, L. and Ntoumanis, N. (2011) The role of athlete narcissism in moderating the relationship between coaches' transformational leader behaviours and athlete motivation. Journal of Sport and Exercise Psychology, 33, 3–19.

Avolio, B.J. (1999) Full leadership development: Building the vital forces in organisations. Thousand Oaks, CA: Sage.

Bandura, A. (1977) Self-efficacy: toward a unifying theory of behavioural change. Psychological Review, 84, 191–214.

Bandura, A. and Walters, R.H. (1986) Social learning and personality development. New York: Holt, Rinehart and Winston.

Barreiros, A., Côté, J. and Fonseca, A.M. (2014) From early to adult sport success: Analysing athletes' progression in national squads. European Journal of Sport Science, 14 (S1), S178–S182.

Bass, B.M. (1985) Leadership: Good, better, best. Organizational Dynamics, 13, 26–40.

Bass, B.M. and Riggio, R.E. (2006) Transformational leadership (2nd ed.), Mahwah, NJ: Lawrence Erlbaum.

Becker, A.J. (2009) It's not what they do, it's how they do it: Athlete experiences of great coaching. International Journal of Sports Science and Coaching, 4(1), 93–119.

Beilock, S.L. and Connell, A.R. (2004) Stereotype threat and sport: Can athletic performance be threatened? Journal of Sport and Exercise Psychology, 26, 597–609.

Biddle, S.J.H., Atkin, A.J., Cavill, N. and Foster, C. (2011) Correlates of physical activity in youth: a review of quantitative systematic reviews. International Review of Sport and Exercise Psychology, 4, 25–49.

Bompa, T.O. and Haff, G.G. (2009) Periodization: Theory and methodology of training (5th ed.). Champaign, IL: Human Kinetics.

Bono, J.E. and Ilies, R. (2006). Charisma, positive emotions and mood contagion. The Leadership Quarterly, 17, 317–334.

Bruce, T. (2016) New rules for new times: Sportswomen and media representation in the third wave. Sex Roles, 74, 361–376.

Burton, L.J. (2015) Underrepresentation of women in sport leadership: A review of research. Sport Management Review, 18, 155–165.

Cambridge English Dictionary (2017) http://dictionary.cambridge.org/dictionary/english/gender [accessed 21 Feb. 2017]

Chalabaev, A., Sarrazin, P., Fontayne, P., Bioche, J. and Clément-Guillotin, C. (2013) The influence of sex stereotypes and gender roles on participation and performance in sports and exercise: Review and future directions. Psychology of Sport and Exercise, 14, 136–144.

Costello, J. T., Bieuzen, F. and Bleakley, C.M. (2014) Where are all the female participants in sport and exercise medicine research? European Journal of Sport Science, 14(8), 847–851.

Côté, J. and Gilbert, W. (2009) An integrative definition of coaching effectiveness and expertise. International Journal of Sports Science and Coaching, 4(3), 307–323.

Cushion, J.C. (2016) Reflection and reflective practice discourses in coaching: a critical analysis. Sport, Education and Society, DOI:

10.1080/13573322.2016.1142961

Deci, E.L. and Ryan, R.M. (1985) *Intrinsic motivation and self-determination in human behaviour.* New York: Plenum.

Deci, E.L. and Ryan, R.M. (2000). The 'What' and 'Why' of Goal Pursuits: Human needs and the self-determination of behaviour. *Psychological Inquiry*, 11(4), 227–268.

Din, C. and Paskevich, D. (2013) An integrated research model of Olympic podium performance. *International Journal of Sports Science and Coaching*, 8(2), 431–444.

Durand-Bush, N. and Salmela, J.H. (2002) The development and maintenance of expert athlete performance: Perceptions of world and Olympic champions. *Journal of Applied Psychology*, 14(3), 154–171.

Dweck, C.S. (2016) *Mindset: The new psychology of success.* NY: https://www.bookdepository.com/publishers/Random-House-USA-Inc

Eagleman, A., Burch, L.M. and Vooris, R. (2014) A unified version of London 2012: New-media coverage of gender, nationality and sport for Olympics consumers in six countries. *Journal of Sports Management*, 28, 457–470.

Erickson, K. and Côté, J. (2016) A season-long examination of the intervention tone of coach-athlete interactions and athlete development in youth sport. *Psychology of Sport and Exercise*, 22, 264–272.

Fasting, K. and Pfister, G. (2000) Female and male coaches in the eyes of female elite soccer players. *European Physical Education Review*, 6(1), 91–110.

Fink, J.S. (2015) Female athletes, women's sport, and the sport media commercial complex: Have we really 'come a long way, baby'? *Sport Management Review* 18, 331–342.

Fleming. S., Hardman, A., Jones, C. and Sheridan, H. (2005) 'Role Models' among elite young male rugby league players in Britain. *European Physical Education Review*, 11(1), 51–70.

Ford, P., De Ste Croix, M., Lloyd, R., Meyers, R., Moosavi, M., Oliver, J., Till, K. and Williams, C. (2011) The long-term athlete development model: Physiological evidence and application. *Journal of Sports Sciences*, 29(4), 389–402.

Fraser-Thomas, J.L., Côté, J. and Deakin, J. (2005) Youth Sport Programmes: An avenue to foster positive youth development. *Physical Education and Sport Pedagogy*, 10, 19–40.

Fraser-Thomas, J., Côté, J. and Deakin, J. (2008) Understanding drop-out and prolonged engagement from a development perspective. *Psychology of Sport and Exercise*, 9, 645–662.

Fredricks, J.A. and Eccles, J.S. (2005) Family socialisation, gender and sport motivation and involvement. *Journal of Sport and Exercise Psychology*, 27, 3–31.

Gibson, D.E. (2004) Role models in career development: New directions for theory and research. *Journal of Vocational Behaviour*, 65, 134–156.

Hilland, T.A., Stratton, G., Vinson, D. and Fairclough, S. (2009) The physical education predisposition scale: preliminary development and validation. *Journal of Sports Sciences*, 27, 1555–1563.

Hively, K. and El-Alayli, A. (2014) 'You throw like a girl': The effect of stereotype threat on women's athletic performance and gender stereotypes. *Psychology of Sport and Exercise*, 15, 48–55.

Hodge, K., Henry, G. and Smith, W. (2014) A case study of excellence in elite sport: Motivational climate in a world champion team. *The Sports Psychologist*, 28, 60–74.

Horn, T.S. (2002) Coaching effectiveness: research findings and future directions. In: *Advances in Sport Psychology* (2nd ed.) (Ed. Horn, T.S.) Champaign, IL: Human Kinetics.

Horn, T.S. (2008) Coaching effectiveness in the sport domain. In: *Advances in Sport Psychology*, (Ed. Horn, T.S.) Champaign, IL: Human Kinetics.

Huntley, E., Cropley, B., Gilbourne, D., Sparkes, A. and Knowles, Z. (2014) Reflecting back and forwards: an evaluation of peer-reviewed reflective practice, 15:6, 863–876, DOI: 10.1080/14623943.2014.969695

Iachini, A.L. (2013) Development and empirical examination of a model of factors influencing coaches' provision of autonomy-support. *International Journal of Sports Science and Coaching*, 8(4), 661–675.

ICCE and ASOIF (2012) International Sport Coaching Framework. Retrieved from http://www.icce.ws/_assets/files/news/ISCF_1_aug_2012.pdf.

Jones, A. and Greer, J. (2011) 'You don't look like an athlete': The effects of feminine appearance on audience perceptions of female athletes and women's sport. Journal of Sport Behaviour, 34(4), 358–377.

Jones, E. and Simmons, G. (2010) Recruit into coaching: Mentoring Guide. The National Coaching Foundation. Retrieved from: https://www.sportscoachuk.org/sites/defa ult/files/mentoring_guide.pdf

Jung, J. (1986) How useful is the concept of role model? A critical analysis. Journal of Social Behaviour and Personality, 1(4), 525–536.

Kao, S. and Tsai, C. (2016) Transformational leadership and athlete satisfaction: The mediating role of coaching competency. Journal of Applied Psychology, DOI: 10.1080/10413200.2016.1187685.

Kavussanu, M., Boardley, I.D., Jutkiewicz, N., Vincent, S. and Ring, C. (2008) Coaching efficacy and coaching effectiveness: Examining their predictors and comparing coaches' and athletes' reports. The Sports Psychologist, 22, 383–4.

Kaye, B. (1997) Up is not the only way: A guide to developing workforce talent, 2nd edn. London: Nicholas Brealy. ISBN: 978-0-891061-63-2.

Knowles, Z., Gilbourne, D., Cropley, B. and Dugdill, L. (2014) Reflective practice in the sport and exercise sciences. Routledge.

Krendl, A., Gainsburg, I. and Ambady, N. (2012) The effects of stereotypes and observer pressure on athletic performance. Journal of Sport and Exercise Psychology, 34, 3–15.

Laios, A., Theodorakis, N. and Gargalianos, D. (2003) Leadership and Power. Two important factors for effective coaching. International Sports Journal, 7, 150–154.

Lloyd, R.S., Oliver, J.L., Faigenbaum, A.D., Howard, R., De Ste Croix, M.B., Williams, C. A., Best, T.M., Alvar, B.A., Michell, L.J., Thomas, D.P., Hatfield, D.L., Cronin, J.B. and Meyer, G.D. (2015) Long-term athletic development – Part I: A pathway for all youth. Journal of Strength and Conditioning Research, 29(5), 1439–1450.

Lowe, K.B., Kroeck, K.G. and Sivasubramaniam, N. (1996) Effectiveness correlates of transformational and transactional leadership: A meta-analytic review of the mlq literature. The Leadership Quarterly, 7, 385–425.

Lyle, J. (2002) Sports coaching concepts: A framework for coaches' behaviour. London: Routledge.

Lyle, J. (2009) Sporting success, role models and participation: A policy related review. (Research report no.101.) Retrieved from www.sportscotland.org.uk.

MacDonald, D.J., Côté, J., Eys, M. and Deakin, J. (2011) The role of enjoyment and motivational climate in relation to the personal development of team and sport athletes. Kinesiology and Physical Education, 25, 32–46.

Mageau, G.A. and Vallerand, R.J. (2003). The coach-athlete relationship: a motivational model. Journal of Sports Sciences, 21, 883–904.

Magnusen, M.J. and Rhea, D.J. (2009) Division I athletes' attitudes towards and preferences for male and female strength and conditioning coaches. Journal of Strength and Conditioning Research, 23(4), 1084–1090.

Mallet, C.J. and Hanrahan, S.J. (2004) Elite athletes: why does the 'fire' burn so brightly? Psychology of Sport and Exercise, 5, 183–200.

Mallet, C.J. (2004) Reflective practices in teaching and coaching. In: Wright, J., MacDonald, D. and Burrows, L. Critical inquiry and problem-solving in physical education, pp.147–158, London: Routledge.

Mallett, C. and Côté, J. (2006) Beyond winning and losing: Guidelines for evaluating high performance coaches. The Sport Psychologist, 20, 213–221.

Mutter, F. and Pawlowski, T. (2014) Role models in sports – Can success in professional sports increase the demand for amateur sports participation? Sport Management Review, 17, 324–336.

Nash, C. S. and D. Collins (2006). 'Tacit knowledge in expert coaching: Science or Art? Quest 58(4): 465-477.

Nash, C.S. and Sproule, J. (2009) Career development of expert coaches. International Journal of Sports Science and Coaching, 4(1), 121–138.

Ntoumanis, N. and Biddle, S.J.H. (1999) A review of motivational climate in physical activity. *Journal of Sports Sciences*, 17, 643–665.

Officer, S.A. and Rosenfeld, L.B. (1985) Self-disclosure to male and female coaches by female high school athletes. *Journal of Sport Psychology*, 7, 360–370.

Parkhouse, B. and Williams, J. (1986) Differential effects of sex and status on evaluation and coaching ability. *Research Quarterly in Exercise and Sport*, 57, 53–59.

Rose, J., Mackey-Kallis, S., Shyles, L., Barry, K., Biagini, D., Hart, C. and Jack, L. (2012) Face it: The impact of gender on social images. *Communications Quarterly*, 60(5), 588–607.

Sarrazin, P., Guillet, E. and Cury, F. (2001) The effect of coach's task- and ego-involving climate on the changes in perceived competence, relatedness, and autonomy among girl handballers. *European Journal of Sports Science*, 1(4), 1–9.

Sheldon, K.M., Turban, D.B., Brown, K.G., Barrick, M.R. and Judge, T.A. (2003). Applying self-determination theory to organizational research. *Research in Personnel and Human Resources Management*, 22, 357–393.

Sosik, J.J. and Godshalk, V.M. (2000) Leadership styles, mentoring functions received, and job-related stress: a conceptual model and preliminary study. *Journal of Organizational Behaviour*, 21, 365–390.

Sports coach UK (a, no date) Coaching female high-performance athletes. Retrieved from http://www.ukcoaching.org/sites/default/files/Coaching-Female-High-Performance-Athletes.pdf [accessed 26 Sept. 2017]

Sports coach UK (b, no date) Female psychology and considerations for coaching practice. Retrieved from https://www.womeninsport.org/wp-content/uploads/2015/04/Female-Psychology-and-Considerations-for-Coaching-Practice.pdf?938151 [accessed 26 Sept. 2017]

Sports coach UK (2015) Gender Equality briefing note. Retrieved from http://www.ukcoaching.org/sites/default/files/Gender per cent20Equality per cent20briefing per cent20note per cent20 per cent20120115_1.pdf [accessed 26 Sept. 2017]

Stenling, A. and Tafvelin, S. (2014) Transformational leadership and wellbeing in sports: The mediating role of need satisfaction. *Journal of Applied Sports Psychology*, 26, 182–196.

Sutton, J. and McIlwain, D.J.F. (2014) Breadth and depth of knowledge in expert versus novice athletes. *The Routledge Handbook of Sports Expertise*: Routledge (eds. Damian Farrow and Joe Baker).

Thelwell, R.C., Lane, A.M., Weston, N.J.V. and Greenlees, I.A. (2008) Examining relationships between emotional intelligence and coaching efficiency. *International Journal of Sport and Exercise Psychology*, 6(2), 224–235.

Turnnidge, J. and Côté, J. (2016) Applying transformational leadership theory to coaching research in youth sport: A systematic literature review. *International Journal of Sports and Exercise Psychology*, DOI: 10.1080/1612197X.2016.1189948

Vallerand, R.J. (2001) A hierarchial model of intrinsic and extrinsic motivation in sport and exercise. *Advances in Motivation in Sport and Exercise* (ed. Roberts, G.C.). Champaign, IL: Human Kinetics.

Vella, S.A., Oades, L.G. and Crowe, T.P. (2010) The application of coach leadership models to coaching practice. *International Journal of Sports Science and Coaching*, 5(3): 425–434.

Vella, S.A., Oades, L.G. and Crowe, T.P. (2013) A pilot test of transformational leadership training for sports coaches: Impact on the development of experience of adolescent athletes. *International Journal of Sports Science and Coaching*, 8(3), 513–530.

Warner, S. and Dixon, M.A. (2015) Competition, gender and the sport experience: an exploration among college athletes. *Sport, Education and Society*, 20(4), 527–545.

Weinberg, R., Reveles, M. and Jackson, A. (1984) Attitudes of male and female athletes towards male and female coaches. *Journal of Sport Psychology*, 6, 448–453.

Williams, J.M. and Parkhouse, B.L. (1988) Social learning theory as a foundation for examining sex bias in evaluation of coaches. *Journal of Sport and Exercise Psychology*, 10, 322–333.

INDEX